PRAISE FOR THE BOOK THAT PARENTS AND DOCTORS TRUST

❖ ❖ ❖ ❖ ❖

"Excellent. I recommend it to all my new patients. I have a 17 month old. This book was a bible even for me—a pediatrician."
—Claudia Somes, M.D.

❖

"**What to Expect When You're Expecting** has been my pregnancy bible."
—Cynthia Cravens Allen,
Kentucky

❖

"Wonderful. Well organized, readable."
—Catherine C. Wiley, M.D.

❖

"Your book . . . has been a godsend. I've faithfully read each chapter prior to beginning that month and have been reassured by your calm and compassionate writing." —Carol Rozner, California

❖

"Contains useful information not available in other books."
—Jim Wiley, M.D.

❖

"Your calm and confident style fills me with courage for our transition to parenthood." —Diane Wheeler, California

❖

"Very reassuring to the new mother." —Ralph Minear, M.D.

❖

"Your books have not left my night table for 18 months (except when they went to the hospital with me)! Your information is always *right on schedule,* clear, concise and unbiased." —Lori Slayton, New Jersey

❖

"Excellent—we used it as our bible during pregnancy." —Bruce Oran, M.D.

❖

"[It] has seen me through my first pregnancy... providing a concise, user-friendly source of information... Thanks to your book, I feel our daughter had a head start on life." —Victoria Schei, Ontario

❖

"Extremely helpful. I've used this book as a valuable resource with my patients." —Saundra Schoichet, Ph.D.
Clinical Psychologist

❖

WHAT TO EXPECT WHEN YOU'RE EXPECTING

❖ ❖ ❖

Arlene Eisenberg

Heidi E. Murkoff

Sandee E. Hathaway, B.S.N.

With a foreword by Dr. Richard Aubry,
Assistant Chairman and Director of Obstetrics, Department of Ob-Gyn,
State University of New York Health Sciences Center at Syracuse

WORKMAN PUBLISHING, NEW YORK

To Emma, who inspired this book while still in the womb, who did her best to keep us from writing it once she was out, and who, we trust, will put it to good use one day.

To Howard, Erik, and Tim, without whom this book would not have been possible—in more ways than one.

To Rachel, Wyatt, and Ethan, who showed up a little late for our first edition, but whose gestations contributed plenty to this one.

Copyright © 1984, 1988, 1991 by Arlene Eisenberg,
Heidi E. Murkoff, and Sandee E. Hathaway

All rights reserved. No portion of this book may be
reproduced—mechanically, electronically, or by any other means,
including photocopying—without written permission of the publisher.
Published simultaneously in Canada by Thomas Allen & Son Limited.

Library of Congress Cataloging-in-Publication Data
Eisenberg, Arlene.
What to expect when you're expecting / by Arlene Eisenberg,
Heidi E. Murkoff, and Sandee E. Hathaway.—2nd ed.
p.   cm.
Includes index.
ISBN 0-89480-829-X
1. Pregnancy. 2. Childbirth. 3. Postnatal care.
I. Murkoff, Heidi Eisenberg. II. Hathaway, Sandee Eisenberg. III. Title.
RG525.E36 1991   618.2′4—dc20   90-50951
                                                          CIP

Book Design: Susan Aronson Stirling
Cover Illustration: Judith Cheng
Book Illustration: Carol Donner

Workman books are available at special discounts when purchased in
bulk for premiums and sales promotions as well as for fund-raising
or educational use. Special editions or book excerpts can also be
created to specification. For details, contact the Special Sales Director
at the address below.

Workman Publishing Company, Inc.
708 Broadway
New York, NY 10003

Manufactured in the United States of America
Second edition first printing, April 1991
25   24   23   22   21   20   19

A MILLION THANKS

Books and babies have a lot in common. Both take plenty of time, hard work, dedication, and care (not to mention a healthy dose of worry) to turn out the best possible product. Both also require the cooperation of a team of concerned people. We've been lucky to have a fine team involved in the creation of our book, all of whom we gratefully thank:

Elise and Arnold Goodman, our agents, for their confidence, advice, support, and friendship.

Suzanne Rafer, our terrific editor at Workman, for her perceptive suggestions, her patience, her sense of humor (she needed it), and her endless capacity for what sometimes seemed endless work.

Shannon Ryan, for a thousand and one things she's taken care of with efficiency, intelligence, and, incredibly, a smile. Kathie Ness, for her astute copy editing of this second edition.

Bert Snyder, Ina Stern, Saundra Pearson, Steve Garvan, Janet Harris, Andrea Glickson, Cindy Frank, Jill Bennett, Nicole Dawkins, Barbara McClain, Tom Starace, Anne Kostick, and everyone else at Workman who helped make our first edition a success and/or contributed to making this one come to fruition. And very special thanks to Peter Workman, for being a very special publisher.

Richard Aubrey, M.D., Professor of Obstetrics and Gynecology and Assistant Chairman and Director of Obstetrics, Department of Ob-Gyn, State University of New York Health Sciences Center at Syracuse, our invaluable medical advisor. Dick's wise, caring, perceptive, informed critique has added immeasurably to the quality of this book. We feel privileged to have worked with such a remarkable physician.

The American College of Obstetricians and Gynecologists (particularly Mort Lebow, Florence Foelak, and Kate Ruddon), the American Academy of Pediatrics (particularly Michelle Weber and Carolyn Kolbaba), and *Contemporary Pediatrics* (and editor Jim Swan) for supplying us with voluminous quantities of information and material, being available to answer our questions, and for helping us to keep our books up-to-date.

The many physicians who clarified points or answered our questions, including John Severs, Irving Selikoff, Michael Starr, Michelle Marcus, Roy Schoen, and the hundreds who answered questionnaires and have given us input at ACOG meetings.

Three men without whom this book (and those that followed) would literally not have been possible: Howard Eisenberg, Erik Murkoff, and Tim Hathaway. It's guys like these that give husbands and fathers a good name, and we thank them for their inspiration and support.

Those who were so instrumental in the success of the first edition, including designer Susan Aronson Stirling, cover illustrator Judith Cheng, and book illustrator Carol Donner; Henry Eisenberg M.D., Ann Appelbaum, and Beth Falk, and, of course, Mildred and Harry Scharaga, better known as Mimi and Gramps.

Friends like Sarah Jacobs who have offered ideas and insights.

The hundreds of readers who have written, phoned, or spoken to us over the years, for all their comments and suggestions.

CONTENTS

Part 1

IN THE BEGINNING

―――――――― *Part 2* ――――――――
NINE MONTHS AND COUNTING:
From Conception to Delivery

--------------------------- *Part 3* ---------------------------

OF SPECIAL CONCERN

--------- *Part 4* ---------

LAST BUT NOT LEAST:
Postpartum, Fathers, and the Next Baby

Another Word From the Doctor

Often, people who notice my name on the front cover of this book call to thank me for writing it. I thank them, in return, for their calls and compliments—and then explain that I *didn't* write it. My role, I tell them, was not author but medical advisor—in charge of the dotting of every anatomic "i" and the crossing of every biologic "t."

Like them, I'm pleased and excited about what these authors have done. What I wrote in my foreword in 1985 is every bit as true today. But with this complete revision, the book that I enthusiastically endorsed then is now even better.

It's even more up-to-date and more comprehensive, dealing in much greater depth with high-risk pregnancies, second pregnancies, and pregnancy loss. These topics are handled with sensitivity, clarity, and accuracy, avoiding the scare-on-every-page approach. The authors take the sensible view that, yes, there are things to be concerned about; any responsible mother-to-be would be concerned.

But then they add what is so often omitted elsewhere: "Here are some commonsense things you can do to avoid that complication."

That constructive approach, I am sure, is what has helped this book, written by non-physicians, win such wide acceptance among doctors and other health care providers in the first place. It's not only recommended (or given) to new patients by many ob/gyns, but used by those physicians and their spouses as well. My young residents read it to learn what patients are wondering and worrying about, so they'll be better prepared when they begin their own practice.

Clearly, expectant parents love this book. Physicians respect it. Those are two good reasons for the resounding success of *What to Expect When You're Expecting*. And if it didn't sound so appallingly unscientific, I'd hypothesize a third: babies appreciate it too.

Richard Aubry, M.D., M.P.H., F.A.C.O.G.

A Word From the Doctor

These are the best years in history to be expecting a baby. In recent decades, there has been a remarkable improvement in the outcome of human pregnancy—for mothers as well as for infants. Women enter pregnancy healthier; they get better, more complete prenatal care; and the hospital maternity wing has replaced the kitchen table and the four-poster as the place to have a baby.

Yet more can be done. To those of us in academic medicine it is becoming increasingly clear that superior doctors and superior equipment aren't enough. Further reductions in pregnancy and childbirth risks will require actively participating expectant couples as well. In order to participate more, couples will have to be more completely and accurately informed, not just about the climactic birth experience, but about the all-important nine months that precede it; not just about the risks that pregnancy presents, but about the steps parents can take to minimize and eliminate risks; not just about the medical aspects of pregnancy, but about psychosocial and lifestyle factors as well.

How can parents become so informed? High schools and colleges, have no time or place in their curricula for Babymaking 101. Professionals who provide obstetrical care have a time problem, too. And, they are sometimes overly scientific in their explanations and insufficiently sensitive to the psychological and emotional needs of expectant parents.

Consumer advocates have vaulted into the void with books, magazine articles, and classroom instruction. They are often tremendously helpful, but almost as often they're medically inaccurate, unnecessarily alarming, and/or disproportionately focused on the inadequacies of the health care profession, driving a wedge of suspicion and doubt between parents and their obstetrical caregivers.

The need for a book that provides accurate, up-to-date, and medically sound information with proper emphasis on nutrition, lifestyle, and the emotional aspects of pregnancy has long been apparent. Now, I believe, that need has been met in a highly readable and eminently practical month-by-month format.

The three authors—each an experienced "consumer" of maternity care—have given us that essential consumer perspective. They have wisely concentrated on giving expectant parents the information that will allow them to intelligently play their central role in the entire process, without threatening the doctors and nurse-midwives with whom they must work closely and congenially.

What to Expect When You're Expecting is lively in style, accurate, current, and well-balanced overall. But four aspects of its structure and content deserve special comment:

❖ The book's thoughtful family-centered approach to childbearing —with involvement of the husband throughout the pregnancy process and with a chapter responding to his special needs and problems—is excellent and important.

❖ Its practical chronological arrangement—sensibly answering all the big and little, trying and troubling questions that come up month after month—makes for timely reassurance and easy bedside-table reference.

❖ The book's emphasis on pre-pregnancy and pregnancy nutrition and lifestyle, and its commonsense approaches to lactation and the psychosocial dimensions of motherhood, make it particularly valuable and unique.

❖ Its accurate and up-to-the-minute medical detail—particularly the clarity of its sections on genetics, teratology, preterm labor, delivery, cesarean section, and again, lactation—is outstanding.

All in all, I believe that this excellent book, should be *required reading* not only for expectant parents, but for doctors and nurses who are training to provide obstetrical care and for professionals already providing it. That is, I know, a long way out on a limb for a generally cautious medical school professor to go. But I say it out of strong conviction: the belief that only with properly informed and responsible consumers and providers working together can we draw near our common goal—healthy babies, mothers, and families. And, ultimately, society.

Richard Aubry, M.D.,
M.P.H., F.A.C.O.G.

Why This Book Was Reborn

Eight years ago, just hours before I delivered Emma, the baby who inspired it, my co-authors and I delivered the proposal for *What to Expect When You're Expecting*. In conceiving it, in researching it, in writing it, our goal was simple and single-minded: to bring reassurance to expectant parents.

Eight years later, our goal hasn't changed. But to help us meet the goal more fully, our book has.

The first copy of *What to Expect* was barely off the presses when we began to collect material in a folder marked "ADD." Though we managed to include the most significant new information, at least briefly, in subsequent printings, squeezing in a line here and a line there, the ADD file soon became a pile of files, then a boxful. When it started to become a

roomful, we decided it was time to begin petitioning our publisher for the opportunity to begin a major revision, so that *all* our ADDs could finally be added.

Much of what we've revised reflects revisions in obstetrical practice. But many more of the changes reflect the input from a source we value as highly as any obstetrical journal or text: expectant parents. On a page at the end of the first edition of *What to Expect,* we asked readers to write and let us know if there was anything they worried about or experienced during pregnancy and postpartum that we didn't cover or didn't cover adequately. And though we received many letters from readers who said they felt we'd covered it all, we received others from readers who'd felt we hadn't.

Planning Ahead

If you aren't pregnant yet but are in the planning phase, turn to the last chapter of this book first. There you will find everything you need to know about getting a head start on a successful pregnancy and a healthy baby.

So, as requested, we've added more on second and subsequent pregnancies, more on chronic medical conditions that affect pregnancy, more on what to do if you get sick, more on coping with common (and not-so-common) pregnancy symptoms, and more on complications that may occur (but please, please, to spare yourself unnecessary worry, do not read this section unless a complication *does* occur).

More important than what we've changed, though, is what has stayed the same—namely, all that readers have told us they've appreciated about *What to Expect*. The practical step-by-step advice. The empathetic approach. The easy-to-read explanation of things medical. And, of course, the reassurance.

No book on pregnancy can anticipate and elaborate on every conceivable concern or situation and still fit comfortably on a single bookshelf. (After all, consider that no two pregnancies are identical and over 3 ½ million pregnancies take place each year in this country.) But we hope you'll find that this edition of *What to Expect When You're Expecting* comes close.

Thanks to you, our readers, for all the support and suggestions you've given us. And do keep those cards and letters coming. We'll do our best to keep responding.

Heidi E. Murkoff
New York City

How This Book Was Born

I was pregnant, which about one day out of three made me the happiest woman in the world. And for the remaining two, the most worried.

Worried about the wine I'd sipped nightly with dinner, and the gin and tonics I'd downed more than a few times before dinner in my first six weeks of pregnancy—after two gynecologists and a blood test convinced me that I wasn't pregnant.

Worried about the seven doses of Provera one of the doctors had prescribed to bring on what she was certain was just a tardy period, but which proved two weeks later to be a nearly two-month gestation.

Worried about the coffee I'd drunk, and the milk I hadn't; the sugar I'd eaten, and the protein I hadn't.

Worried about the cramps in my third month, and the four days in my fifth month when I felt not even a flicker of fetal movement.

Worried about the time I fainted while touring the hospital I was to deliver in (I never did get to see the nursery), my middle-of-the-street belly-flop in the eighth month, and a bloody vaginal discharge in the ninth.

Worried, even, about feeling *good* ("But I'm not constipated.... I don't have morning sickness.... I'm not urinating more frequently—something must be wrong!").

Worried that I wouldn't be able to tolerate the pain during labor, or stand the sight of blood at delivery. And worried that because I couldn't squeeze out a drop of the colostrum all my books told me should fill my breasts by the ninth month, I wouldn't be able to breastfeed.

Where could I turn to find reassurance that all would be well? Not to the ever-growing stack of pregnancy books piled high on my bedside table. As common and normal as a few days of no fetal activity is in the fifth month, I couldn't find a single reference to it. As often as pregnant women take a tumble—almost always without harming their babies—I could find no mention of accidental falls.

When my symptoms, problems, or fears *were* discussed, it was usually in an alarming way which only compounded my concern. *Never* take Provera unless you would "absolutely abort," warned one volume—without adding that a woman who has taken the drug has so slight an increased risk of birth defects in her baby that an unwanted abortion need never be considered. "There is evidence that a single drinking 'binge' during pregnancy may affect some babies, depending on the stage of development they have reached," cautioned another book ominously—disregarding studies which show that a few drinking sprees in early pregnancy, when many women indulge unknowingly, appear to have no effect on a developing embryo.

I certainly couldn't find relief for my worries by opening a newspaper, flipping on the radio or television, or browsing through magazines. According to the media, threats to the pregnant lurked everywhere: in the air we breathed, in the food we ate, in the water we drank, at the dentist's office, in the drugstore, even at home.

My doctor offered some solace, of course, but only when I was able to summon up the courage to phone. (I was either afraid my worries would sound silly or afraid of what I would hear. Besides, how could I spend two days out of three on the phone badgering her?)

Was I (and my husband, Erik—who worried about everything I worried about, and then some) alone in my fears? Far from it. Worry, according to one study, is one of the most common complaints of pregnancy, affecting more expectant women than morning sickness and food cravings combined. Ninety-four out of every hundred women worry about whether their babies will be normal, and 93% worry about whether they and their babies will come through delivery safely. More women worry about their figures (91%) than their health (81%) during pregnancy. And most worry that they worry too much.

But though a little worry is normal for pregnant women and their mates, a lot of worry is an unnecessary waste of what should be a blissfully happy time. Despite all that we hear, read, and worry about, never before in the history of reproduction has it been safer to have a baby—as Erik and I discovered some seven and a half months of worrying later, when I gave birth to a healthier and more beautiful baby girl than I'd dared to dream possible.

Thus, out of our concerns, *What to Expect When You're Expecting* was born. It is dedicated to expectant couples everywhere (especially to my co-author and sister, Sandee, and her husband, Tim, whose first baby will be in a tight race with this book for publication), and written with the hope that it will help fathers- and mothers-to-be worry less and enjoy their pregnancies more.

Heidi E. Murkoff

Part 1

IN THE BEGINNING

1
Are You Pregnant?

Am I really pregnant? This is the first preoccupation of the hopeful expectant parent, and it arises the first moment one or another of the signs of pregnancy appears. Happily, it's a question that can very soon be answered, via the combination of a pregnancy test and a medical examination.

WHAT YOU MAY BE CONCERNED ABOUT

SIGNS OF PREGNANCY

'I only have some of the signs of pregnancy—can I still be pregnant?''

You can have all of the signs and symptoms of early pregnancy and not be pregnant. Or you can have only a few of them and be very definitely pregnant. The various signs and symptoms of pregnancy are only clues—important to pay attention to, but not to be relied upon for absolute confirmation.

Some of the pregnancy signs you may notice suggest the *possibility* you are pregnant, others the *probability*. *No* early signs are positive indications of pregnancy. In fact, the first sign that is proof positive of your pregnancy is your baby's heartbeat, which is audible at about 10, or more often 12, weeks with the sensitive ultrasound Doppler device, or with an or-dinary stethoscope at 18 to 20 weeks.[1] Earlier signs only indicate the possibility or probability that you're carrying a child. Combined with a reliable pregnancy test and your doctor's examination, they can help provide an accurate diagnosis.

PREGNANCY TESTS

'My doctor said the exam and pregnancy test indicated I wasn't pregnant, but I really feel I am.''

As remarkable as modern medical science is, when it comes to pregnancy diagnosis, it still sometimes takes a backseat to a woman's intuition. The accuracy of the different

---

1. Verification of a pregnancy can be made earlier through ultrasound or via a blood test, but these are not routine procedures.

pregnancy tests varies, and none are accurate as early as some women begin to "feel" that they are pregnant—sometimes within a few days after conception. There are basically three kinds of pregnancy tests available today—and a rabbit needn't give its life for any of them.

POSSIBLE SIGNS OF PREGNANCY

SIGN	WHEN IT APPEARS	OTHER POSSIBLE CAUSES
Amenorrhea (absence of menstruation)	Usually entire pregnancy	Travel, fatigue, stress, fear of pregnancy, hormonal problems or illness, extreme weight gain or loss, going off the Pill, breastfeeding
Morning sickness (any time of day)	2–8 weeks after conception	Food poisoning, tension, infection, and a variety of diseases
Frequent urination	Usually 6–8 weeks after conception	Urinary tract infection, diuretics, tension, diabetes
Tingling, tender, swollen breasts	As early as a few days after conception	Birth control pills, impending menstruation
Changes in color of vaginal and cervical tissue*	First trimester	Impending menstruation
Darkening of areola (area around nipple) and elevation of tiny glands around nipple	First trimester	Hormonal imbalance or effect of prior pregnancy
Blue and pink lines under skin on breasts and later on abdomen	First trimester	Hormonal imbalance or effect of prior pregnancy
Food cravings	First trimester	Poor diet, stress, imagination, or impending menstruation
Darkening of line from navel to pubis	4th or 5th month	Hormonal imbalance or effect of prior pregnancy

*Signs of pregnancy looked for in medical examination.

The Home Pregnancy Test. This test is much more accurate than in the past, and a lot simpler to use. Like the urine test done in the lab or the doctor's office, it diagnoses pregnancy by detecting the presence of the hormone hCG (human Chorionic Gonadotropin) in the urine. Some tests can tell you if you're pregnant as early as the first day of your missed menstrual period (about 14 days after conception), and in as little as five minutes, with an any-time-of-the-day urine sample.

If it's done correctly—and this is increasingly possible as tests become less complicated to carry out and evaluate—an at-home test is now almost as accurate as a urine test done in a doctor's office or laboratory (the accuracy is close to 100%, according to the manufacturers), with a positive result much more likely to be correct than a negative one. Home tests offer the advantage of privacy and virtually immediate results. And because they provide an accurate diagnosis very early in pregnancy—earlier than you would probably consider consulting a physician—they can give you the opportunity to start taking optimum care of yourself within days of conception, actually at about the same time as the pregnancy is implanting in your uterus. But they can be relatively expensive, and because you're less likely to feel confident in the results, you're more apt to want a retest, increasing the cost. (Some brands include a second test in the package.) Let your practitioner know which brand and type of test you used so that he or she can decide whether or not a retest is needed.

The major drawback with home pregnancy tests is that if a test produces a false-negative result and you actually are pregnant, you may postpone seeing a doctor and taking appropriate care of yourself. And even

PROBABLE SIGNS OF PREGNANCY

SIGN	WHEN IT APPEARS	OTHER POSSIBLE CAUSES
Softening of uterus and cervix*	2–8 weeks after conception	A delayed menstrual period
Enlarging uterus* and abdomen	8–12 weeks	Tumor, fibroids
Intermittent painless contractions	Early in pregnancy, increasing in frequency as pregnancy advances	Bowel contractions
Fetal movements	First noted at 16–22 weeks of pregnancy	Gas, bowel contractions

*Signs of pregnancy looked for in medical examination.

POSITIVE SIGNS OF PREGNANCY

SIGN	WHEN IT APPEARS	OTHER POSSIBLE CAUSES
Visualization of embryo or gestational sac through ultrasound*	As early as 4–6 weeks after conception	None
Fetal heartbeat*	At 10–20 weeks**	None
Fetal movements felt through abdomen*	After 16 weeks	None

*Signs of pregnancy looked for in medical examination.
**Depending on device used.

with a positive result, you may postpone the office visit because you assume that getting a diagnosis is the only reason to see your doctor at this point. So if you use such a test, keep in mind that it is not designed to take the place of a consultation with and examination by a medical professional. Medical follow-up to the test is essential. If the result is positive, you should have it confirmed by a physical exam and then get a complete prenatal checkup. If it is negative and your period still hasn't started, you and your doctor need to find out why.

The Lab or In-Office Urine Test. Like the at-home variety, this test can detect hCG in the urine with an accuracy of close to 100%—and as early as seven to ten days after conception. Unlike the home test, it is performed by a professional, who is, at least theoretically, more likely to do it correctly. If you plan on taking a urine test, call the doctor's office or lab the day before and ask if there are any instructions. The in-office test (which usually yields results in minutes) will probably not require first-morning urine; the lab version (you'll have to wait until they phone the news to the doctor's office) may. Urine tests are usually less expensive than blood tests, but they aren't used as often because they don't provide as much information; see below.

The Blood Test. The more sophisticated serum, or blood, pregnancy test can detect pregnancy with virtually 100% accuracy as early as one week after conception (barring lab error). It can also help to date a pregnancy by measuring the exact amount of hCG in the blood, since hCG values alter as pregnancy progresses. Occasionally a practitioner may order both a urine and a blood test to be doubly certain of the diagnosis.

No matter which test you use, the chances of the diagnosis being correct are enhanced when the test is followed by a medical examination. The physical signs of pregnancy—an enlarging and softening of the uterus, and a change in the texture of the cervix—may be apparent to your doc-

Testing Smart

To improve the chances that your home pregnancy test will be accurate, be sure to:

❖ Read test package directions carefully and thoroughly before use and follow them precisely. No matter how eager you are for results, if first-of-the-morning urine is required, wait until morning to perform the test.

❖ Have an easy-to-read clock or watch ready so that you can time the test precisely.

❖ Be sure containers, dipsticks, or any other equipment to be used with the test are clean and uncontaminated when you begin the test. Don't reuse containers if you want to try again.

❖ If a waiting period is required, place the sample away from the heat where it won't be disturbed.

❖ If the kit you've purchased contains a second test, or if you buy a second kit, wait a few days before trying a retest.

---

tor or midwife by the sixth week of pregnancy. But as with tests, a practitioner's diagnosis of "pregnant" is more likely to be correct than one of "not pregnant"—though false-negative results are fairly uncommon. False negatives are most likely to occur early in pregnancy, when a woman's body may not be producing enough hCG to test positive.

If you are experiencing the symptoms of early pregnancy (a missed period or two, breast fullness and tenderness, morning sickness, frequent urination, fatigue) and feel, test or no test, exam or no exam, that you are pregnant, act as though you are, taking all prenatal precautions, until you find out definitely otherwise. Neither tests nor medical practitioners are infallible. You know your own body—at least externally—better than your practitioner does. Ask for a retest (preferably a blood test) and another exam in a week or so; it may just be too early for an accurate diagnosis. More than one baby has arrived seven and a half or eight months after a pregnancy test and/or a doctor concluded that its mother wasn't pregnant.

If the tests continue to be negative but you still haven't begun to menstruate, be sure to check with your doctor to rule out an ectopic pregnancy, one that takes place outside of the uterus. (See page 109 for warning signs of this kind of pregnancy.)

It is possible, of course, to experience all the signs and symptoms of early pregnancy and not be pregnant at all. None of them alone or in combination is proof positive of pregnancy. After a second pregnancy test and physical exam determine that you are not pregnant, you must consider that the "pregnancy" may have psychological roots—possibly because you very strongly do, or don't, want to have a baby. In which case professional counseling is probably a good idea. Or it may be that the symptoms have some other biological cause that should be investigated by your doctor.

DUE DATE

"I am trying to plan my pregnancy leave. How do I know if my due date is really correct?"

L ife would be a lot simpler if you could be certain that your due date is actually the day you will deliver. But life isn't that simple very often. According to some studies only 4 women in 100 give birth on their due date. Most, because a normal full-term pregnancy can last anywhere from 38 to 42 weeks, deliver within two weeks either way of that date.

That's why the medical term for "due date" is EDD, or the *estimated* date of delivery. The date your practitioner gives you is only an educated estimate. It is usually calculated this way: Take the date of the first day of your last normal menstrual period (LNMP) and add 7 to it. From that date, count back three months and you have your due date—a year later, of course. For example, say your last menstrual period began on April 11. Add 7 to 11, which gives you 18; then count back three months. Your EDD would be January 18, the following year.

If your periods come predictably every 28 days, you are more likely to deliver close to your estimated due date. If your cycles are longer than 28 days, you are more likely to deliver later than your EDD, and if they are shorter, earlier.

But if your cycle is irregular, this dating system may not work for you at all. Say you haven't had your period in three months and suddenly you're pregnant. When did you conceive? Because a reliable EDD is important, you and your practitioner will have to try to come up with one. Even if you can't pinpoint conception or are unaware of your most recent ovulation (some women recognize the release of an ovum by flank pain and cramping that lasts a few hours, clear stringy vaginal mucus, and if they're keeping track, the characteristic temperature drop just before and the rise afterward), there are clues that can help.

The very first clue, the size of your uterus, will be noted when your initial internal pregnancy examination is performed. It should conform to your suspected stage of pregnancy. Later on there are other milestones that together can more accurately gauge just how pregnant you are: the first time the fetal heartbeat is heard (at about 10 to 12 weeks with a Doppler device, or at about 18 to 22 weeks with a stethoscope); when the first flutter of life is felt (at about 20 to 22 weeks with a first baby, or 16 to 18 with subsequent ones); the height of the fundus (the top of the uterus) at each visit (for example, it will reach the navel at about the 20th week). If all of these indications seem to correspond to the due date you and your practitioner have calculated, you can be pretty sure that it is close to accurate—that is, that you are quite likely to deliver within two weeks of that date. But if they don't correspond, the doctor may decide to do a sonogram sometime between the 12th and 20th weeks (the best information, some believe, can be garnered between weeks 16 and 20), which can more closely pinpoint the gestational age of your fetus. Some doctors will do a sonogram routinely, to obtain the most accurate date possible.

As delivery nears, there will be other clues to the date of the big event: painless contractions may become more frequent (and possibly uncomfortable), the fetus will drop into the pelvis (engagement), your cervix will begin to thin and shorten (effacement), and last of all, your cervix will begin to dilate. These clues will be helpful, but not definitive—only your baby knows for sure what his or her birthday will be. (For more information, see Lightening and Engagement, page 260; When You Will Deliver, page 261.)

WHAT IT'S IMPORTANT TO KNOW:
CHOOSING (AND WORKING WITH)
YOUR PRACTITIONER

While it takes two to conceive a baby, it takes a minimum of three—mother, father, and at least one health care professional—to make that transition from fertilized egg to delivered infant a safe and successful one. Assuming you and your husband have already taken care of conception, the next challenge you face is selecting that third member of your pregnancy team. And making sure that it's a selection you can live with—and labor with.[2]

A LOOK BACK

The selection of a pregnancy caregiver wasn't a major consideration for mothers-to-be 30 years ago. Those were the days of no-questions-asked obstetrical care, when the few choices there were in childbirth were left up to the doctor. As far as selecting an obstetrician was concerned, one seemed pretty much like the next. And besides, since you were likely to be unconscious during delivery, it didn't ultimately matter much whether you had rapport with your doctor. Instead of being a participating team member, the mother-to-be was more or less a spectator, sitting obediently on the bench while her obstetrical captain called the plays.

Today there are almost as many choices in childbirth—yours for the choosing—as there are doctors in the Yellow Pages. The trick is in matching yourself up with a compatible practitioner.

2. Of course you can and ideally should make this selection even before you conceive.

WHAT KIND OF PATIENT ARE YOU?

Your first step in figuring out the kind of practitioner that is right for you is to give some thought to the kind of patient you are.

Do you believe that "doctor knows best" (after all, he or she's the one who went to medical school)? Would you prefer your physician to make all the decisions without consulting you, and do you feel safest when all the latest medical technology is being used in your care? In your medical fantasies, does the man in the white lab coat taking your pulse fit the description of Dr. Welby or Dr. Kildare? Then you may feel most comfortable with an obstetrician who has a traditional practice, a godlike aura, and an unswerving dedication to his or her own obstetrical philosophy.

Or do you believe that your body and your health are your business and no one else's? Do you have definite ideas about pregnancy and childbirth and feel you'd like to run the show, from conception to delivery, with minimal interference from your health professional? Then skip over the Welbys and Kildares, and look for a physician or midwife who's willing to relinquish the starring role and serve as your consultant on the production of your baby. Someone who will let you make as many of the childbirth decisions as is medically practical, who is dogmatic only when it comes to giving the patient a controlling vote. Don't assume, however, that a doctor who leans toward "New

Wave" obstetrics is going to be any less doctrinaire in his or her beliefs than a traditional physician.

Or perhaps you're somewhere in the middle and would prefer a practitioner who makes you a partner in your own care, one who makes decisions based on his or her experience and knowledge but always includes you in the process. If so, the practitioner for you is probably one who sees his or her role in your pregnancy as somewhere between star and consultant—who is neither a slave to medical gospel nor putty in your hands; who would like to give you the "natural" delivery you want but won't hesitate to do a cesarean if your baby's safety (or yours) requires it; who doesn't routinely either give or withhold medication; who sees nothing incongruous in using a fetal monitor and a birthing room at the same time; and who's more interested in a healthy mother and a healthy baby than in your personal preferences or his or her own. The practitioner for you sees the doctor-patient relationship as one in which each partner contributes what he or she does best.

Whatever your patienting style, if you believe that the father-to-be should have equal billing in the pregnancy-childbirth drama, you'll also need to determine if the caregiver you're considering does too. A practitioner's attitude is usually apparent at the first visit, sometimes even when you make the first appointment. Is the father invited to both the examination and the interview? Are his questions given full consideration? Does the practitioner direct comments to both the mother and father? Is it clear that, when the time comes, the father will be welcome to share in both labor and delivery?

OBSTETRICIAN? FAMILY PRACTITIONER? NURSE-MIDWIFE?

Narrowing your ideal practitioner down to one of three general personality types makes your job of finding him or her easier, but exam-table-side manner and philosophy aren't everything. You'll also have to give some thought to the kind of medical credentials that would best meet your requirements.

The Obstetrician. If yours is a high-risk pregnancy,[3] then you will very likely need and want a specialist who is trained to handle every conceivable complication of pregnancy, labor, and delivery: an obstetrician. You may even want to find a specialist's specialist, an obstetrician who specializes in high-risk pregnancies, or even a subspecialist in maternal-fetal medicine.

If your pregnancy looks pretty routine from an obstetrical point of view, you may still want to select an obstetrician (more than 8 out of 10 women do), or you can choose between a physician who is a family practice specialist (about 10% to 12% of women use one) and a certified nurse-midwife (selected by 1% to 2%).

The Family Physician. The family practitioner (FP), a relatively new specialist, is actually an updated version of the old-fashioned general practitioner (GP), who once provided one-stop medical service for the whole

---

3. Traditionally, a high-risk pregnancy is one in which the expectant mother has had a problem pregnancy before; has a medical problem, such as diabetes, hypertension, or heart disease; has an Rh or a genetic problem; or is under 17 or over 35 (though there is some question as to whether women in their 30s are really high risk).

family. The major difference between the GP and the family physician is training: the FP, unlike the GP, has had several years of specialty training in primary care, including obstetrics, after receiving an MD. If you decide on an FP, he or she can serve as your internist, obstetrician/gynecologist, and when the time comes, pediatrician. Ideally, an FP will become familiar with the dynamics of your family, will be interested in all aspects of your health, not just your pregnancy, and will view pregnancy as just a normal part of the life cycle, not an illness. If complications occur, your FP may call in a specialist for consultation, but may remain in charge of your case.

The Certified Nurse-Midwife.[4] If you are looking for a practitioner whose emphasis is on you the person and not you the patient, who will take extra time to talk with you about your feelings and problems, who will be oriented toward the "natural" in childbirth, then a certified nurse-midwife (CNM) may be right for you (though, of course, many physicians meet these requirements too). Although a nurse-midwife is a medical professional, thoroughly trained to care for women with low-risk pregnancies and to attend uncomplicated births (having received special education, training, and certification in midwifery), she is more likely to treat your pregnancy as a human, rather than a medical, condition. If you choose a midwife, be sure she's certified; a lay midwife cannot provide you and your baby with optimal care.

---

4. Today, some midwives are being trained and certified without first becoming nurses. So, in some parts of the country, you may find the Certified Midwife (CM) in addition to, or instead of, the CNM.

TYPE OF PRACTICE

You've decided on an obstetrician, a family practitioner, or a nurse-midwife. Next you've got to decide which kind of medical practice you would be most comfortable with. The most common kinds of practices, and their possible advantages and disadvantages, are:

Solo Medical Practice. In such a practice, a doctor works for him- or herself, using another doctor to cover when he or she is away or otherwise unavailable. An obstetrician or a family physician might be in solo practice; a nurse-midwife, in almost all states, must work in a collaborative practice with a physician. The major advantage of solo practice is that you see the same practitioner at each visit, one you can get to know and hopefully feel more comfortable with before delivery. The major disadvantage is that if your doctor is not available, a physician you don't know may deliver your baby.[5] A solo practice may also be a problem if, midway during your pregnancy, you find you're not really crazy about the doctor. You're stuck unless you can afford to pick up and change to another without worrying about the investment you've already made.

Partnership or Group Medical Practice. Two or more doctors in the same specialty care jointly for patients, seeing them on a rotating basis. Again, you can find both obstetricians and family doctors in this type of practice—sometimes both in one group. The advantage of this arrangement is that by seeing a different doctor each time, you will get to know them all, and when those labor pains

---

5. You can remedy this by asking to meet the covering physician in advance.

are coming strong and fast there will be a familiar face in the room with you. The disadvantage is that you may not like all of the doctors in the practice equally, and you usually won't be able to choose the one who attends your birthing. Also, depending on whether you find it reassuring or unsettling, hearing different points of view from the various partners may be an advantage or a disadvantage.

Combination Practice. A group practice that includes one or more obstetricians and one or more nurse-midwives. The advantages and disadvantages are similar to those of any group practice. In addition, there is the advantage of having at some of your visits the extra time and attention a midwife may offer and at others the security of a physician's expertise. You may have the option of a midwife-coached delivery, assured that if a problem develops, a physician you know is in the wings.

Maternity or Birth Center–Based Practice. These are facilities in which certified nurse-midwives provide the bulk of the care, and physicians are on call as needed. Some maternity centers are based in hospitals with special birthing rooms, and others are separate units. All maternity centers provide care for low-risk patients only.

The obvious advantage of this type of practice is to those women who prefer certified midwives as their primary practitioners. The major disadvantage is the fact that if a complication arises during pregnancy (as it does 20% to 30% of the time), you may have to switch to a physician and start developing a relationship all over again; if one arises during labor or delivery (as occurs 10% to 15% of the time), you may need to be delivered by the doctor on call, who may be a perfect stranger. If complications arise at a free-standing maternity center,

you may have to be transported to the nearest hospital for emergency care.

Independent Certified Nurse-Midwife Practice. In the few states in which they are permitted to practice independently, CNMs offer the advantage of personalized pregnancy care and a low-tech natural delivery at home for those who desire such an experience. However, sometimes an unpredictable emergency arises that requires medical help in a matter of minutes. So, unless a nurse-midwife has an association with a physician who can quickly step in in emergency situations and have emergency transport on call, the risk to both mother and child can be significant.

FINDING A CANDIDATE

When you have a good idea of the kind of practitioner you want and the type of practice you'd prefer, where can you find some likely candidates? The following are all good sources:

❖ Your gynecologist or family doctor (if he or she doesn't do deliveries) or your internist, assuming you're happy with his or her style of practice. (Doctors tend to recommend others with philosophies similar to their own.)

❖ Friends who have recently had babies and whose childbearing philosophies are similar to yours.

❖ An obstetrical nurse, if you're lucky enough to know one.

❖ The county medical society, which can give you a list of names of physicians who deliver babies, along with information on their medical training, specialties, special interests, type of practice, and board certification. The society may also be able to tell you whether or not a specialist will be helpful in your situation, and if so, what kind of specialist.

❖ The *Directory of the American Medical Association* or the *Directory of Medical Specialties,* often available at your public library or doctor's office.

❖ The local La Leche League, if you're strongly interested in breastfeeding.

❖ A nearby hospital with facilities that appeal to you; for example, a neonatal intensive care unit, birthing rooms, rooming-in, father participation. They can give you the names of attending physicians.

❖ The International Childbirth Education Association, P.O. Box 20852, Milwaukee, WI 53220, or the American Society for Prophylaxis in Obstetrics (ASPO) / Lamaze, 1411 K Street NW, Suite 200, Washington, DC 20005, if you are interested in a practitioner who emphasizes prepared childbirth.

❖ A local maternity or birth center, or the American College of Nurse-Midwives, 1522 K Street NW, Suite 1120, Washington, DC 20005, if you are looking for a CNM.

❖ The Yellow Pages, if all else fails, under Physicians—Obstetrics and Gynecology, Maternal-Fetal Medicine, or Family Physicians.

BIRTHING ALTERNATIVES

Never before have women had so much control over the process of having a baby. For millennia it was largely nature's whims that decided a woman's obstetrical fate; then early in this century it became the physician who decided how she was to deliver. Now, at last, though nature still holds a few cards and physicians still have a

say, more and more of the decisions are falling to women and their spouses. It is becoming increasingly possible for a woman to choose the best time to conceive (thanks to better birth control methods and ovulation prediction kits) and often, barring complications, how she will give birth. Among birthing options the array is dizzying, even in a hospital setting. Leave the hospital, and there's yet more to select from.

Though your preliminary preferences for delivery shouldn't be your only criteria in choosing a practitioner, they should certainly come into play. (Keep in mind, however, that no firm decisions can be made until further into your pregnancy, and many can't be finalized until the delivery itself.) The following birthing options are among those that expectant mothers today can consider and might want to ask about before making a final decision on a practitioner and hospital:

Family-Centered Care. What many feel is the ideal in hospital maternity care, complete family-centered care is not yet a reality in many hospitals, though there's definitely a trend in that direction. ASPO/Lamaze has set criteria for this ideal, which include an official hospital policy of family-centered maternity care; childbirth education programs that reflect such a policy; management of labor without unnecessary technological interference and with attention to psychosocial needs; an atmosphere in which questions, self-help, and self-knowledge are encouraged, in which adaptations are made for cultural differences, and in which breastfeeding is encouraged within one hour of birth unless medically contraindicated; and a program that assesses a mother's basic infant care skills and determines satisfactory initiation of breastfeeding, if applicable, prior to discharge. Patient rooms should have a door (for privacy), comfortable furnishings, private toilet and bath/shower facilities, as well as sufficient space to accommodate family (siblings included) and other support persons, professional personnel and medical equipment, personal possessions, a newborn crib and supplies, and a sofa bed for family members staying overnight. There should also be an area nearby for support persons to take relaxation breaks away from the scene of the labor.

Birthing Rooms. At one time, every woman about to have a baby labored in a labor room, delivered in a delivery room, and recovered in a postpartum room. Her newborn was immediately whisked from her after birth and tucked away in a nursery to be cared for behind glass windows. Today, the availability of birthing rooms in many hospitals makes it possible for women to stay in the same bed from labor through recovery, sometimes even for their entire hospital stay, and for their babies to remain by their sides from birth on. Birthing rooms are fully equipped for uncomplicated deliveries and for unexpected emergencies (in most hospitals, cesareans and other complications must be handled in a delivery or operating room), but they look much like a cozy bedroom or hotel room (with soft lighting, pictures on the wall, curtains on the windows, an arm or rocking chair, and a comfortable bed—which usually converts to a birthing bed).

In most hospitals, a newly delivered mother (and her baby, if she's rooming in) is moved from the birthing room to a postpartum room after an hour or so of largely uninterrupted family togetherness. In a few more progressive hospitals, she can plan to stay in the birthing room straight through to check-out—sometimes with daddy, and even siblings, sharing the room.

Birthing rooms are usually available only for women who are at low risk for childbirth complications. Since the supply of birthing rooms at some hospitals is far exceeded by the demand, and they are often assigned on a first-come, first-served basis, there's the possibility that you won't get one. Fortunately, you may be able to experience unrushed, family-oriented, noninterventionist labor and delivery in some more traditional hospital settings, too.

Birthing Bed. The hard, flat delivery table on which your mother probably delivered you is losing out to a soft, roomy bed that is comfortable for labor and then, with a flip of a lever, becomes ideal for delivery. Usually the back can be raised to support the mom in a squatting or semi-squatting position and the foot of the bed can snap off to make way for the birthing attendant. After delivery, a change of linens, a few switches flipped, and presto, you're back in bed.

Birthing Chairs. Advocates of squatting deliveries prefer the birthing chair over the birthing bed. This chair is designed to support a woman in a sitting position during delivery. Since this position allows for an assist from gravity, theoretically speeding labor, it is appealing to some mothers and their birth attendants. Occasionally, however, the increased pressure of the baby's head against the pelvis when the mother is squatting in a birthing chair can lead to excessive tearing of the perineum. Though such tears can be repaired, they can prolong postpartum recuperation and discomfort.

Leboyer Births. When the French obstetrician Frederick Leboyer first propounded his theory of childbirth without violence, the medical community scoffed. Today many of the procedures he proposed, aimed at making a newborn's arrival in the world more tranquil, are common practice. Many babies are delivered in birthing rooms, without the aid of the bright lights once deemed necessary, on the theory that gentle lighting can make the transition from the dark uterus to the bright outside world more gradual and less jolting. Upending and slapping the newborn is no longer routine anywhere, and less violent procedures are preferred for establishing breathing when it doesn't start on its own. In some hospitals, the umbilical cord isn't cut immediately; instead, this last physical bond between mother and baby remains intact while they get to know each other for the first time. And though the warm bath Leboyer recommended for soothing the new arrival (and smoothing the transition from a watery home to a dry one) isn't common, being put immediately into mother's arms is.

In spite of the growing acceptance of many Leboyer theories, a full-blown Leboyer birth—with soft music, soft lights, and a warm bath for baby—isn't widely available. If you're interested in one, ask about it when you're interviewing practitioners.

Underwater Births. The concept of delivering underwater to simulate the environment in the womb is one that is not widely accepted in the medical community. Though many women who have experienced such a birth report that it was exhilarating, most physicians and hospitals feel that the risk of the fetus drowning, though probably remote, is still too great to make the procedure an acceptable one.

Home Births. For some women, the idea of being hospitalized when they aren't sick isn't appealing, but delivering at home is. And sometimes such a birth is very successful. The newborn arrives amid family and friends in a warm and loving atmosphere. The risk, of course, is that if something goes wrong, the facilities for an emergency cesarean or resuscitation of the newborn will not be close at hand. For many women a maternity center or a hospital birthing room is an ideal compromise, combining homey atmosphere with the security of high-tech backup. Those low-risk women who insist on a home birth need to be certain they will be attended by a qualified physician or certified nurse-midwife, and that emergency transportation to a nearby hospital will be available at a moment's notice. In Great Britain home births are not uncommon, but a fully equipped ambulance or "flying squad" is usually standing by, ready to transport the mother and, if delivery has already taken place, her baby to the hospital in case of emergency.

MAKING YOUR SELECTION

Once you've secured your prospective practitioner's name, call and make an appointment for an interview. Go armed with questions that will enable you to sense if your philosophies are in sync and if your personalities mesh comfortably. But don't expect that you will agree on everything—that doesn't happen even in the happiest of marriages. If it's important that your doctor be a good listener or a careful explainer, does this one seem to fulfill those requirements? If you're concerned with the emotional aspects of pregnancy, will this ·practitioner take your concerns seriously? Ask about his or her positions on any of the following issues that you feel strongly about: natural childbirth vs. anesthetized childbirth vs. pain relief as needed in childbirth; breastfeeding; induction of labor; use of fetal monitoring; enemas; forceps; cesarean sections; or anything else that concerns you. That way there won't be any unpleasant last-minute surprises.

Perhaps the most important thing you can do at this first meeting is to let the practitioner know what kind of patient you are. You can judge from the response whether he or she will be comfortable with you.

You will probably also want to know something about the hospital the doctor is affiliated with. Does it have features that are important to you, such as birthing rooms, birthing chairs, facilities for Leboyer birth, rooming-in, a neonatal intensive care unit, the latest fetal monitoring equipment? Are they flexible about routines that concern you, such as shaving and enemas? Do they allow fathers in the labor, delivery, and operating rooms even during a cesarean? Will you have to keep your legs in stirrups during delivery?

Before you make a final decision, think about whether the practitioner inspires a feeling of trust. Pregnancy is one of the most important voyages you'll ever make—you'll want a skipper (or first mate) in whom you have complete faith.

MAKING THE MOST OF THE PATIENT-PRACTITIONER PARTNERSHIP

Choosing the right practitioner is only the first step. For the vast majority of women, those who are ready neither to cede all responsibility to the physician nor to take over entirely themselves, the next step is nurturing a good working partnership with that professional. Here's how:

❖ When a question or concern you think is worth mentioning crops up between visits, write it down on a list that you will take to your next appointment. (It helps to keep a few notepads in convenient places—the refrigerator door, your purse, your desk at work, your bedside table—so that you'll always be within jotting distance of one; consolidate the lists before each doctor's visit.) That's the only way you can be sure that you won't forget to ask all your questions and report all your symptoms. And that you won't be wasting your time, or your practitioner's, while you try to remember what it was you wanted to ask.

❖ Along with your list of questions, bring a pen and pad to each office visit so you can make a note of your practitioner's recommendations. Many people are too nervous in a medical setting to remember directions accurately. If your practitioner doesn't volunteer adequate information, make inquiries before you leave, so there's no confusion once you get home. Ask about such things as side effects of treatments, when to stop taking a medication if one is prescribed, when to check back about a problem situation.

❖ Though you don't want to call your physician at every pelvic twinge, you shouldn't hesitate to call about worries that you can't resolve by checking in a book such as this one, and that you feel can't wait until the next visit. Don't be afraid that your concerns will sound silly. Unless your practitioner is just out of training, he or she's heard them all before. Be prepared to be very specific about your symptoms. If you are experiencing pain, be precise about its location, duration, quantity (is it sharp, dull, crampy?), and severity. If possible, explain what makes it worse or better—changing positions, for example. If you have a

Protecting Yourself Against Malpractice

Recognizing that the modern obstetrical practitioner-patient relationship is a partnership, and that when there is a less than perfect outcome it isn't always the physician who's at fault, doctors are no longer allowing themselves to be sitting ducks while patients take malpractice pot shots at them. They're fighting back and even in rare instances turning the tables and charging with malpractice the very same patients who are hurling malpractice charges at them. Still, though a few doctor vs. patient countersuits are actually coming to trial, you needn't worry that you will have to pay your doctor a million dollars if you don't take the vitamins he or she prescribes. What you do need to worry about, however, if you are guilty of malpractice, is that you and your baby will pay the price in possibly more devastating ways—with health and even life being the cost.

If you want to be a patient whom no one can charge with malpractice, take the following precautions:

❖ Tell the whole truth, and nothing but the truth. Don't give your practitioner a false or incomplete medical history. Make sure he or she knows about any drugs—prescription or non-, legal or illegal, medicinal or recreational, including alcohol and tobacco—that you are currently taking as well as about any past or present illnesses or operations.

❖ Don't reject necessary x-rays, tests, or medications unless you have an authoritative second opinion that backs up your decision.

❖ Follow instructions carefully when undergoing a medical procedure. You can't blame the radiologist for a blurred x-ray if you moved when you were told to stand still.

❖ Follow your practitioner's recommendations as to appointment schedule, weight gain, bed rest, exercise, medication, vitamins, and so on—unless, again, you have respected medical opinion that advises you otherwise.

❖ Do not allow anyone who is clearly under the influence of drugs or alcohol to treat you. Doing so makes you an accomplice to his or her crime.

❖ Always alert a practitioner to an obvious adverse effect of a medication or treatment, as well as to any other worrisome symptoms that you experience in your pregnancy. Also speak up if you believe your practitioner's instructions may be incorrect (see page 15).

❖ Never threaten or otherwise alarm a physician in a manner that could interfere with the treatment you are receiving.

❖ Take good care of yourself, following the Best-Odds Diet (see page 80), getting adequate rest and exercise, and absolutely avoiding alcohol, tobacco, and other nonprescribed drugs and medications, once you find out you're pregnant, or better still, once you start trying to conceive.

If you feel you can't follow your practitioner's instructions or go along with his or her recommended course of treatment, right or wrong, you clearly have little faith in the person you've chosen to care for you and your baby during your pregnancy, labor, and delivery. In such a case, all sides will be better served if you find a replacement.

vaginal discharge, describe its color (bright red, dark red, brownish, pinkish, yellowish), when it started, and how heavy it is. Also report accompanying symptoms (such as fever, nausea, vomiting, chills, diarrhea). (See When to Call the Practitioner, page 117.)

❖ When you read about something new in obstetrics, don't brandish the clipping in front of the practitioner at your next visit saying, "I must have this." Instead ask if he or she feels there is any value to this new procedure or validity to that new theory. Often the media report medical advances prematurely, before they are proven safe and effective through controlled studies. If indeed it is a legitimate advance, your practitioner may already be aware of it or may want to find out more about it. Whether it is or not, you may both learn something through the exchange.

❖ When you hear something that doesn't correspond with what your practitioner has told you, ask for an opinion on what you've heard. Not in a challenging way, just in order to get more information.

❖ If you suspect that the practitioner may be mistaken about something (for example, okaying intercourse when you have a history of miscarriage), speak up. You can't assume that he or she, even with your chart in hand, will always remember every aspect of your medical and personal history—and you share the responsibility of making sure errors are not made. The best approach in such a situation is to lay out your understanding of the situation and your concerns in a noncombative way. Almost invariably you will find that your provider really cares and will be glad for your candid input.

❖ If you have a gripe about anything (from being kept waiting to not getting answers to your questions), air it. Letting it fester will jeopardize the practitioner-patient relationship.

❖ If your relationship with your practitioner breaks down irreparably, think about changing doctors. He or she probably doesn't enjoy the bad feelings any more than you do. Don't, however, expect to get good obstetrical care if you regularly switch from doctor to doctor, trying to find one who will follow *your* orders. Consider, instead, that the problem with the care you've been receiving may originate with you.

2
Now That You Are Pregnant

WHAT YOU MAY BE CONCERNED ABOUT

Now that you no longer have to worry about what the result of the pregnancy test will be, you're sure to come up with a whole new set of concerns: What effect will my age or my husband's age have on my pregnancy and on our baby? How will chronic medical problems or family genetic problems affect him or her? Will our past lifestyles make a difference? Can my previous obstetrical history repeat? What can I do to lower any risks my history may present?

YOUR GYNECOLOGICAL HISTORY

"I haven't mentioned a previous pregnancy to my obstetrician because it occurred before I was married. Is there any reason I should?"

Your past gynecological history can be as important to your practitioner as the information he or she gains at each checkup during this pregnancy. Previous pregnancies, miscarriages, abortions, surgery, or infections may or may not have an impact on what happens in this pregnancy, but any information you have about them should be passed on to your practitioner. It will be handled with confidentiality. And don't worry about what your doctor will think. It's the job of the physician to help mothers and babies, not to judge them.

PREVIOUS ABORTIONS

"I've had two abortions. Will they affect this pregnancy?"

Probably not, if they were done in recent years and during the first trimester. Though abortions performed before 1973 have been linked to an increased risk of midtrimester miscarriage (because of damage in the course of the procedure that weakened the cervix, making it "incompetent"), improved techniques in first-trimester abortions since that time appear to have eliminated the risk of this type of cervical injury.

Multiple second-trimester abortions (14 to 26 weeks), however, do appear to increase the risk of premature delivery. If you had your abortions after the third month, see page 218 for reducing the risks of premature birth.

In either case, be sure your practitioner knows about the abortions. The more familiar he or she is with your gynecological history, the better care you will receive.

FIBROIDS

"I've had fibroids for several years, and they've never caused me any problem. But now that I'm pregnant, I'm worried that they will."

Fibroids occur most commonly in women over 35, and since the ranks of women in that age group who are having babies are swelling, fibroids are becoming relatively common in pregnancy (estimates range from 1 to 2 women in 100). The vast majority of pregnant women with fibroids can expect to go to term without added complications related to this condition. Occasionally, however, these small nonmalignant growths in the inner walls of the uterus do cause problems, increasing slightly the risk of ectopic pregnancy, miscarriage, placenta previa (a low-lying placenta), abruptio placenta (a premature separation of the placenta from the uterine wall), premature labor, premature rupture of membranes, stalled labor, fetal malformation, and breech and other more-difficult-to-deliver fetal posi-

tions. To minimize these risks, you should: be under the care of a physician; discuss the fibroids with your physician so that you become better informed on the condition in general and the risks in your particular case; reduce other pregnancy risks (see page 50); and be particularly attentive to symptoms that could signal impending trouble (see page 117).

Sometimes a woman with fibroids notices pressure or pain in the abdomen. And though it should be reported to the doctor, it usually isn't anything to worry about. Bed rest and safe pain relievers (see page 320) for four or five days usually bring relief. Sometimes the fibroids degenerate or twist, causing abdominal pain often accompanied by fever. Rarely, surgery may be needed to remove such a degenerating fibroid or one that is otherwise causing problems. If doctors suspect that the fibroids could interfere with a safe vaginal delivery, they may opt to deliver by cesarean section.

"I had a couple of fibroids removed a few years ago. Will this cause problems now that I'm pregnant?"

In most cases, surgery for the removal of small uterine fibroid tumors doesn't affect a subsequent pregnancy. Extensive surgery for large fibroids could, however, weaken the uterus enough so that it would be unable to tolerate labor. If, on reviewing your surgical records, your physician decides this might be true of your uterus, a cesarean delivery will be planned. You should become familiar with the signs of early labor in case contractions begin before the planned surgery (see page 221). And you should have an emergency plan for getting to the hospital immediately if you do go into labor.

INCOMPETENT CERVIX

"I had a miscarriage in my fifth month in my first pregnancy. The doctor said it was caused by an incompetent cervix. I just had a positive home pregnancy test and I'm terrified that I will have the same problem again."

Now that your incompetent cervix has been diagnosed, your physician should be able to take steps to prevent it from causing you to miscarry again. An incompetent cervix, one that opens prematurely under the pressure of the growing uterus and fetus, is estimated to occur in 1 or 2 of every 100 pregnancies; it is believed responsible for 20% to 25% of all second-trimester miscarriages. An incompetent cervix can be the result of genetic weakness of the cervix (the neck of the uterus); exposure of the mother to DES (diethylstilbestrol; see page 40) when she was in her mother's womb; extreme stretching of or severe lacerations to the cervix during one or more previous deliveries; cervical surgery or laser therapy; or traumatic D and Cs or abortions (particularly those performed before 1973). Carrying more than one fetus can also lead to incompetent cervix, but if it does, the problem will not usually recur in subsequent single-fetus pregnancies.

Incompetent cervix is usually diagnosed when a woman miscarries in the second trimester after experiencing progressive painless effacement (thinning) and dilatation of the cervix without apparent uterine contractions or vaginal bleeding. Ideally, doctors would like to be able to diagnose the problem before the miscarriage occurs so that steps can be taken to save the pregnancy. Recent attempts at diagnosing an opening cervix early on with ultrasound look promising.

If you lost a prior pregnancy because of an incompetent cervix, tell your obstetrician about it immediately if he or she is not already familiar with that fact. It is likely that cerclage (suturing, or stitching closed, the opening of the cervix) can be performed early in the second trimester (12 to 16 weeks) to prevent a repeat of this tragedy. The simple procedure is performed in the hospital after a normal pregnancy has been confirmed by ultrasound. After surgery and 12 hours of bed rest, the patient is usually allowed to get up to go to the bathroom and 12 hours later can resume normal activities. Sexual intercourse may be prohibited for the duration of the pregnancy, and frequent exams by the doctor may be necessary. Rarely, complete bed rest and the use of a specially designed appliance called a pessary to support the uterus may be substituted for cerclage. Treatment may also be initiated when ultrasound or a vaginal examination shows the cervix is opening, even if there was no previous late miscarriage.

When or whether the sutures will be removed will depend partly on the doctor's preference and partly on the type of sutures. Usually they are removed a few weeks before the estimated due date; in some cases they may not be removed until labor begins unless there is infection, bleeding, or premature rupture of the membranes.

Regardless of which course of treatment is taken, your chances of carrying to term are good. Still, you will have to be alert for signs of an impending problem in the second or early third trimester: pressure in the lower abdomen, vaginal discharge with or without blood, unusual urinary frequency, or the sensation of a lump in the vagina. If you experience any of these, go immediately to the doctor's office or the emergency room. (For more on midtrimester miscarriage, see page 177.)

YOUR OBSTETRICAL HISTORY REPEATING ITSELF

"My first pregnancy was very uncomfortable—I must have had every symptom in the book. Will I be that unlucky again?"

In general, your first pregnancy is a pretty good predictor of future pregnancies, all things being equal. So you are a little less likely to breeze comfortably through pregnancy than someone who already has. Still, there's always the hope that your luck will change for the better. All pregnancies, like all babies, are different. If, for example, morning sickness or food cravings plagued you in your first pregnancy, they may be barely noticeable in the second (or vice versa, of course). While luck, genetic predisposition, and the fact that you've experienced certain symptoms before have a lot to do with how comfortable or uncomfortable this pregnancy will be, other factors—including some that are within your control—can alter the prognosis to some extent. The factors include:

General Health. Being in good all-round physical condition gives you a better shot at having a comfortable pregnancy. Ideally, attend to chronic conditions (allergies, asthma, back problems) and clear up lingering infections (such as urinary tract infections or vaginitis) before conception (see Chapter 15). Once you become pregnant, continue to take good care of yourself as well as your pregnancy.

Diet. While it can't offer any guarantees, following the Best-Odds Diet gives every pregnant woman the best odds of having a comfortable pregnancy. Not only can it better your chances of avoiding or minimizing the miseries of morning sickness and indigestion, it can help fight excessive fatigue, combat constipation and hemorrhoids, prevent urinary tract infections and iron-deficiency anemia, and give you a leg up against leg cramps. (And even if your pregnancy turns out to be uncomfortable anyway, you'll have bestowed on your baby the best odds of developing well and being born healthy.)

Weight Gain. Gaining weight at a steady rate and keeping the gain within the recommended boundaries (between 25 and 35 pounds) can improve your chances of escaping or minimizing such pregnancy miseries as hemorrhoids, varicose veins, stretch marks, backache, fatigue, indigestion, and shortness of breath.

Fitness. Getting enough and the right kind of exercise (see page 189 for guidelines) can help improve your general well-being. Exercise is especially important in second and subsequent pregnancies because abdominal muscles tend to be laxer, making you more susceptible to a variety of aches and pains, most notably backache.

Lifestyle Pace. Leading a harried and frenetic life, as so many women do today, can aggravate or sometimes even trigger one of the most uncomfortable of pregnancy symptoms—morning sickness—and exacerbate others such as fatigue, backache, and indigestion. Getting some help around the house, taking more breaks away from whatever frazzles your nerves (including older children, if any), cutting back on job responsibilities, or letting low-priority tasks go undone for the time being can bring some relief (see page 102 for more tips).

Other Children. Some pregnant women with other children at home find that keeping up with their off-spring keeps them so busy that they barely have time to notice pregnancy discomforts, major or minor. But for many others, having one or more older children tends to aggravate pregnancy symptoms. For example, morning sickness can increase during times of stress (the getting-to-school or the getting-dinner-on-the-table rush, for instance); fatigue can be heightened because there doesn't seem to be any time to rest; backaches can be aggravated if you're doing a lot of child toting; even constipation becomes more likely if you never have a chance to use the bathroom when the urge strikes. The key to lessening the toll that caring for your other children can take on your pregnant body is sometimes elusive, but worth seeking: more time to take care of yourself. Take advantage of any potential helper you can find (paid or volunteer) to lighten your load and to help free up personal time.

"My first pregnancy was rough, with several serious complications. I'm very nervous now that I'm pregnant again."

O ne complicated pregnancy doesn't necessarily predict another. Often a woman who weathered high seas the first time around is rewarded with smooth sailing the next. If it was a one-time event, such as an infection or an accident, that caused the complications, then they aren't likely to recur. Nor will they recur if they were caused by lifestyle habits that you've now changed (like smoking, drinking, or using drugs), an exposure to an environmental hazard (such as lead) to which you are no longer exposed, or by failure to seek medical care early in pregnancy (assuming you've sought such care early on this time).

If the cause was a chronic health problem, such as diabetes or high blood pressure, correcting or controlling the condition prior to conception or very early in pregnancy can greatly reduce the risk of repeat complications.

If you had a specific complication during your first pregnancy that you would like to avoid the second time around, it's a good idea to discuss it with your practitioner now to see if anything can be done to prevent a repeat. No matter what the problem or its cause (even if it's been labeled "cause unknown"), the tips in the response to the previous question can help make your pregnancy more comfortable and safer for both you and your baby.

"With my first child, I had a very comfortable and uneventful pregnancy. That's why the 42-hour labor with 5 hours of pushing I had came as such a shock. I'm glad I'm pregnant again, but I dread another labor like the first one."

R elax, enjoy your pregnancy, and put thoughts of another difficult labor out of your mind. Second and subsequent deliveries are, barring a less than ideal fetal position or some other unforeseen complication, almost always easier than first ones, thanks to a more experienced uterus and a laxer birth canal. All phases of labor tend to be shorter, and the amount of pushing necessary to deliver generally decreases dramatically.

REPEAT CESAREANS

"When I had my first baby by cesarean I was told I could never deliver vaginally because of my abnormal pelvis. I want to have six kids just like my mother did, but I understand three cesareans is the limit."

Tell that to Ethel Kennedy, the indomitable wife of Robert F. Kennedy, who is reported to have had 11 cesareans in an era when the procedure was neither as safe nor as easy as it is today. Of course, sometimes having numerous cesareans isn't possible. Much depends upon the kind of incision that was made and the kind of scar that formed. Talk to your obstetrician about your concern, because only someone fully familiar with your clinical history can predict whether or not you can do an "Ethel Kennedy" (or even half an "Ethel Kennedy"). You may be pleasantly surprised.

If you do have multiple cesareans, however, you may, because of numerous scars, be at increased risk for uterine rupture caused by labor contractions. For this reason, you should be particularly alert for the signs of oncoming labor (contractions, bloody show, ruptured membranes; see page 269) in the final months of pregnancy. Should they occur, notify your doctor and go to the hospital immediately. You should also notify him or her at *any* time in your pregnancy if you have bleeding or unexplained, persistent abdominal pain.

"I had my last baby by cesarean. I'm pregnant again and I'm wondering what the chances are of my having a vaginal delivery."

"Once a cesarean always a cesarean" was, until very recently, an obstetrical edict engraved in stone, or rather in the uteruses of women who'd had one or more surgical deliveries. Today the American College of Obstetricians and Gynecologists has turned that theory upside-down. The new position: Repeat cesareans should not be considered routine; Vaginal Birth After Cesarean (VBAC) should be the norm. Experience shows that between 50% and 80% of women who have had cesareans are able to go through a normal labor and a vaginal delivery in subsequent deliveries. Even women who have had more than one cesarean or are carrying twins have a good chance of being able to successfully deliver vaginally.

Whether or not you will be able to try VBAC will depend on the type of uterine incision (which may be different from your abdominal incision) made in your previous c-section and on the reason your baby was delivered surgically. If you had a low-transverse incision (across the lower part of the uterus), as 95% of women do today, your chances of succeeding at VBAC are good; if you had a classic vertical incision (down the middle of your uterus), as was popular in the past and is still occasionally needed, you will not be allowed to attempt a vaginal delivery because of the risk of uterine rupture. If the reason for your c-section was one that isn't likely to repeat (fetal distress, premature separation of the placenta, faulty placement of the placenta, infection, breech, toxemia), it's very possible you can have a vaginal delivery this time. If it was a chronic disease (diabetes, high blood pressure, heart disease) or an uncorrectable problem (a badly contracted pelvis, for example), you will probably require a repeat cesarean. Don't rely on your recollection of the type of uterine incision you had or the reason you needed a cesarean last time—check, or have your physician check, the medical records of your prior delivery.

If you feel strongly about wanting a vaginal delivery this time, then discuss the possibility with your physician now. Some doctors still cling to the old adage and will not permit a woman with a cesarean-scarred uterus to go through a trial of labor. If you are to succeed at VBAC, you will need to find an amenable doctor who is willing to be with you from the very beginning of labor through delivery. And for safety's sake, you must plan on delivering in a hospital fully equipped and staffed for emergency cesarean sections, should one become necessary.

Your role in ensuring a safe vaginal delivery is as important as your doctor's. You should:

❖ Take childbirth education classes, and take them seriously, so that you will be able to labor as efficiently as possible to minimize the stress on your body.

❖ Notify your doctor when the first signs of labor (see page 269) occur.

❖ Agree to use little or no medication during labor and delivery, since medication could mask signs of an impending rupture.

❖ Tell your doctor immediately if *between* contractions you notice any unusual abdominal pain or tenderness.

Though your chances of having a normal vaginal delivery are good, even the woman who has never had a cesarean has a 20% or better chance of needing one. So don't be disappointed if you end up with a repeat. After all, the safest possible birth of that wonderful baby of yours is what this is all about.

"I had a cesarean my first time after an agonizing, long labor. My doctor said I should try to have a vaginal delivery this time, but I would rather have a cesarean and avoid another ordeal."

To read what staunch cesarean opponents have to say about it, one would quickly conclude that the medical establishment is solely responsible for the high rate of cesareans in this country. But there's another side of the story that isn't often told, and that

is that many repeat cesareans (and repeats make up at least one-third of the total performed each year) are performed at the request of the expectant mother. And the most common reason these mothers give for opting for the planned surgical delivery over VBAC is the desire to avoid another prolonged and painful labor.

It's normal for the human being not to want to suffer—it's an automatic reflex designed to protect against injury. Your eyelid blinks when a sharp object approaches; you pull your hand away from a flame. Those actions make sense. But though it might seem that choosing a cesarean just to avoid the pain of labor also makes sense, it doesn't. It's true that labor may cause more pain than a cesarean, but it isn't as likely to inflict injury. Your risks actually increase with a surgical delivery, and though the risks remain minute (with the chances of dying during a vaginal delivery at 1 in 10,000 and the chances of dying during a surgical delivery at 4 in 10,000), increasing risk without reason never makes sense.

Remember, too, that your labor this time is likely to be much easier and shorter. And if the VBAC is successful, you'll avoid the two or three days of abdominal pains that often follow a c-section. You owe it to yourself to give it a try.

YOUR FAMILY HISTORY

"I recently discovered that my mother and one of her sisters both lost babies shortly after delivery. No one knows why. Could that happen to me?"

It used to be that family histories of infant illness or death were often concealed, as though losing a baby or a child were somehow sinful or something to be ashamed of. But now we realize that exposing the history of past generations can help keep today's generation healthy. Though the deaths of the two babies under similar circumstances may just be coincidental, it would certainly make sense to see a genetic counselor or maternal-fetal subspecialist to get some advice. Your practitioner can recommend one.

Any couple that does not have information on possible hereditary defects in their families might be wise to make an effort to learn more, possibly by questioning older family members. Because prenatal diagnosis is possible for many hereditary disorders, being armed with such information beforehand may make it possible to prevent problems before they occur or to treat them when they do.

"There are several stories in our family about babies who seemed fine at birth but then started to get sicker and sicker. Eventually they died in early infancy. Should I be concerned?"

A mong the major causes of infant illness and death in the first few days and weeks of life are what are known as inborn errors of metabolism. Babies born with this type of genetic defect are missing an enzyme or other chemical substance, making it impossible for them to metabolize a particular dietary element; which element depends on which enzyme is missing. Ironically, the baby's life is in jeopardy as soon as feeding begins.

Fortunately most such disorders can be diagnosed prenatally, and many can be treated. So consider yourself lucky if you turn out to have this information available to you in advance, and be sure to act on it. Discuss this information with your practitioner and, if it's recommended, with a genetic counselor.

PREGNANCIES TOO CLOSE TOGETHER

"I became pregnant again just ten weeks after I delivered my first child. I'm worried about what effect this might have on my health and on the baby I'm now carrying."

C onceiving again before you've fully recovered from a recent pregnancy and delivery puts enough strain on your body without adding the debilitating effects of worry. So first of all, *relax*. Though conception in the first three postpartum months is rare (almost a miracle if the new baby is exclusively breastfed), it's taken other women by surprise too. And most have delivered normal, healthy infants, little the worse for wear themselves.

However, it's essential to be aware of the toll two quickly consecutive pregnancies can take, and to do everything possible to compensate. Conception within three months of delivery puts the new pregnancy in a high-risk category, which in this case isn't as ominous as it sounds, particularly with the proper care and precautions, including:

❖ The best prenatal care, starting as soon as you think you're pregnant. As with any high-risk pregnancy, you're probably best off with an obstetrician, or with a nurse-midwife who practices with one. You should be scrupulous about following doctor's orders and not missing office visits.

❖ The Best-Odds Diet (see page 80), adhered to, if not religiously, at least faithfully. It's possible your body has not had a chance to rebuild its stores and you may still, even some time after delivery and particularly if you are nursing, be at a nutritional disadvantage. That means you may need to overcompensate nutritionally to be sure both you and the baby you are carrying will not be deprived. Pay particular attention to protein (have at least 100 grams or four Best-Odds servings daily) and iron (you should take a supplement).

❖ **Adequate weight gain.** Your new fetus doesn't care whether or not you've had time to shed the extra pounds his or her sibling put on you. The two of you need the same 25-to-35-pound gain this pregnancy. So don't even think about losing weight, not even early on. A carefully monitored gradual weight gain will be relatively easy to take off afterward, particularly if it was gained on the highest-quality diet, and especially once you have two children to keep up with.

Be certain, too, that you don't let lack of time or energy keep you from eating enough. Feeding and caring for the child you already have shouldn't keep you from feeding and caring for your child-to-be. Watch your weight gain carefully, and if you're not progressing as you should (see page 147), monitor your calorie intake more closely and follow the suggestions given on page 81 for aid in increasing weight gain.

❖ **Weaning your older baby immediately if you're nursing.** He or she's already reaped many of the benefits of breastfeeding, and weaning at this stage should be neither difficult nor traumatic for your baby, though it may be uncomfortable for you. Some women do continue nursing, but trying to rally the nutritional forces for both nursing and pregnancy can be a losing battle for all concerned. For tips on weaning at any age, see *What to Expect the First Year.*

❖ **Rest**—more than is humanly (and new-motherly) possible. This will require not only your own determination but help from your husband and possibly others as well. Set priorities: let less important chores or work go undone, and force yourself to lie down when your baby is napping. Have Daddy take over as many nighttime feedings as he can rise to the occasion for, as well as much of the cooking, housework, and baby care (particularly tasks that involve a lot of heavy lifting or carrying).

❖ **Exercise**—just enough to keep you in shape and relax you, but not enough to overtax your system. If you can't seem to find the time for a regular pregnancy exercise routine, build physical activity into your day with your baby. Take him or her for a brisk walk in the stroller or in a baby carrier. Or enroll in a pregnancy exercise class (see page 194 for tips on choosing one) or swim at a club or Y that offers baby-sitting services. But avoid jogging or other strenuous exercise.

❖ **Eliminating or minimizing all other pregnancy risk factors,** such as smoking and drinking (see page 50). Your body and your baby shouldn't be subjected to any additional stress.

TEMPTING FATE THE SECOND TIME AROUND

"I had a perfect first baby. Now that I'm pregnant again, I can't get rid of the fear that I won't be so lucky this time."

A million-dollar lottery winner isn't likely to hit the jackpot again, though his or her odds remain as good as any other player's. A mother who has had a "perfect" baby, however, is not only likely to win again, her odds are better than they were before she had a successful pregnancy under her belt. In addition, with each subsequent pregnancy, she has the chance to improve her odds a little—by eliminating any existing negatives (smoking, drinking, drug use) and accentuating all positives (proper diet, exercise, and medical care).

HAVING A BIG FAMILY

"I'm pregnant for the sixth time. Does this pose any additional risk for my baby or for me?"

Time-honored medical theory has it that not only does practice in childbearing not make perfect, it may make imperfect. It has long been believed in medical circles that women who have five or more children are putting both themselves and their babies at increased risk with each additional pregnancy. This may have been true before the advances in modern obstetrical care—and it is probably true today for women who receive inadequate care—but the fact is that women getting good prenatal care have an excellent chance of having healthy, normal babies even in fifth or later pregnancies. In a recent study the only increased risk discovered for fifth and subsequent pregnancies was a small jump in the incidence of multiple births (twins, triplets, and so on) and in babies born with trisomy 21, a chromosomal disorder.[1] So enjoy your pregnancy *and* your large family. But do take a few precautions:

---

1. Though according to this study having a large family doesn't seem to be particularly risky for the babies, another study has shown that with each baby the mother's risk of developing noninsulin-dependent diabetes later in life increases.

❖ Consider prenatal testing if you are 30 years old or older (rather than waiting until you're 35), since the incidence of offspring with chromosomal problems appears to increase earlier in women with many pregnancies.

❖ Be sure to get all the help you can solicit or pay for. And drop nonessential chores for the duration. Teach your older children to be more self-sufficient (even toddlers can dress and undress themselves, put away toys, and so on). Exhaustion isn't good for any pregnant woman, particularly not one with a large brood to look after.

❖ Watch your weight. It's not uncommon for women who've had several pregnancies to put on a few extra pounds with each baby. If that's been the case with you, be particularly careful to eat efficiently and not gain too much (see page 147). Overweight does increase some risks, particularly that of having a difficult labor, and it can complicate cesarean delivery and recovery. On the other hand, make sure you're not so busy you don't eat enough to gain adequate weight.

❖ Keep all other pregnancy risks to a minimum—see page 50.

❖ Be particularly aware of signs that something may be wrong during pregnancy, labor, or postpartum (see pages 117 and 381). One study showed that, although there was no increased risk of either the many-time mother or her baby dying during pregnancy or delivery, there was an increased risk of such complications as breech or other unusual presentations, premature separation of the placenta, rupture of the uterus, and postpartum hemorrhage, and of the need for forceps and cesarean deliveries.

BEING A SINGLE MOTHER

"I'm single, I'm pregnant, and I'm happy about it—but I'm also a little nervous about going through this alone."

Just because you don't have a husband doesn't mean you'll have to go through pregnancy alone. The kind of support you'll need can come from other sources besides a spouse. A good friend or a relative you feel close to and comfortable with (a mother, aunt, sibling, or cousin) can step in to hold your hand, emotionally and physically, throughout pregnancy. That person can, in many ways, play the role of the father during the nine months and beyond—accompanying you to prenatal visits and childbirth education classes, lending an ear when you need to talk about your concerns and fears as well as your joyous anticipation, helping you get both your home and life ready for the new arrival, and acting as coach, supporter, and advocate during labor and delivery.

Something you might want to keep in mind when reading this book: the many references to "husband" and "father-to-be" aren't meant to exclude you. Since the majority of our readers are in traditional families, it's just simpler to use these terms consistently than try to include all the other possibilities that exist. We hope that you'll understand, and that as you read this book you'll find that it's meant as much for you as for married mothers-to-be.

HAVING A BABY AFTER 35

"I'm 38 and pregnant with my first—and probably last—baby. It's so important that it be healthy, but I've read so much about the risks of pregnancy after 35."

Becoming pregnant after 35 puts you in good—and growing—company. While the pregnancy rate has been dropping among women in their 20s, it has been zooming among women over 35. Nowadays, it isn't unheard of for a woman to have her first child, or start a second family, after 40 or even 45.

If you've lived for more than 35 years, however, you know that nothing one does in life is completely risk-free. Pregnancy, at any age, certainly isn't. And though these days the risks are very small to begin with, they do increase slightly as age advances. Most older mothers, however, feel that the benefits of starting a family at the time that is right for them far outweigh any risks. And they are buoyed by the fact that new medical discoveries are rapidly reducing these risks.

The major reproductive risk faced by a woman in your age group is not becoming pregnant at all because of decreased fertility. Once she's overcome that and become pregnant, the most common and most notorious risk is that of having a baby with Down syndrome. This risk increases with age: 1 in 10,000 for 20-year-old mothers, about 3 in 1,000 for 35-year-old mothers, and 1 in 100 for 40-year-old mothers. It's speculated that this and other chromosomal abnormalities, though still relatively rare, are more common in older women because their ova are older too (every woman is born with a lifetime supply of eggs) and have had more exposure to x-rays, drugs, infections, and so on. (It is now known, however, that the egg is not always responsible for such chromosomal abnormalities. An estimated minimum of 25% of Down syndrome cases have been linked to a defect in the father's sperm. See page 30.)

While Down syndrome (characterized by mental retardation, a flat face, and slanting eyes) isn't preventable at this time, it can, like many other genetic disorders, be diagnosed in utero, through prenatal diagnosis (see page 42). Such diagnostic testing is now routine for mothers over 35 and others in high-risk categories, including those who have low MSAFP readings (see page 47). Often, so is a sonogram (page 45). Should Down syndrome or another abnormality be discovered, the parents then must decide, with input from genetic counselors, pediatricians, maternal-fetal subspecialists, and other professionals, whether to terminate or continue the pregnancy. In making the decision about having a Down syndrome baby, it is important for expectant parents to keep in mind that such children have the potential for living fulfilling, if somewhat suboptimal, lives. They are exceptionally loving and lovable, and most can, with early intervention[2], learn to take care of themselves, even to read and write.

In addition to an increased risk of a baby with Down syndrome, mothers who are 35-plus are also slightly more likely to develop high blood pressure (especially if they are overweight), diabetes, and cardiovascular disease—all of which are more common in older groups in general and are usually controllable. Older mothers are also somewhat more subject to miscarriage, often due to a blighted embryo that is too defective to develop further. Because studies are contradictory, it isn't clear whether or not labor and delivery are on the average longer, more difficult, or more complicated in older mothers than in younger ones. But if they are, the differences are probably small. In some older

---

2. Such intervention, which includes training of parents as well as daily exposure of the infant to a specially designed program, can have a remarkable effect on children with mental handicaps.

women, a decrease in muscle tone and joint flexibility may contribute to labor difficulties, but in many others, thanks to excellent physical condition resulting from healthy lifestyles, this is not a problem.

In spite of the risks—which, as you can see, are far less threatening than most people suppose—today's older mothers have a lot going for them. Medical science, for example. Screening for birth defects can be done in utero through amniocentesis, chorionic villous sampling, ultrasound, and other newer procedures (see About Prenatal Diagnosis, page 42) and can potentially reduce the risk of bearing an infant with a severe birth defect to a level comparable to that of younger women. Drugs and close medical supervision can sometimes forestall preterm labor. Electronic fetal monitoring during labor can warn of fetal distress, allowing speedy measures to be taken to protect the fetus from further trauma.

As successful as these advances have been in reducing the risks of pregnancy after 35, they pale next to the strides older mothers have taken—and can take—to improve the odds for themselves and their babies through exercise, diet, and quality prenatal care. Advanced reproductive age alone does not necessarily put a mother in a high-risk category. But an accumulation of many individual risks can. When the older mother makes a concerted effort to eliminate or minimize as many risk factors as possible, she can take years off her pregnancy profile—making her chances of delivering a healthy baby virtually as good as those of a younger mother. (See Reducing Risk in Any Pregnancy, page 50.)

And there may be some additional pluses. It's been theorized that this new breed of woman—better educated (more than half of older mothers have gone to college), career-oriented, and more settled—make better parents, thanks to their maturity and stability. Because they are older and have probably had their share of the fast lane, they are now less likely to resent being tied down by a baby. One study showed that these mothers were generally more accepting of parenting and displayed more patience and other strengths that were beneficial to the development of their children. And though they may have less physical stamina than when they were younger, are separated by a wide generation gap from their children, and often find the lifestyle change more stressful because they're more set in their ways, few regret having become parents. Most, in fact, are thrilled about it.

AGE AND TESTING FOR DOWN SYNDROME

"I'm 34, and I'm due to deliver just two months before my 35th birthday. Should I consider testing for Down syndrome?"

The chances of having a baby with Down syndrome don't escalate suddenly on a woman's 35th birthday. The risk increases gradually from the early 20s on, with the greatest jump coming as a woman passes 40. So there is no clear scientific answer to whether or not it makes sense to resort to prenatal diagnosis when you are just shy of 35. The 35 cutoff is simply an arbitrary age, selected by doctors trying to detect as many fetuses with Down syndrome as possible without exposing more mothers and babies than necessary to the slight risk of some types of prenatal diagnosis. Some practitioners do advise women who will turn 35 during pregnancy to consider prenatal diagnosis; others don't.

In many cases, the practitioner will suggest that an MSAFP test (see page 47) be evaluated first, before a woman under 35 undergoes amniocentesis. A low reading on this simple blood test indicates the possibility, but not the probability, of Down syndrome in the fetus and suggests that a follow-up amniocentesis is a good idea. And though the test doesn't catch all cases of the syndrome, it is a useful screening tool. If the MSAFP reading is normal, on the other hand, amniocentesis becomes somewhat less essential— assuming there are no indications for it other than advanced age. Discuss the options, and your concerns, with your practitioner or genetic counselor.

THE FATHER'S AGE

"I'm only 31, but my husband is over 50. Does advanced paternal age pose risks to a baby?"

Throughout most of history, it was believed that a father's responsibility in the reproductive process was limited to fertilization. Only during this century (too late to help those queens who'd lost their heads for failing to produce a male heir) was it discovered that a father's sperm held the deciding genetic vote in determining his child's sex. And only in the last few years has it begun to be postulated that an older father's sperm might contribute to birth defects such as Down syndrome. Like the older mother's ova, the older father's primary oocytes (undeveloped sperm) have had longer exposure to environmental hazards and might conceivably contain altered or damaged genes or chromosomes. And from the isolated studies that have been done, there is some evidence that in about 25% or 30% of Down syndrome cases, the faulty chromosome can be traced to the father. It also appears that there is an increase in the risk of Down syndrome when the father is over 50 (or 55, depending on the study), though the association is weaker than in the case of maternal age.

But the evidence remains inconclusive—mostly because of the inadequacy of the existing research. Setting up the kind of large-scale studies required to obtain conclusive results has been difficult so far, for two reasons. First of all, Down syndrome is relatively rare (about 1 or 2 in 1,000 live births). Second, in the majority of cases, older fathers are married to older mothers, making it tricky to clarify the independent role of paternal age.

So the question of whether or not Down syndrome and other birth defects can be linked to advanced paternal age remains largely unanswered. Experts believe that there probably is some connection (although it's not clear at what age it begins), but that the risk is almost certainly very small. At this time, genetic counselors do not recommend amniocentesis on the basis of paternal age alone. If, however, you're going to spend the rest of your pregnancy worrying about the possible—though unlikely—effects of your husband's age on your baby, you might discuss your fears with your practitioner to see if amniocentesis is at all warranted.

IN-VITRO FERTILIZATION (IVF)

"I conceived my baby through in-vitro fertilization. Are my chances of having a healthy baby as good as anyone else's?"

T he fact that you conceived in a laboratory rather than in bed apparently doesn't affect your chances of having a healthy baby.[3] Recent studies have shown that all other factors being equal (age, DES exposure, the condition of the uterus, the number of fetuses, for example), there is no significant increase in such complications as prematurity, pregnancy-induced hypertension, prolonged labor, delivery complications, or the need for c-sections in IVF mothers. Nor does there appear to be more risk of a baby being born with abnormalities. There is a slightly higher miscarriage rate, but this is probably due to the fact that women who have IVF are so closely monitored that every pregnancy is diagnosed and therefore every miscarriage noted. This, of course, is not the case in the general population, in which many miscarriages occur before diagnosis and go unobserved or unreported.

There will, however, be some differences between your pregnancy and others, at least in the beginning. Because a positive test doesn't necessarily mean a pregnancy, because trying again can be so emotionally and financially draining, and because it's not known right off how many of the test-tube embryos are going to develop into fetuses, the first six weeks of an IVF pregnancy are usually more nervewracking than most. In addition, if an IVF mother has miscarried in previous tries, intercourse and other physical activities may be restricted, or complete bed rest may even be ordered. And the hormone progesterone may be prescribed to help support the developing pregnancy during the first two months. But once this period is past, you can expect that your pregnancy will be pretty much like everyone else's—unless you're carrying more than one fetus, as 5% to 25% of

---

3. Although less information is available on GIFT (gamete intrafallopian transfer) and intratubal insemination, it is assumed that the picture is pretty much the same for babies conceived through these newer methods.

IVF mothers do. If you are, see page 143.

And as with everyone else, your odds of having a healthy baby can be improved significantly by good medical care, excellent diet, moderate weight gain, a healthy balance of rest and exercise, and avoidance of alcohol, tobacco, and unprescribed drugs. See page 50 for tips on reducing pregnancy risk.

LIVING AT A HIGH ALTITUDE

"I'm concerned because we live at a high altitude, and I've heard that this can cause problems in pregnancy."

Since you're accustomed to breathing the thinner air where you live, you're far less likely to encounter an altitude-induced problem in your pregnancy than if you'd just moved there after thirty years at sea level. Though women who live at high altitudes run a *very slightly* increased chance of developing such pregnancy complications as hypertension and water retention, and of giving birth to a somewhat smaller than average baby, good prenatal care coupled with sensible self-care (eating a top-notch diet, gaining adequate weight, abstaining from alcohol and other drugs) can greatly minimize these risks. So can avoiding tobacco smoke—yours and/ or anybody else's. Smoking, which deprives babies of oxygen and optimum development at any altitude, appears to do still further damage at higher elevations, more than doubling the decrease in average birthweight. Strenuous exercise can also rob your baby of oxygen in high altitudes, so choose brisk walking over jogging, for example, and (of course this goes for all pregnant women) quit before you reach exhaustion.

Though you should be able to handle the high altitude without any trouble, women accustomed to living at low altitudes may have difficulty handling pregnancy high above sea level. Some doctors suggest postponing a contemplated move or visit (see page 180) from low altitude to high until after delivery. And of course attempting Mt. Rainier is definitely out.

RELIGIOUS OBJECTIONS TO MEDICAL CARE

"Because of my religious beliefs, I am opposed to seeking medical care. That holds especially for pregnancy, which after all is a natural process. My in-laws insist this is dangerous."

They're right. One study shows that women who refuse prenatal care on religious grounds are 100 times more likely to die in childbirth than women who get prenatal care, and that their babies are 3 times as likely to die at birth. You have to decide if these are risks you want to take for yourself and your child-to-be. And beyond the personal risk, are you willing to subject yourself to the legal risk if any injury that you might have prevented befalls your baby? Some courts are holding mothers responsible for behavior potentially damaging to the fetus they are carrying.

It's not likely that your in-laws are saying that your religious principles aren't important, rather that human life, not religious principle, is what is at stake here. Not only yours, but that of your precious baby.

Finally, it may help you to know that almost all religious convictions are fully compatible with good and safe obstetrical care. Discuss your convictions with two or three prospective practitioners. It's very possible that you can find a physician or nurse-midwife who will be able to find ways to safely adapt your pregnancy care to your religious rules.

RH INCOMPATIBILITY

"My doctor said my blood tests show I am Rh negative and my husband is Rh positive. He said not to worry, but my mother lost her second child because of Rh disease."

Every human being inherits a blood type that is either Rh positive (has the dominant Rh factor) or negative (lacks the factor). All pregnant women are tested for the Rh factor early in pregnancy. If a woman turns out to be Rh positive (85% are), or if both she and her husband are negative, there is no cause for concern. If, however, she is Rh negative and her husband Rh positive, she is a candidate for Rh incompatibility problems and her pregnancy must be kept under careful obstetrical surveillance.

When your mother had children, the problem of Rh incompatibility was indeed an ominous one. But thanks to several medical advances, your worry about losing a child to this condition is now largely unnecessary.

First of all, if this is your first pregnancy, there is very little threat to the baby. Trouble doesn't start brewing until the Rh factor enters the Rh-negative mother's circulatory system during the delivery (or abortion or miscarriage) of a child who has inherited the Rh factor from his or her father. The mother's body, in a natural protective immune response to the "foreign" substance, produces antibodies against it. The antibodies themselves are harmless—until she becomes pregnant again with another Rh-positive baby. Then the antibodies cross the placenta and attack the fetal red blood cells, causing very mild (if maternal antibody levels are low) to very serious (if they are high) anemia in the fetus. Only very rarely do these antibodies form in first pregnancies, in reaction to fetal blood leaking back through the placenta into the mother's circulatory system.

Today, prevention of the development of Rh antibodies is the key to protecting the fetus when there is Rh incompatibility. Most doctors use a two-pronged attack. At 28 weeks, an expectant Rh-negative woman who shows no antibodies in her blood is given a dose of Rh-immune globulin. Another dose is administered within 72 hours after delivery, if the baby is Rh positive. (A dose of vaccine is also administered after a miscarriage, an abortion, an amniocentesis, or bleeding during pregnancy.) Giving immune-globulin as required now can head off serious problems in future pregnancies.

If tests determine that a woman has developed Rh antibodies previously, amniocentesis (see page 44) can be used to check the blood type of the fetus. If it is Rh positive, and thus incompatible with the mother's, the maternal antibody levels are monitored regularly. If the levels become dangerously high tests will be done to assess the condition of the fetus. If at any point the safety of the fetus is threatened, indicating the development of erythroblastosis fetalis (also known as hemolytic or Rh disease), a transfusion of Rh negative blood may be necessary. When the incompatibility is severe, which is rare, the fetal transfusion can take place while the fetus is still in the uterus. More often it can wait until immediately after delivery. In mild cases, when antibody levels are low, a transfusion may not be needed. But doctors will be ready to do one at delivery if necessary.

The use of Rh vaccines has reduced the need for transfusions in Rh-incompatible pregnancies to less than

1%, and in the future may make this lifesaving procedure a medical miracle of the past.

OBESITY

"I'm about 60 pounds overweight. Does this put me and my baby at higher risk during pregnancy?"

M ost overweight mothers and their babies come through pregnancy and delivery safe and sound. Still, health risks do multiply as the pounds do, in pregnancy as well as out of it. The risk of both hypertension and diabetes, for example, is increased when you are overweight, and both of these conditions can complicate pregnancy (in the form of preeclampsia and gestational diabetes). Accurate dating of a pregnancy may be tricky because ovulation is often erratic in obese women and because some of the yardsticks doctors traditionally use to estimate the date (the height of the fundus, the size of the uterus) may be made indecipherable by layers of fat. An overly padded abdomen can also make it impossible for the doctor to determine a fetus's size and position manually, so that technological assistance might be necessary to avoid surprises during delivery. And delivery difficulties can result if the fetus is much larger than average, which is often the case in obese mothers (even those who don't overeat during pregnancy). Finally, if a cesarean delivery is necessary, the ample abdomen can complicate both the surgery and recovery from it.

As with other high-risk pregnancies, top-notch medical care can greatly increase the odds in favor of mother and baby. Right from the start you will probably undergo more tests than the typical low-risk pregnant woman: ultrasound early on to more accurately date your pregnancy, and later to determine the baby's size and position; at least one glucose tolerance test or screening for gestational diabetes, probably late in the second trimester, to determine if you are showing any signs of developing diabetes; and toward the end of your pregnancy, nonstress and other diagnostic tests to monitor your baby's condition.

Self-care will also be important. Your doctor will probably warn you not to smoke and to reduce all the other pregnancy risks that are within your control (see page 50). You will be cautioned against dieting, but also warned not to gain excessive weight. Most of the time, obese women can gain less than the recommended 25 to 35 pounds during pregnancy without adversely affecting the weight or health of their fetus.[4] But their lower-calorie diets must contain at least 1,800 calories and be packed with foods that are dense with vitamins, minerals, and protein (see Best-Odds Diet, page 80). Making every bite count is especially important for you, as is taking a pregnancy vitamin and mineral supplement. Getting regular exercise, within the guidelines recommended by your doctor, will also help keep your weight gain in check without your having to reduce food intake drastically.

For your next pregnancy, if you are planning on one, try to get as close as possible to your ideal weight *prior* to conception. It will make the course of your pregnancy easier.

---

4. Definitions vary, but usually a woman is considered obese if her weight is 120% of her ideal weight, very obese if it measures 150%. Thus a woman who should weigh 100 pounds is obese at 120 and very obese at 150 pounds.

HERPES

"I was anxious for a positive pregnancy test; but now that I am definitely pregnant, I'm terrified because I have genital herpes."

With the notable exception of AIDS (acquired immune deficiency syndrome), herpes has had the dubious distinction of generating more frightening headlines in recent years than any other sexually transmitted disease (STD). And many of the accompanying stories have emphasized that not only can adults contract the disease through sexual intercourse, but babies can contract it by passing through an infected birth canal. Though the disease is merely annoying in adults, it can be serious in newborns, whose immune systems are immature.

Certainly concern is warranted, but hysteria, in spite of alarmist headlines, isn't. First of all, neonatal infection is quite rare—occurring in an estimated 1 in 3,000 to 1 in 20,000 deliveries. Second, though still very serious, the disease seems to be somewhat milder in newborns than it was in the past.

Third, a baby has only a 2% to 3% chance of infection if its mother has a recurrent herpes infection during pregnancy—and recurrent infections are much more common than primary ones. Even among those babies at greatest risk, those whose mothers have their first herpes outbreak as delivery nears, 60% to 75% will escape infection. And though a primary infection earlier in pregnancy increases the risk of miscarriage and premature delivery, such infection is relatively rare.

So if you picked up your herpes infection before pregnancy, which is most likely, the risk to your baby is low. And with proper diagnosis and good medical care it can be lowered still further.

The best way to prevent most herpes infections in newborns would be to routinely screen all mothers for the disease prior to delivery, and to deliver those who test positive by cesarean section, which greatly reduces the chance of the infection being passed to the baby. But since an inexpensive screening test is not yet available, testing is usually reserved for women who have a history of genital herpes.

Signs and Symptoms of Genital Herpes

Since it is during a primary, or first, episode that genital herpes is most likely to be passed on to the fetus, your doctor should be informed if you experience the following symptoms of the disease: fever, headache, malaise, achiness for two or more days, accompanied by genital pain, itching, pain with urination, vaginal and urethral discharge, and tenderness in the groin (inguinal adenopathy), as well as lesions that blister and then crust over. Healing generally takes place within two to three weeks, during which time the disease can be transmitted.

If you have genital herpes, be careful not to pass it to your partner (and he should likewise be careful if he's infected). Avoid intercourse when either of you has lesions; wash hands thoroughly with mild soap and water after using the toilet or having sexual relations; shower or bathe daily; keep lesions clean, dry, and dusted with cornstarch; and wear cotton underpants and avoid wearing clothes that are constricting in the crotch area.

Many doctors only test when a woman develops genital lesions close to her delivery date. If the culture is positive, then the test is usually repeated weekly so that when labor begins it is known whether the infection is still present.[5]

If the most recent culture was positive, or more important, if genital lesions are present as labor begins or the membranes rupture, a c-section is usually performed. Because of the slight chance that infection could spread to the fetus once the protection of the amniotic sac is removed, cesarean delivery is usually carried out within four to six hours after the membranes rupture, unless the fetus is not mature enough for immediate delivery.

Newborns at risk for herpes infection are usually isolated from other newborns at birth to prevent the possible spread of infection. In the unlikely event that infection does occur, treatment with an antiviral drug will reduce the risk of permanent damage. If the mother has an active infection, she can still care for her baby and even breastfeed if she takes special precautions to avoid transmitting the virus.

OTHER STDs (SEXUALLY TRANSMITTED DISEASES)

'I've heard that herpes can harm the fetus. Is this also true of other sexually transmitted diseases?"

The bad news: Yes, there are other STDs that present a hazard to the fetus. The good news: Most are easily diagnosed and treated.

5. Since antiviral drugs haven't yet been approved for use in pregnancy, their use is reserved for life-threatening situations.

Gonorrhea. Gonorrhea has long been known to cause conjunctivitis, blindness, and serious generalized infection in the fetus delivered through an infected birth canal. For this reason, pregnant women are routinely tested for the disease, usually at their first prenatal visit (see page 101). Sometimes, particularly in women at high risk for STDs, the test is repeated late in pregnancy. If infection with gonorrhea is found, it is treated immediately with antibiotics. Treatment is followed by another culture, to be sure the woman is infection-free. As an added precaution, drops of silver nitrate or an antibiotic ointment are squeezed into the eyes of every newborn at birth. (This treatment can be delayed for as long as an hour—but no longer—if you want to have some eye-to-eye contact with your baby first.)

Syphilis. The fetal bone and tooth deformities, the progressive nervous system damage, the stillbirths, and the eventual brain damage caused by syphilis have long been recognized too. And testing for this disease is also routine at the first prenatal visit. Antibiotic treatment of infected pregnant women before the fourth month, when the infection usually begins to cross the placental barrier, will almost always prevent damage to the fetus.

Chlamydia. More recently recognized as a potential danger to the fetus, chlamydia is now reported to the Center for Disease Control more often than gonorrhea. It is the most common infection passed from mother to fetus—which is why chlamydia screening in pregnancy is a good idea, particularly if you have had multiple sexual partners in the past (which increases your chance of infection). Since about half the women with chlamydial infection experience no symptoms, it often goes undiagnosed when not tested for.

Prompt treatment of chlamydia prior to or during pregnancy can prevent chlamydial illness (pneumonia, which fortunately is most often mild, and eye infections, which are occasionally severe) from being transmitted by the mother to the baby during delivery. Though the best time for treatment is prior to conception, administering antibiotics to the pregnant infected mother can also effectively prevent infant infection. Antibiotic ointment used at birth protects the newborn from chlamydial eye infection.

Nonspecific vaginitis (NSV). NSV, also known as bacterial vaginosis or Gardnerella vaginitis, can cause such pregnancy complications as premature rupture of the membranes and intra-amniotic infection, which may lead to premature labor. Some experts believe pregnant women should be screened for NSV, so it may be among the infections you are tested for at your first visit.

Venereal, or genital, warts. These sexually transmitted warts may appear anywhere in the genital area and are caused by the human papilloma virus. Their appearance can vary from a barely visible lesion to a soft, velvety, flat bump or a cauliflower-like growth. The warts range in color from pale to dark pink. Highly contagious, venereal warts are particularly important to treat not only because they can be transmitted to the baby or even block delivery, but because 5% to 15% of cases go on to produce inflammation of the cervix, which can progress to cervical cancer. Treatment usually includes a prescribed topical medication—*do not* use over-the-counter wart medicines for venereal warts. If necessary, large warts may be removed late in pregnancy by freezing, electrical heat, or laser therapy.

Acquired Immune Deficiency Syndrome (AIDS). Infection in pregnancy by the HIV virus, which causes AIDS, is a threat not just to the expectant mother but to her baby as well. A large proportion (estimates range from 20% to 65%) of babies born to mothers who are HIV positive develop the infection within six months, and it is suspected that pregnancy itself could speed up the progress of the disease in the mother. For these reasons, some infected women choose to terminate their pregnancies. Before taking any action, anyone who tests HIV positive should consider retesting (tests are not always accurate and can sometimes be positive in someone who does not have the virus).[6] If a second test is positive, then formal counseling about AIDS and the treatment options is absolutely imperative. Although it isn't known whether treating the mother for AIDS will prevent the development of disease in the fetus, it might be wise to inquire about experimental treatment for pregnant women with AIDS.

If you suspect that you may have been infected with any sexually transmitted disease, check with your practitioner to see if you've been tested; if you haven't, ask to be. If a test turns out to be positive, be sure that you—and your partner, if necessary—are treated. Treatment will protect not only your health, but that of your baby.

FEAR OF AIDS

"Both my husband and I had a number of partners before we met. Since I heard that AIDS sometimes doesn't show up for

---

6. Occasionally, a woman who has had several children will test false-positive for HIV. If you have a large family and test positive, discuss this possibility with your physician.

years, I can't get rid of the fear that I might have it and give it to my baby."

T he chance that you or your husband contracted AIDS before you met is slight if neither one of you is in a high-risk group (hemophiliacs, IV drug users, those who've had sex with bisexual or homosexual males or with intravenous drug users), even if you've had multiple partners. But if that's not enough to shake your nagging fear, or if that fear is becoming a debilitating focus of your pregnancy, discuss with your practitioner the possibility of having your blood tested for the HIV virus.

"I was surprised when my doctor asked if I wanted to be tested for HIV—I don't think I'm in a high-risk category."

I t is becoming increasingly common for all pregnant women to be offered a test for HIV, whether or not they have a prior history of high-risk behavior. So don't be offended; be glad your practitioner cares enough to give you the opportunity to take the test.

HEPATITIS B

"I'm a carrier of hepatitis B, and just found out that I'm pregnant. Will my being a carrier hurt my baby?"

K nowing you're a carrier for hepatitis B is the first step in making sure that your condition won't hurt your baby. Though babies born to some carriers (those with a certain antigen) are at high risk for infection, treating them within 12 hours of birth with hepatitis B vaccine and immune globulin can almost always prevent such infection. So be sure that your practitioner knows that you're a carrier, that a titer is taken to determine

how contagious you are, and that your baby is treated as needed. For more information on hepatitis infections, see page 318.

AN IUD STILL IN PLACE

"I've been wearing an IUD for two years and just discovered that I'm pregnant. We want to be able to keep the baby; is it possible?"

G etting pregnant while using birth control is always a little unsettling, but it does happen. The odds of it happening with an IUD are 1 to 5 in 100, depending on the type of device used and whether or not it has been properly inserted. A woman who conceives with an IUD in place and doesn't want to terminate her pregnancy has two choices—which she should discuss as soon as possible with her doctor: leaving the IUD in place or having the IUD withdrawn. Which is preferable usually depends on whether or not the removal cord is found, on examination, to be visibly protruding from the cervix. If it isn't visible, the pregnancy has a very good chance of proceeding uneventfully with the IUD in place. The IUD will simply be pushed up against the wall of the uterus by the expanding amniotic sac surrounding the baby, and during childbirth, will usually deliver with the placenta. If, however, the IUD string is visible early in pregnancy, the chances of a safe and successful pregnancy are greater if the IUD is removed as soon as feasible, once conception is confirmed. If it isn't, there is a significant chance that the fetus will spontaneously miscarry; when it's removed, the risk is only 20%. If that doesn't sound reassuring, keep in mind that the rate of miscarriage in all known pregnancies is estimated to be about 15% to 20%.

If you do continue your pregnancy with the IUD left in, you should, during the first trimester, be especially alert for bleeding, cramps, or fever, because the IUD puts you at higher risk for early pregnancy complications (see Ectopic Pregnancy, page 109, and Miscarriage, page 111.) Notify your doctor of such symptoms promptly.

BIRTH CONTROL PILLS IN PREGNANCY

"I got pregnant while using birth control pills. I kept taking them for over a month because I had no idea I was pregnant. Now I'm worried about the effect this may have on my baby."

Ideally, you should stop using oral contraceptives three months, or for at least two normally occurring menstrual cycles, before you want to become pregnant. But conception doesn't always wait for ideal conditions, and occasionally a woman becomes pregnant while taking the Pill. In spite of warnings you might have read on drug inserts, there's no reason for alarm. Statistically, there is no good evidence of an increased risk of fetal malformation when the mother has conceived while on oral contraceptives. A discussion of the subject with your practitioner should further relieve your concern.

SPERMICIDES

"I conceived while using a spermicide with my diaphragm, and used it several times again before I knew I was pregnant. Could the chemicals have damaged the sperm before conception, or the embryo after it?"

It is estimated that between 300,000 and 600,000 women who become pregnant each year used spermicides around the time of conception and in the early weeks of pregnancy before finding out that they'd conceived. So the question of what effects spermicides may have during conception and pregnancy is of great significance to a great many expectant couples—and to those choosing a method of birth control.

Fortunately, the answers so far have been reassuring. No more than a tentative link has ever been suggested between the use of spermicides and the incidence of certain birth defects, specifically Down syndrome and limb deformities. And the most recent and most convincing studies have found no increase in the incidence of such defects even with the repeated use of spermicides in early pregnancy. So according to the best information available, you and the other 299,999 to 599,999 mothers-to-be can relax—there appears to be nothing to worry about.

You may, however, be more comfortable with a different, and perhaps more reliable, method of birth control in the future. And because any chemical exposure of embryo or fetus is suspect, if you do continue to use a spermicide, you should plan on discontinuing its use before you decide to become pregnant again—assuming your next pregnancy is planned.

PROVERA

"Last month my doctor gave me Provera to bring on a late period. It turns out that I was pregnant. The package insert warns that pregnant women should never take this drug. Could my baby be malformed? Should I consider an abortion?"

Having taken the progesterone drug Provera during pregnancy, though it isn't recommended, is no reason to consider an abortion—as your obstetrician will probably tell you. It's not even a reason to worry. The drug company's warnings are not only for your protection but for theirs: in case of a lawsuit. It's true that some studies show a 1 in 1,000 risk of certain birth defects when an embryo or fetus has been exposed to Provera, but that risk is only minimally higher than for the risk of the same defects occurring in any pregnancy.

Whether Provera actually does cause birth defects or not isn't even certain. Some physicians who prescribe Provera to prevent miscarriage believe that it only *appears* to cause defects—by occasionally enabling a woman to sustain a blighted pregnancy that would have otherwise miscarried. It will probably take years more study on hundreds of thousands of pregnant women to definitely determine the effects—if any—of progesterone drugs on the fetus. But from what is presently known, it is believed that if Provera is actually a teratogen (a substance that can harm an embryo or fetus), it is a very weak one (see Playing Baby Roulette, page 76). Cross this one off your worry list.

DES

"My mother took DES when she was pregnant with me. Can this affect my pregnancy or my baby in any way?"

B efore the dangers of using the synthetic estrogen drug diethylstilbestrol (DES) to prevent miscarriage were known, more than a million pregnant women took it. Now that their daughters, many of whom were born with structural abnormalities of the reproductive tract (the majority so minor that they are of no gynecological or obstetrical signifi-

cance), are of childbearing age, they are concerned about the effects DES exposure will have on their own pregnancies. Happily, these effects appear to be minimal for most women—it is estimated that at least 80% of DES-exposed women have been able to have children.

The women with the most severe abnormalities, however, do appear to have an increased risk of certain pregnancy problems: ectopic pregnancy (probably because of malformed fallopian tubes), and midtrimester miscarriage and preterm birth (usually because of a weakened, or incompetent, cervix, which under the weight of a growing fetus can open prematurely). Because of the risks involved with all of these complications, it's important that you advise your physician of your DES exposure.[7] It is also important for you to be aware of the symptoms of these pregnancy mishaps and, should they occur, to report them to your doctor at once. If an incompetent cervix is suspected, one of two courses will probably be taken. Either a preventive stitch will be placed around the cervix between the 12th and 16th weeks of your pregnancy or your cervix will be examined regularly for signs of premature opening; if such signs are noted, steps will be taken to prevent further progression toward premature delivery.

GENETIC PROBLEMS

"I keep worrying that I might have a genetic problem and not know it. Should I get genetic counseling?"

---

7. Because of the slightly increased risk of pregnancy complications, DES-exposed women are probably better off with an obstetrician overseeing their pregnancy care.

P robably all of us carry one or more deleterious gene for mild or serious genetic disorders. But fortunately, because most disorders (Tay-Sachs or cystic fibrosis, for example) require a matching one-from-mom, one-from-dad pair of genes, they rarely manifest themselves in our children. One or both parents can be tested for some of these disorders before or during pregnancy. But testing makes sense only if there is a better-than-average possibility that both parents are carriers of a particular disorder. The clue is often ethnic or geographic. For example, Jewish couples whose forebears came originally from Eastern Europe should be tested for Tay-Sachs. (In most cases, a practitioner will recommend a test for one parent; testing the second parent becomes necessary only if the first test is positive.) Similarly, black couples should be tested for the sickle-cell anemia trait.

Diseases that can be passed on via a single gene from one carrier parent (hemophilia, for example) or by one affected parent (Huntington's chorea) have usually turned up in the family before, but this may not be common knowledge. That's why it's important to keep records of family health histories.

Most expectant parents, happily, are at low risk for transmitting genetic problems and need never see a genetic counselor. In many cases an obstetrician will talk to a couple about the most common genetic issues, referring to a genetic counselor or a maternal-fetal subspecialist those with a need for more expertise:

❖ Couples whose blood tests show them both to be carriers of a genetic disorder.

❖ Parents who have already borne one or more children with genetic birth defects.

❖ Couples who know of a hereditary disorder on any branch of either of their family trees. In some cases, as with certain thalassemias (hereditary anemias common among Mediterranean peoples), doing DNA testing of the parents before pregnancy makes interpreting later testing of the fetus much easier.

❖ Couples in which one partner has a congenital defect (such as congenital heart disease).

❖ Pregnant women who have had positive screening tests for the presence of a fetal defect.

❖ Closely related couples, because the risk of inherited disease in offspring is greatest when parents are related (for example, 1 in 8 for first cousins).

❖ Women over 35.

A genetic counselor is a sort of heredity bookmaker, trained to give such couples the odds of their having a healthy child and to guide them in deciding whether or not to have children. If they are already pregnant, the counselor can suggest appropriate prenatal testing.

Genetic counseling has saved hundreds of thousands of high-risk couples from the heartbreak of bearing children with serious problems. The best time to see a genetic counselor is before getting pregnant, or in the case of close relatives, before getting married. But it's not too late even after pregnancy is confirmed.

If testing uncovers a serious defect in a fetus, the expectant parents are faced with the decision of whether or not to continue with the pregnancy. Though the decision is theirs, a genetic counselor can provide important input.

YOUR OPPOSITION TO ABORTION

"My husband and I don't believe in abortion. Why should I have to go through amniocentesis?"

Amniocentesis isn't only appropriate for those couples who would consider abortion should a serious fetal defect be detected via the procedure. For the vast majority of expectant parents the best reason for prenatal diagnosis is the reassurance it almost always brings.

And although many couples opt for terminating the pregnancy when the news is bad, testing can also be valuable when abortion is not an option. When the defect discovered is a fatal one, it gives the parents time to grieve before the birth and eliminates the sense of shock later. When other kinds of defects are present, it provides parents a head start on preparing for life with a sick or handicapped child.

Rather than having to work out the inevitable reactions that come with discovering that their baby has a defect (such as denial, resentment, and guilt) after delivery, when such feelings can seriously compromise parent-child bonding, parents can start working them out during the pregnancy. Instead of starting at delivery to learn about the child's particular handicap, parents can research it in advance and be prepared to take steps to ensure the best possible life for their new baby. It is even conceivable that discovering a defect prenatally will allow for treatment in the uterus or special precautions at or after birth that will improve the chances that the baby will be okay.

So, if prenatal diagnosis is indicated, don't reject it out-of-hand. Talk to your practitioner, a genetic counselor, or a maternal-fetal subspecialist to help you clarify your options before you make your decision. And don't let your opposition to abortion deprive you and your doctors of potentially valuable information.

What It's Important to Know:
ABOUT PRENATAL DIAGNOSIS

Is it a boy—or a girl? Will it have blond hair like Grandma, green eyes like Grandpa? Daddy's voice and Mommy's flair for figures or—heaven forbid!—the other way around? The questions of pregnancy far outnumber the answers, providing lively material for nine months of dinner table debate, neighborhood speculation, and office pools.

But there's one question that isn't a topic for casual wagering. It's one most parents hesitate to talk about at all: "Is my baby okay?"

Until recently, that question could be answered only at birth. Today it can to some extent be answered as early as six weeks after conception, through prenatal diagnosis.

Because of inherent risks, small as they are, prenatal diagnosis isn't for everyone. Most parents will continue to play the waiting game, with the happy assurance that the odds are overwhelming that their babies are indeed "okay." But for those whose concerns represent more than normal expectant-parent jitters, the benefits of prenatal diagnosis can far outweigh the risks. Women who are good candidates for prenatal diagnosis include those who:

❖ Are over 35.

❖ Have a family history of genetic disease and/or have been shown to be carriers of such a disease.

❖ Have been exposed to infection (such as rubella or toxoplasmosis) that could cause a birth defect.

❖ Have been exposed since conception to a substance or substances that they fear might have been harmful to their developing baby. (Consultation with a physician can help determine whether prenatal diagnosis is warranted in a particular case.)

❖ Have had unsuccessful pregnancies previously, or have had babies with birth defects.

In more than 95% of cases, prenatal diagnosis turns up no apparent abnormalities. In the remainder, the expectant couple's discovery that something is wrong with their baby isn't comforting. But, teamed with expert genetic counseling, the information can be used to make vital decisions about this and future pregnancies. Possible options include:

Continuing the Pregnancy. This option is often chosen when the defect uncovered is one the family feels that both they and the baby they are awaiting can live with, or when the parents are opposed to abortion under any condition. Having some idea of what is to come allows the family to make preparations (both emotional and practical) for either receiving a child with special needs into the family or for coping with the birth of an infant who is unlikely to survive.

Terminating the Pregnancy. If testing suggests a defect that will be fatal or extremely disabling, and retesting and/or interpretation by a genetic counselor confirms the diagnosis, many parents opt for terminating the pregnancy. In such a case, careful examination of the products of the pregnancy for abnormalities is a must, and may be helpful in determining the chances of a repeat in future pregnancies. Most couples, armed with this information and the guidance of a physician or genetic counselor, do try again, with the hope that prenatal test results—and thus pregnancy outcome—will turn out favorable the next time around. And most often, they do.

Prenatal Treatment of the Fetus. This option is available in only a few instances, though in the future it can be expected to become more and more common. Treatment may consist of blood transfusion (as in Rh disease), surgery (to drain an obstructed bladder, for instance), or administration of enzymes or medication (such as steroids to accelerate lung development in the fetus who must be delivered before term). As technology advances, more kinds of prenatal surgery, genetic manipulation, and other fetal treatments may also become commonplace.

Donating the Organs. If diagnosis indicates that the fetal defects are not compatible with life, as when all or most of the brain is missing, it may be possible to donate one or more of the other organs to an infant in need. Some parents find that this provides at least some small consolation for their own loss. A neonatologist at a local medical center may be able to provide helpful information in such a situation.

Of course it's important to remember that nothing is perfect, not even high-tech prenatal diagnosis. For that reason, all results that indicate there is something wrong with the fetus should be confirmed by further testing or consultation with additional professionals. Acting too quickly to terminate a pregnancy has on occasion resulted in the aborting of a normal fetus.

The most commonly used methods of prenatal diagnosis follow.

AMNIOCENTESIS

The fetal cells, chemicals, and microorganisms in the amniotic fluid surrounding the fetus provide a wide range of information—genetic makeup, present condition, level of maturity—about the new human being. Thus being able to extract and examine some of the fluid through amniocentesis has been one of the most important advances in prenatal diagnosis. It is recommended when:

❖ The mother is over age 35. Between 80% and 90% of all amniocentesis is performed solely on the basis of advanced maternal age, primarily to determine if the fetus has Down syndrome, which is most prevalent among children of older mothers.

❖ The couple has already had a child with a chromosomal abnormality, such as Down syndrome, or with a metabolic disorder, such as Hunter's syndrome.

❖ The couple has already had a child or has a close relative with a neural tube defect. (A test to determine maternal-serum alpha-fetoprotein, or MSAFP, levels in the mother's blood will probably be performed first.)

❖ The mother is a carrier of an x-linked genetic disorder, such as hemophilia (which she has a 50-50 chance of passing on to any son she bears). Amniocentesis can identify the sex of the fetus, although not whether the baby has inherited the gene.

❖ Both parents are carriers of an au-

tosomal recessive inherited disorder, such as Tay-Sachs disease or sickle-cell anemia, and thus have a 1 in 4 chance of bearing an affected child.

❖ It is necessary to assess the maturity of the fetal lungs (among the last organs ready to function on their own).

❖ A parent is known to have a condition such as Huntington's chorea, which is passed on by autosomal dominant inheritance, giving the baby a 1 in 2 chance of inheriting the disease.

❖ Results of screening test (usually MSAFP, sonogram, estriol, and/or hCG) turn out to be abnormal, and evaluation of the amniotic fluid is necessary to determine whether or not there actually is a fetal abnormality.

When Is It Done? Diagnostic second-trimester amniocentesis is usually performed between the 16th and 18th weeks of pregnancy, though occasionally as early as the 14th or as late as the 20th week. The feasibility of earlier amniocentesis—between the 10th and 14th weeks—is presently being investigated. Most tests, because cells must be cultured in the laboratory, take from 24 to 35 days to be completed, though a few, such as those for Tay-Sachs disease, Hunter's syndrome, and neural tube defects, can be performed immediately.

Amniocentesis can also be performed in the last trimester to assess the maturity of fetal lungs.

How Is It Done? After changing into an examination gown and emptying her bladder, the expectant mother is positioned on the examining table on her back, her body draped so that only her abdomen is exposed. The fetus and placenta are then located via ultrasound, so that the doctor will be able to steer clear of them during the procedure. (A more detailed ultrasound will have previously been done to identify any easily visible fetal abnormalities.) The abdomen is swabbed with antiseptic solution, and in some cases, numbed with an injection of a local anesthetic, similar to the novocaine used by dentists. (Because this injection is as painful as the passage of the amniocentesis needle itself, some practitioners omit it.) Then a long, hollow needle is inserted through the abdominal wall into the uterus and a small amount of fluid is withdrawn. The slight risk of accidentally pricking the fetus during this part of the procedure is further reduced by the use of simultaneous ultrasound guidance. The mother's vital signs and the fetal heart tones are checked before and after the procedure, which, from start to finish, shouldn't take more than 30 minutes. Rh-negative women are usually given an injection of Rh-immune globulin after an amniocentesis to be sure the procedure does not result in Rh problems.

Unless it is a necessary part of the diagnosis, parents have the option not to be told their baby's sex when the report comes back, but to find out the old-fashioned way, in the delivery room. (Keep in mind that mix-ups, though rare, do happen.)

How Safe Is It? Most women experience no more than a few hours of mild cramping after the procedure; rarely there is slight vaginal bleeding or amniotic fluid leak. Although fewer than 1 in 200 women experience an infection or other complication that may lead to miscarriage, amniocentesis, like most other prenatal diagnostic tests, should be performed only when the benefits outweigh the risks.

ULTRASOUND

The advent of ultrasonography has made obstetrics a much more precise science and pregnancy a much less worrisome experience for many expectant parents. Through the use of sound waves that bounce off internal structures, it allows visualization of the fetus without the hazards of x-ray. If the apparatus used has a TV-like viewing screen, it provides a unique opportunity to "see" your baby—and maybe even get a sonogram photo to show to friends and family—though it may take an expert to make out a head or buttocks in the blurry image.

A level 1 ultrasound is usually done to date a pregnancy. A more detailed, or level 2, ultrasound is used for more sophisticated diagnostic purposes. Ultrasound may be recommended when the mother has a poor obstetrical history; for example, when she's had an ectopic (tubal) pregnancy, a hydatidiform mole (the placenta develops into a bunch of grapelike cysts that can't support a developing embryo); a ce-

Amnio Complication

Although complications with amniocentesis are rare, it is estimated that following about 1 in 100 procedures there is some leakage of amniotic fluid. If you should notice such leakage from your vagina, report it to your practitioner at once. The odds are very good that the leakage will stop after a few days, but bed rest and careful observation are usually recommended until it does.

sarean section; or a baby with a birth defect or genetic disease. It may also be used to:

❖ Verify a due date by checking to see if it correlates with the baby's size.[8]

❖ Determine the condition of the fetus when there is a greater than average risk of an abnormality, or when there is greater than average concern. This can be done earlier and often more accurately with transvaginal (through the vagina) ultrasound.

❖ Rule out pregnancy by the seventh week if there's been a suspected false-positive pregnancy test.

❖ Determine the cause of bleeding or spotting in early pregnancy, such as a tubal pregnancy or a blighted ovum (an embryo that has stopped developing and is no longer viable).

❖ Locate an IUD that was in place at the time of conception.

❖ Locate the fetus prior to amniocentesis and during chorionic villus sampling biopsy.

❖ Determine the condition of the fetus if no heartbeat has been detected by the 14th week with a Doppler device, or if there has been no fetal movement by the 22nd week.

❖ Diagnose the existence of multiple fetuses, usually when the mother has taken fertility drugs and/or the uterus is larger than expected for the date.

❖ Determine if abnormally rapid uterine growth is being caused by

an excess of amniotic fluid.

❖ Determine the condition of the placenta, when deterioration might be responsible for retarded fetal growth or fetal distress.

❖ Visualize the placenta to determine if bleeding late in pregnancy is due to the placenta being located low in the uterus (placenta previa) or to its separating prematurely (abruptio placenta). Blood clots behind the placenta can also be visualized.

❖ Determine the size of the fetus when preterm delivery is being contemplated or when the baby is believed to be late.

❖ Evaluate the condition of the fetus through observation of fetal activity, breathing movements, amniotic fluid volume (see Biophysical Profile, page 263).

❖ Verify breech presentation or other uncommon fetal or cord position prior to delivery.

When Is It Done? Depending on the reason for it, ultrasound can be used any time from the fifth week of gestation through delivery. Transvaginal ultrasound may be used earlier than the transabdominal (through the abdomen) procedure to determine whether there is a multiple gestation or abnormal fetal development.

How Is It Done? Ultrasound examination may be through the abdomen or through the vagina; sometimes, when there's a special need, the doctor may have a look both ways. The procedures are quick (five to ten minutes) and painless, except for the discomfort of the full bladder necessary for the transabdominal exam (which is probably why most women appear to prefer the transvaginal). During either exam, the expectant mother lies on her back. For the transabdominal, her

---

8. Some physicians believe this should be done routinely because verifying the date early on reduces the possibility of unnecessarily inducing labor when a baby is (incorrectly) believed to be late; this in turn reduces the need for cesareans for failed induction.

bare abdomen is spread with a film of oil or gel that will improve the conduction of sound. A transducer is then moved slowly over the abdomen. For the transvaginal, a probe is inserted into the vagina. The instruments record echoes of sound waves as they bounce off parts of the baby. With the help of a technician or doctor, you may be able to differentiate the beating heart; the curve of the spine; the head, arms, and legs. You may even catch sight of your baby sucking its thumb. Sometimes even the genital organs are distinguishable and the sex can be surmised, although with less than 100% reliability. (If you don't want to know your baby's sex yet, inform the doctor in advance.)

How Safe Is It? In 25 years of clinical use and study, no known risks and a great many benefits have been associated with the use of ultrasound photography. Still, because of the slim possibility that side effects may show up in the future, it's generally recommended by U.S. experts that ultrasound be used in pregnancy only when valid indications exist. Recent research in Great Britain, however, suggests that the benefits of routine ultrasound examinations in pregnancy may be great enough to outweigh any potential risk.

FETOSCOPY

Fetoscopy is science fiction turning fast into medical fact. In a voyage as fantastic as any penned by Isaac Asimov, a miniaturized telescope-like instrument, complete with lights and lenses, is inserted through tiny incisions in the abdomen and uterus into the amniotic sac, where it can view and photograph the fetus. At the same time, fetoscopy makes it possible to diagnose, through blood and tissue sampling, several blood and skin diseases that amniocentesis can't detect. Because it's a relatively high-risk procedure, however, and because other safer techniques are becoming available to detect the same disorders, fetoscopy is not widely used.

When Is It Done? Usually after the 16th week.

How Is It Done? After the abdomen is swabbed with antiseptic and numbed with a local anesthetic, tiny incisions are made in the abdomen and uterus. With ultrasound monitoring to guide the instrument, a fiber-optic endoscope is passed through the incisions and into the uterus. With this miniature telescope, the fetus, placenta, and amniotic fluid can be observed, blood samples can be taken from the junction of the umbilical cord and the placenta, and/or a tiny bit of fetal or placental tissue can be removed for examination.

How Safe Is It? Fetoscopy is, at this point, still a relatively risky procedure, carrying between a 3% and 5% chance of fetal loss. Though this risk is greater than that of other diagnostic tests, it is outweighed for the occasional woman who needs it by the benefit of discovering, and possibly treating or correcting, a defect in her fetus.

MATERNAL-SERUM ALPHA-FETOPROTEIN SCREENING

Elevated levels in the mother's blood, or serum, of alphafetoprotein (MSAFP), a substance produced by the fetus, can indicate a neural tube defect such as spina bifida (a deformity of the spinal column) or anencephaly (the absence of all or part of the brain). Abnormally low levels suggest an increased risk of Down syndrome or other chromosomal defect. This is only a screening test, and any abnormal result requires further testing to confirm the existence of a problem.

When Is It Done? Between the 16th and 18th weeks.

How Is It Done? This simple test requires only a maternal blood sample. If MSAFP levels are found to be abnormally high, a second test is run. If the second test duplicates the initial results, then a variety of other procedures—including genetic counseling; ultrasound to date the pregnancy, check for multiple fetuses, or look for abnormalities in the fetus; and/or amniocentesis to determine MSAFP and acetylcholinesterase levels in the amniotic fluid—are performed to confirm or rule out the presence of a neural tube defect. Only 1 or 2 out of 50 women with high initial readings will eventually be shown to have an affected fetus. In the other 48, further testing will reveal that the reason MSAFP levels are elevated is that there is more than one fetus, or that the pregnancy is further along than at first believed, or that the original readings were inaccurate. Still, though elevated MSAFP levels are not usually a cause for alarm, practitioners may recommend extra rest and vigilance for women with high readings because they may be at a slightly increased risk of having low-birthweight or preterm babies.

If MSAFP levels are abnormally low, ultrasound, genetic counseling, and/or amniocentesis will be offered to determine whether or not the fetus actually does suffer from Down syndrome or another chromosomal defect.

How Safe Is It? The initial screening test itself poses no more risk to

mother or baby than does any other standard blood test. The major risk of the test is that a false-positive result may lead to follow-up procedures that present greater risk—and in rare cases, to therapeutic or accidental abortion of perfectly normal fetuses. Before you consider taking any action on the basis of prenatal testing, be sure the results have been evaluated by an experienced physician or genetic counselor. Get a second opinion if you have any doubts. A maternal-fetal medicine subspecialist may be particularly helpful.

CHORIONIC VILLUS SAMPLING (CVS)

Unlike amniocentesis, chorionic villus sampling can detect defects in the fetus very early in pregnancy, at a stage when abortion is a less complicated and less traumatic procedure. Though still less common than amniocentesis, CVS is gaining in popularity. It is also being used experimentally in the second trimester in the place of amniocentesis because it can yield more rapid results, and because it is useful when amnio is not possible, as when there is very little amniotic fluid (oligohydramnios).

It is believed that chorionic villus sampling will eventually be able to detect virtually all of the 3,800 or so disorders for which defective genes or chromosomes are responsible. And in the future it may make possible the treatment or correction in utero of many of these conditions. At present, CVS is useful only to detect disorders for which the technology exists, such as Tay-Sachs, sickle-cell anemia, most types of cystic fibrosis, the thalassemias, and Down syndrome. Testing for specific diseases (other than Down syndrome) is usually done only when there is a family history of the disease or the parents are known to be carriers. The indications for doing the test are the same as those for amniocentesis, though CVS is not used to assess fetal lung maturity. Occasionally, both CVS and amniocentesis may be needed.

When Is It Done? Usually between the 8th and 12th weeks for transvaginal, between the 9th and 11th weeks for transabdominal CVS. The transabdominal procedure is also being used experimentally in the second and third trimesters.

How Is It Done? CVS may someday be an office procedure, but at the moment it is performed in medical centers only. Though originally the sampling of cells was always taken via the vagina and cervix (transcervical CVS), it is now sometimes taken through an incision in the abdominal wall (transabdominal CVS). Neither procedure is entirely pain-free; the discomfort can range from very mild to severe.

In the transcervical procedure, the expectant mother lies on an examining table and a long thin tube is inserted through the vagina into the uterus. Guided by ultrasound imaging, the doctor positions the tube between the uterine lining and the chorion, the fetal membrane that will eventually form the fetal side of the placenta. A sampling of the chorionic villi (finger-like projections of the chorion) is then snipped or suctioned off for diagnostic study.

In the transabdominal procedure, the patient also lies on an examining table, tummy up. Ultrasound is used to determine the location of the placenta and to view the uterine walls.[9] It

also helps the physician to find a safe spot in which to insert the needle. This area is washed and disinfected, then injected with a local anesthetic to numb it. Still under ultrasound guidance, a guide needle is inserted through the abdomen and the uterine wall to the edge of the placenta. then a narrower needle, which will draw up the cells, is inserted through the guide needle. The narrow needle is rotated and pushed in and out 15 or 20 times per sampling, then withdrawn with the sample of cells to be studied.

Since the chorionic villi are of fetal origin, examining them can give a complete picture of the genetic makeup of the developing fetus. Because many cells are collected in CVS, diagnostic study can begin almost immediately rather than after weeks of growing the cells in a lab, as is usually the case with amniocentesis. Depending on the cells that are sampled, results may be available within a day or two (when cells from the middle of the chorion are used), or in up to a week (when inner cells are used).

How Safe Is It? Though most studies so far conclude CVS is safe and reliable, there have been reports from at least one testing center linking it to limb deformities in the fetus. The procedure also increases the risk of miscarriage slightly (more so than amniocentesis). And there is a slim risk that a pregnancy could be terminated on the basis of incorrect information, since an abnormality called mosaicism may be detected in the villi when it doesn't exist in the fetus. This problem can be eliminated by always rechecking such a diagnosis with amniocentesis. These risks have to be weighed against the benefit of earlier diagnosis with CVS. Risks can be reduced by choosing a testing center with a good safety record.

Some vaginal bleeding can occur af-

---

9. Women who have a placenta that is located deep in the back of the uterus or who have fibroids in the uterine walls are not good candidates for this type of ultrasound.

Reducing the Risk in Any Pregnancy

Good Medical Care. Even a low-risk pregnancy is put at high risk if prenatal care is absent or poor. Seeing a qualified practitioner regularly, beginning as soon as pregnancy is suspected, is vital for all expectant mothers. (Choose an obstetrician experienced in your particular condition if you are in a high-risk category.) But just as important as having a good doctor is being a good patient. Be an active participant in your medical care—ask questions, report symptoms—but don't try to be your own doctor. (See page 15.)

Good Diet. The Best-Odds Diet (see page 80) gives every pregnant woman the best odds of having a successful and comfortable pregnancy and a healthy baby.

Fitness. It's best to begin pregnancy with a well-toned, fit body, but it's never too late to start deriving the benefits of exercise. Regular exercise can prevent constipation and improve respiration, circulation, muscle tone, and skin elasticity, contributing to a more comfortable pregnancy and an easier, safer delivery. (See page 189).

Sensible Weight Gain. A gradual, steady, and moderate weight gain may help prevent a variety of complications, including diabetes, hypertension, varicose veins, hemorrhoids, low birth weight, and difficult delivery due to an overly large fetus. (See page 147.)

No Smoking. Or quitting as early in pregnancy as possible to reduce its many risks to mother and baby, including prematurity and low birth weight. (See page 54.)

Abstinence from Alcohol. Drinking very rarely or not at all will reduce the risk of birth defects, particularly fetal alcohol syndrome (the result of heavy drinking) and fetal alcohol effect (the result of moderate drinking). See page 52.)

Avoidance of Drugs. All illicit drugs are dangerous to the fetus and should be avoided during pregnancy. Medication should be used only when its benefits outweigh its risks, and only when it has been approved or prescribed by a physician who is aware that you are pregnant. (See page 58.)

Avoidance of Environmental and Occupational Toxins. Though everything we touch, breathe, eat, and drink isn't as hazardous as newspaper headlines would have us believe, avoiding known hazards (such as excessive x-rays, lead, and so on; see individual topics) is prudent.

Prevention of and Prompt Treatment for Infection. All infections—from the common cold to urinary tract and vaginal infections to the increasingly common sexually transmitted diseases—should be avoided whenever possible. When contracted, however, infection should be treated promptly by a physician who knows you are pregnant.

Being Wary of the Superwoman Syndrome. Often well established in their careers and highly motivated in everything they do, today's mothers tend to be overachievers and overdoers. Getting enough rest during pregnancy is far more important than getting everything done, especially in high-risk pregnancies. Don't wait until your body starts pleading for relief before you slow down. If your doctor recommends that you begin your maternity leave earlier than you'd planned, take the advice. Some studies have suggested a higher incidence of premature delivery among women who work up until term, if their job entails physical labor or long periods of standing.

ter CVS and should not be a cause for concern, though it should be reported to your doctor. Your doctor should also be informed if the bleeding lasts for three days or longer. Since there is also a very slight risk of infection, be sure to report any fever in the first few days following the procedure.[10]

Since many women feel physically and emotionally drained following CVS (it's not unusual to fall into bed and sleep around the clock), it's generally recommended that those undergoing the procedure arrange to have someone drive them home afterward and that they make no other plans for the rest of the day.

OTHER TYPES OF PRENATAL DIAGNOSIS

The field of prenatal diagnosis is expanding so rapidly that new methods are constantly being evaluated. In addition to the standard methods listed above, there are others that are being used experimentally or only occasionally. These include:

❖ **Maternal blood screening for hCG** (human chorionic gonadotropin), which may eventually turn out to surpass age as the most important criterion for determining who should have amniocentesis to detect Down syndrome. Researchers have found that a high level of hCG in a pregnant woman's blood means she is at greater than normal risk for having a baby with Down syndrome. She then becomes a good candidate for amniocentesis. Even more accurate screening

might be possible by combining this test with tests for alpha-fetoprotein (see page 47) and estriol blood levels (low levels may be predictive of Down syndrome), and then factoring in maternal age.

❖ **Fetal blood sampling,** or cordocentesis, in which blood is drawn from the umbilical cord or the fetal hepatic vein for study. It is somewhat safer than fetoscopy when done under ultrasound guidance, and can detect the same conditions.

❖ **Fetal skin sampling,** in which a tiny sample of fetal skin is taken and studied. This method is particularly useful in detecting certain skin disorders.

❖ **Magnetic resonance imaging,** a method that is still investigational but offers some promise of being able to give a clearer picture than ultrasound of what the newborn will be like, inside and out.

❖ **Radiography (x-ray),** once the predominant way of visualizing an infant prenatally, has been almost entirely replaced by ultrasound.

❖ **Echocardiography,** with which defects in the fetal heart can be detected.

❖ **Maternal blood testing to determine the gender** of a fetus, though still experimental, could be valuable in screening for certain hereditary diseases that affect male offspring only.

---

10. Since there is the potential for leakage of fetal red blood cells into the mother's circulatory system, some doctors believe all Rh-negative women should be given an immune globulin called anti-D-globulin prior to CVS.

3
Throughout Your Pregnancy

WHAT YOU MAY BE CONCERNED ABOUT

Pregnant women have always worried. What they worry about, however, has changed considerably over the generations, as obstetrical medicine—and expectant parents—have learned more and more about what does and does not affect the health and well-being of the unborn. Our grandmothers, vulnerable to a variety of old wives' tales, feared that seeing a monkey while pregnant would result in monkey-like offspring, or that slapping their bellies in fright would leave their babies with hand-shaped birthmarks. We, vulnerable instead to a daily deluge of modern media tales (usually as frightening, sometimes as unfounded), have other fears: Is the air I'm breathing polluted? Is my drinking water safe? Is my job, or my husband's smoking, or that cup of coffee I had this morning hazardous to my baby's health? What about that x-ray I had at the dentist's? As a basis for worry, these concerns can make pregnancy unnecessarily nervewracking. As a basis for action,

they can give you an enhanced sense of control and greatly improve the odds of your having a healthy baby.

ALCOHOL

"I had a few drinks on several occasions before I knew I was pregnant. I'm afraid that the alcohol may have harmed my baby."

"Behold, thou shalt conceive, and bear a son; now beware, drink no wine or strong drink," an angel tells Samson's mother in the Book of Judges. Lucky lady. She was able to start ordering Evian when her son was just a gleam in his father's eye. Not many of us receive such advance notice of our pregnancies. And because we're often unaware that we're pregnant until we are into our second month, we're apt to have done things we wouldn't have done if only we had known. Like having a few, a few times too often. Which is why your concern is one of the most common brought to the first prenatal visit.

Fortunately, it's also one of the concerns that can most easily be put aside. There's no evidence that a few drinks on a couple of occasions early in pregnancy will prove harmful to a developing embryo. In fact, one recent study showed that women who'd had two or three such drinking episodes early in pregnancy weren't any more likely to have babies with structural defects or growth retardation than were teetotalers.

Continuing to drink heavily throughout pregnancy, however, is associated with a wide variety of problems in the offspring. That's not surprising when you consider that alcohol enters the fetal bloodstream in approximately the same concentrations present in the mother's blood; each drink a pregnant woman takes is shared with her baby. Since it takes the fetus twice as long as its mother to eliminate the alcohol from its system, the baby can be at the point of passing out when the mother is just pleasantly high.

Heavy drinking (generally considered to be the consumption of five or six drinks of wine, beer, or distilled spirits a day) throughout pregnancy can result, in addition to many serious obstetrical complications, in what is known as fetal alcohol syndrome (FAS). Described as the hangover that lasts a lifetime, this condition produces infants who are born undersized, usually mentally deficient, with multiple deformities (particularly of the head and face, limbs, heart, and central nervous system), and a high neonatal mortality rate. Later in life, those with FAS find it difficult to learn from experience.

The risks of continued drinking are certainly dose-related: the more you drink, the more potential danger to your baby. But even moderate consumption (three or four drinks daily or occasional heavy binging on five or more drinks) throughout pregnancy is related to a variety of serious problems, including the increased risk of miscarriage, prematurity, low birthweight, and complications during labor and delivery. It has also been linked to the somewhat more subtle fetal alcohol effect (FAE), which is characterized by numerous developmental and behavioral problems. Even one or two drinks daily apparently increases the risk of miscarriage, stillbirth, growth abnormalities, and developmental problems.

Although some women drink lightly during pregnancy—one glass of wine nightly, for instance—and still manage to deliver an apparently healthy baby, there is no assurance that this is a wise practice. The safe daily alcohol dose in pregnancy, if there is one, is not known.

All that is known about alcohol and pregnancy leads us to suggest that although you shouldn't worry about what you drank before you knew you were pregnant, it would be prudent to stop drinking for the rest of your pregnancy—except perhaps for a celebratory half glass of wine on a birthday or anniversary (taken *with* a meal, since food reduces the absorption of alcohol).

That's as easily done as said for some women—especially those who develop a distaste for alcohol in early pregnancy, which may linger through delivery. For others, particularly those who are accustomed to "unwinding" with cocktails at the end of the day or to taking wine with dinner, abstinence may require a concerted effort, possibly including a lifestyle change. If you drink to relax, for example, try substituting other methods of relaxation: music, warm baths, massage, exercise, reading. If drinking is part of a daily ritual that you don't want to give up, try a Virgin Mary (a Bloody Mary without the vodka) at brunch, sparkling cider or grape juice or nonalcoholic malt beer at dinner, juice spritzer (half juice, half seltzer, with a twist) or a Mock Strawberry Daiquiri or Virgin Sangria (see page 98) at cocktail hour—served at the accustomed time, in the accustomed glasses, with the accustomed ceremony.[1] If your husband joins you on the wagon (at least while in your company), the ride will be considerably smoother.

In the United States, alcohol use during pregnancy is the major cause of mental retardation and a leading cause of birth defects generally; but these defects are preventable. The sooner a heavy drinker stops drinking during pregnancy, the less risk to her baby. The heavy drinker who refuses to abstain or to seek help from Alcoholics Anonymous, a certified alcohol counselor or physician, or an alcohol treatment program may want to consider terminating her pregnancy and postponing childbearing until her illness is under control.

CIGARETTE SMOKING

"I've been smoking for ten years. Will this hurt my baby?"

Happily, there's no clear evidence that any smoking you've done prior to pregnancy—even if it's been for 10 or 20 years—will harm a developing fetus. But it's well documented that continuing to smoke during pregnancy—particularly beyond the fourth month—can increase the chances of a wide variety of pregnancy complications. In fact, tobacco use is one of the leading causes of prenatal problems. Among the more serious of these are vaginal bleeding, miscarriage, abnormal placental implantation, premature placental detachment, prematurely ruptured membranes, and early delivery. It has been suggested that as many as 14% of preterm deliveries in the United States are related to cigarette smoking.

There is also strong evidence that an expectant mother's smoking adversely and very directly affects her baby's development in utero. The most widespread risk is low birthweight. In industrialized nations, such as the United States and Britain, smoking is blamed for as many as a third of all the babies who are born too small. And being born too small is the major cause of infant illness and perinatal death (those that occur just before, during, or after birth).

But there are other potential risks as well. Babies of smoking moms are more likely to suffer from apnea (breathing lapses) and are twice as likely to die of SIDS (sudden infant death syndrome, or crib death) as babies of nonsmokers. In general, babies of smokers aren't as healthy at birth as babies of nonsmokers, with three-pack-a-day maternal smoking associated with a quadrupled risk of low Apgar scores (the standard scale used to evaluate an infant's condition at birth). And there's evidence that, on the average, they may never catch up to the children of nonsmokers, that they may have long-term physical and intellectual deficits, and that they may also be hyperactive. At age 14, one study showed, children of smokers tended to be more prone to respiratory disease, to be shorter than children of nonsmokers, and to be less successful in school.

It was once believed that the reason

---

1. Though substituting nonalcoholic look-alikes for favorite alcoholic beverages during pregnancy can work for the occasional drinker, the heavy drinker may find that these beverages serve to trigger a desire for alcohol. If they do in you, avoid any drink, or even setting, that reminds you of alcohol.

Breaking the Smoking Habit

Identify Your Motivation for Smoking. For example, do you smoke for pleasure, stimulation, or relaxation? To reduce tension or frustration, to have something in your hand or mouth, to satisfy a craving? Perhaps you smoke out of habit, lighting up without thinking about it. Once you understand your motivations, you should be able to find substitutes.

Identify Your Motivation for Quitting. When you're pregnant, that's easy.

Choose Your Method of Withdrawal. Do you want to go cold turkey or to taper off? Either way, pick a "last day" that isn't far off. Plan a full day of activities for that date—those you don't associate with smoking.

Try to Sublimate Your Urge to Smoke. Use any and all of the following that you think will help:

❖ If you smoke mainly to keep your hands busy, try playing with a pencil, beads, a straw; knit, polish silver, create a new nutritious recipe, write a letter, play the piano, learn to paint, make rag dolls, do jigsaw or crossword puzzles, challenge someone to a game of chess or Scrabble—anything that might make you forget to reach for a cigarette.

❖ If you smoke for oral gratification, try a substitute: sorbitol- or aspartame-sweetened gum, raw vegetables, popcorn, a whole-wheat breadstick, a toothpick, an empty cigarette holder. Do avoid empty-calorie nibbles.

❖ If you smoke for stimulation, try to get your lift from a brisk walk, an absorbing book, good conversation. Be sure your diet contains all essential nutrients and that you eat frequently, to avoid feeling draggy because of low blood sugar.

❖ If you smoke to reduce tension and relax, try exercise instead. Or relaxation techniques. Or listening to soothing music. Or a long walk. Or a massage. Or making love.

❖ If you smoke for pleasure, seek pleasure in other pursuits, preferably in no-smoke situations. Go to a movie, visit baby boutiques, tour a favorite museum, attend a concert or a play, have dinner with a friend who is allergic to smoke. Or try something more active, like tennis doubles.

❖ If you smoke out of habit, avoid the settings in which you habitually smoke and friends who smoke; frequent places with no-smoking rules instead.

❖ If you associate smoking with a particular beverage, food, or meal, avoid the food or beverage, eat the meal in a different location. (Say you smoke with breakfast but you never smoke in bed. Have breakfast in bed for a few days.)

❖ When you feel the urge to smoke, take several deep breaths with a pause between each. Hold the last breath while you strike a match. Exhale slowly, blowing out the match. Pretend it was a cigarette and crush it out.

If You Do Slip Up and Have a Cigarette, Don't Despair. Just get right back on your program, knowing that every cigarette you *don't* smoke is going to help your baby.

Look at Smoking as a Non-Negotiable Issue. When you were a smoker, you couldn't smoke in a theater, subway, or department store, even in some restaurants. That was that. Now you have to tell yourself that you can't smoke, period. That is that.

for the difficulties these children display was poor prenatal nutrition: their mothers smoked rather than ate during their pregnancies. But recent studies disprove this theory; smoking mothers who eat as much and gain as much weight as nonsmoking mothers still give birth to smaller babies. This seems to be the result of carbon monoxide poisoning and a reduction of oxygen to the fetus through the placenta. Gaining weight in excess of 40 pounds may somewhat reduce the risk of a smoking mother having an undersized baby, but that kind of weight gain poses other risks to the mother and child.

In effect, when you smoke, your baby is confined in a smoke-filled womb. His heartbeat speeds, he coughs and sputters, and worst of all, due to insufficient oxygen, he can't grow and thrive as he should.

Studies show that the effects of tobacco use, like those of alcohol use, are dose-related: tobacco use reduces the birthweight of babies in direct proportion to the number of cigarettes smoked, with a pack-a-day smoker 130% more likely to give birth to a low-birthweight child than a nonsmoker. So cutting down on the number of cigarettes you smoke may help some. But cutting down can be illusory because the smoker often compensates by taking more frequent and deeper puffs and smoking more of each cigarette. This can also happen when she tries to reduce the risk by using low-tar or low-nicotine cigarettes.

The news, however, isn't all bad. Some studies show that women who quit smoking early in pregnancy—no later than the fourth month—can reduce the risk of damage to the fetus to the level of the nonsmoker. Sooner is better, but quitting even in the last month can help preserve oxygen flow to the baby during delivery. For some smoking women, quitting will never be easier than in early pregnancy, when they develop a sudden distaste for cigarettes—probably the warning of an intuitive body. If you're not lucky enough to develop such a natural aversion, try quitting with the help of Smoke Enders or another smoking-cessation group. Or ask your practitioner to recommend other local resources. You may even want to try hypnosis.

Most people experience withdrawal symptoms when they quit smoking, though the symptoms and their intensity vary from person to person. Some of the most common include a craving for tobacco, irritability, anxiety, restlessness, tingling or numbness in the extremities, lightheadedness, fatigue, and sleep and gastrointestinal disturbances. Some people also find that both physical and mental performance are impaired at first. Most find that for a while they are coughing more, rather than less, because their bodies are suddenly better able to bring up all the secretions that have accumulated in the lungs.

To try to slow the release of nicotine and the nervousness that may result, increase your intake of fruit, fruit juice, milk, and mixed greens and temporarily cut back on meat, poultry, fish, and cheese; avoid caffeine, which can add to the jitters. Get plenty of rest (to counter fatigue) and exercise (to replace the kick you used to get from nicotine). Let your mind go fallow for a few days, if necessary and if possible, doing mindless tasks or going to the movies or other places where smoking is prohibited.

The worst effects of withdrawal will last a few days to a few weeks. The benefits, however, will last a lifetime—for you and your baby. (For more tips on improving your pregnancy lifestyle, see page 63.)

"My sister-in-law smoked two packs a day through three pregnancies, and had no

complications and big healthy babies. Why should I quit?"

Everyone has heard inspiring stories of someone beating the odds—a cancer patient given a 10% chance of survival living to a ripe age, or a quake victim found alive after being trapped under rubble without food or drink for days. But there's something much less inspiring about an expectant mother who consciously stacks the odds against her unborn babies by choosing to smoke, yet manages to beat the odds and produce healthy offspring anyway.

There are no sure things when it comes to making a baby, but there are many ways of bettering the odds. And giving up smoking is one of the most tangible ways you can improve the odds of your having an uncomplicated pregnancy and delivery and a healthy baby. Though there's the chance that you, too, can have a vigorous full-term baby even if you smoke your way through your pregnancy, there's also a significant risk that your baby would suffer some or all of the effects detailed on page 54. Your sister-in-law was lucky (and to a certain extent, this luck could have gotten a boost from heredity or other factors that might not hold for you)[2]; but do you really want to take the gamble that you will be lucky too? And then again that luck may not be all that it seems to be. Some of the deficits—physical and intellectual—that afflict babies of smokers aren't apparent immediately. The seemingly healthy infant can grow into a child who is often sick, who is hyperactive, or who has trouble learning.

In addition to the effect smoking could have on your baby while you're still pregnant, there is the effect it would have once he or she has moved from your smoke-filled womb to your smoke-filled rooms. Babies of parents (mothers and/or dads) who smoke are sick more often than the babies of nonsmokers and are more likely to be hospitalized through infancy and childhood.

So as you can see, quitting is your best bet.

WHEN OTHER PEOPLE SMOKE

"I quit smoking, but my husband still goes through two packs a day, and a couple of my co-workers smoke like chimneys. I keep worrying that somehow this may hurt our baby."

Smoking, it is becoming more and more apparent, doesn't just affect the person who is puffing away—it affects everyone around him. Including a developing fetus whose mother happens to be nearby. So if your husband (or anyone else who lives in your home or works at the next desk) smokes, your baby's body is going to pick up nearly as much contamination from tobacco smoke by-products as if *you* were lighting up.

If your husband says he can't quit smoking, ask him to at least do all his smoking out of the house or in a different room, away from you and the baby. Quitting, of course, would be better, not just for his own health but for the baby's long-term well-being. Studies show that parental smoking—mother's or father's—can cause respiratory problems in their children, impairing lung development even into

---

2. It's possible that the reason her babies were not undersized is that she gained an excessive amount of weight by consuming an excessive number of calories. Taking in more calories than are usually required can, in some cases, reduce the risk of a smoker's baby being born smaller than average—but can present other problems.

adulthood. It can also increase the odds that the children themselves will end up becoming smokers.

You probably won't be able to get your friends and co-workers to kick the habit, but you may be able to get them to curtail smoking around you. If there are laws protecting non-smokers where you live or work, then it will be relatively easy to do this. If there are no such laws, try tactful persuasion—show them the material in this book on the danger of tobacco smoke to a fetus. If that fails, try to get a regulation passed where you work that limits smoking to certain areas, such as a lounge, and prohibits smoking in the vicinity of nonsmokers. If all else fails, then try to move your office for the duration of your pregnancy.

MARIJUANA USE

"I've been a social smoker of marijuana —indulging only at parties—for about ten years. Could this have caused harm to the baby I'm now carrying? And is smoking pot during pregnancy dangerous?"

As it was with cigarette smoking over 20 years ago, all the evidence on the effects of marijuana use is not yet in. Consequently, those who choose to smoke it today are guinea pigs testing a substance whose dangers may not be fully documented for some time to come. And since marijuana crosses the placenta, mothers who smoke it during pregnancy make guinea pigs out of their unborn children as well.

It is usually recommended that couples trying to conceive abstain from marijuana use, since it can interfere with conception. But if you are already pregnant, you needn't worry about your past smoking—there is no present evidence that it will harm your fetus.

Continuing to smoke marijuana now that you've found out you're pregnant, however, might well be a story with a less happy ending. Some, though not all, studies show that women who use marijuana even as infrequently as once a month throughout pregnancy are more likely to: gain inadequate weight; suffer from hyperemesis (severe and chronic vomiting), which can interfere seriously with prenatal nutrition if not treated; have dangerously rapid labor, prolonged or arrested labor, or a cesarean section; have a low-birthweight baby (though the increased risk is small); show meconium staining of the amniotic fluid during labor (a complication that can indicate fetal distress); and have a baby that needs resuscitation after delivery. Although there is no clear-cut evidence of an increased incidence of malformations in the babies of marijuana users, there have been reports of Fetal Alcohol Syndrome–like characteristics (see page 53) as well as tremors, vision abnormalities, and a withdrawal-like cry during the newborn period. Marijuana has also been shown to adversely affect placental function and the fetal endocrine system, potentially interfering with the successful completion of pregnancy. Based on the available evidence, the United States surgeon general has warned that marijuana use by a pregnant woman may be hazardous to the health of the fetus she is carrying.

So treat marijuana as you would any other drug during pregnancy: Don't take it unless it is medically required and prescribed. If you have already smoked early in your pregnancy, don't worry. Since most of the negative effects of marijuana appear to occur as pregnancy progresses, it's very unlikely any harm was done. Any pregnant woman who can't seem to break her marijuana habit should tell her practitioner or seek other professional help as soon as pregnancy is confirmed.

COCAINE AND OTHER DRUG USE

"I did some cocaine a week before I found out I was pregnant. Now I'm worried about what that could have done to my baby."

D on't worry about past cocaine use; just make sure it was your last. While the good news is that using the drug before you found out you were pregnant isn't likely to have had any effect, the bad news is that continuing to use it during pregnancy could

be catastrophic. Cocaine not only crosses the placenta, it can damage it, reducing blood flow to the fetus and retarding fetal growth. It can also result in a variety of serious pregnancy complications, including miscarriage, premature labor, and stillbirth. In the baby who survives, there's the risk of stroke at birth and numerous long-term effects. Among them are chronic diarrhea, irritability, excessive crying and other behavioral problems, and abnormal breathing patterns and brain waves. It's also suspected, though not yet confirmed, that babies born to cocaine users are at an increased risk of SIDS.

Certainly, the more often the expectant mother uses cocaine, the greater the risk to her baby. But even very occasional use later on in pregnancy can be hazardous. For instance,

---

Perils in Perspective

Open a newspaper or turn on the television or radio, and chances are you'll encounter yet another report on the hazards of being pregnant in modern times. To hear the media tell it, an expectant mother can't eat, drink, breathe, or work without exposing her fetus to potential harm. Yet the reassuring truth is that pregnancy has never been so safe; never before in the history of reproduction have babies had a better chance of being born alive and well. Most environmental risks are theoretical, and those that are substantiated account for only a tiny fraction of all birth defects and pregnancy complications.

What's a mother-to-be to do? Read about the environmental risks listed in this chapter, eliminate some of them, minimize some of them, learn to live with some of them, and most important, put all of them in sensible perspective. The fact is that all of the

environmental factors that are not within your control when you're pregnant—a job that has you sitting in front of a video display terminal, a hometown that's polluted with carbon monoxide, incidental brief exposures to paint fumes, hair dyes, insecticides—have far less impact on the outcome of your pregnancy than the factors you have complete control over, such as getting good, regular medical care, eating an excellent diet, and not drinking, smoking, or taking nonprescribed drugs once you find out you're pregnant. The woman who worries about the permanent she had before she found out she was pregnant but continues to smoke a pack a day is misdirecting her concern. She'd be much wiser to concentrate on those factors that will almost definitely have an effect on her baby's well-being instead of worrying about those that almost certainly will not.

a single use in the third trimester can trigger contractions and an abnormal fetal heartbeat.

Tell your practitioner about any cocaine use since you've conceived. As with every aspect of your medical history, the more your doctor knows, the better care you and your baby will receive. If you have any difficulty giving cocaine up entirely, seek professional help immediately.

Pregnant women who use drugs of any kind—other than those that have been prescribed by a physician who knows they are pregnant—are also putting their babies in jeopardy. Every known illicit drug (including heroin, methadone, crack, "ice," LSD, and PCP), and every prescription drug of abuse (including narcotics, tranquilizers, sedatives, and diet pills) can cause serious harm to a developing fetus and/or to the pregnancy with continued use. Check with your practitioner or another knowledgeable doctor about any drugs you've used during pregnancy, or call one of the hotlines listed in the Appendix to see what effect they could have had. Then, if you are still using drugs, get professional support (from a certified addiction counselor, an addictionologist, or a treatment center) to help you quit now.

CAFFEINE

"I find it difficult to start the day without my two cups of coffee. I've read, though, that caffeine can cause birth defects and low-birthweight babies. Is this true?"

According to the most recent scientific studies, probably not. Caffeine (found in coffee, tea, colas and other soft drinks) and its cousin theobromine (found in chocolate) do cross the placenta and enter the fetal circulation. But, though early animal studies showed numerous harmful effects from caffeine on developing animal fetuses, human studies to date have shown no harm from moderate use—up to three cups of coffee or the equivalent in other caffeinated beverages in a 24-hour period—throughout pregnancy.

Still, there are some valid reasons to give up caffeinated coffee (and tea and colas) during pregnancy, or at least to cut down consumption. First of all, caffeine has a diuretic effect, drawing fluid and calcium—both vital to maternal and fetal health—from the body. If you're having a problem with frequent urination anyway, caffeine intake will compound it. Second, coffee and tea, especially when taken with cream and sugar, are filling and satisfying without being nutritious and can spoil your appetite for the nutritious food you need. Colas are not only filling but may contain questionable chemicals in addition to unneeded sugar. Third, caffeine can exacerbate your normal pregnancy mood swings and also interfere with adequate rest. Fourth, caffeine may interfere with the absorption of the iron both you and your baby need. Fifth, research suggests excessive caffeine use could result in temporary abnormal heartbeat, rapid respiration, and tremors in the newborn and the development of diabetes[3] later in life. Finally, the fact that many women lose their taste for coffee early in pregnancy suggests that mother nature herself considers the substance to be unsuitable for pregnant women.

How Do You Break the Caffeine Habit? The first step, finding your motivation, is easy in pregnancy: giving your

---

3. In countries where caffeine consumption is highest, the incidence of diabetes is highest too; it is suspected that caffeine builds up in the fetal pancreas and eventually damages the cells that produce insulin.

baby the healthiest possible start in life. Next you need to determine why you indulge, and which beverages you can safely substitute to satisfy this need. If it's the taste of coffee or tea, or the comfort of a warm drink, that appeals to you, then switch to a naturally decaffeinated replacement (but don't let it take the place of your milk, orange juice, or other nutritious beverages).[4] If you drink cola for the taste, you can substitute caffeine-free soft drinks occasionally, but soft drinks have no regular place in a pregnancy diet; instead explore the varied flavors of unsweetened 100% fruit juices (papaya, passion fruit, mango, cherry, berry, cran-apple, and so on, in the countless combinations available) and flavored seltzers. If it's refreshment you're thirsting for, you'll find that juices and plain or carbonated water are better thirst quenchers than colas, anyway. If it's the caffeine lift you crave, you'll get a more natural, longer-lasting boost from exercise and good food, especially complex carbohydrates and protein, or from doing something that exhilarates you: dancing, jogging, making love. Though you'll doubtless sag for a few days after giving up caffeine, you'll soon feel better than ever. (Of course, you will still experience the normal fatigue of early pregnancy.)

If you drink coffee, tea, or cola for something to do, do something else—something good for your baby. Knit him or her a sweater, go for a walk or shop for a crib, scrub a bunch of vegetables for dinner. If you drink your caffeinated beverage as part of a daily ritual (the coffee break, reading the paper, watching TV), change the location of that ritual, and change the beverage that accompanies it.

---

4. Though decaffeinated teas are okay, beware of medicinal or heavy use of herbal teas; see page 323.

Minimizing Caffeine Withdrawal Symptoms. As any coffee, tea, or cola addict is well aware, it is one thing to want to give up caffeine and another thing to do it. Caffeine is an addictive drug; heavy imbibers who quit cold turkey can expect to experience withdrawal symptoms, including headache, irritability, fatigue, and lethargy. Which is why it's probably a better idea to ease off the caffeine gradually—starting by cutting down to an almost certainly safe level of two cups (taken with food to buffer the effect on your system) for a few days. Then, once you've adjusted to two cups, gradually reduce your daily intake, a quarter of a cup at a time, down to one cup, and finally, as the need for the drug lessens, to none. Or switch temporarily to a half caffeinated–half decaffeinated brew during the withdrawal period, gradually increasing the proportion of decaffeinated until your mug is completely caffeine-free. (If your taste buds miss the flavor of coffee, continue to satisfy them by using a brewed decaffeinated coffee. It isn't necessary to spring for the costlier water-processed varieties—the chemically processed coffees appear to pose no health risks. Even espresso lovers can be appeased with decaffeinated espressos, which are nearly as rich and flavorful as the caffeinated ones.)

Withdrawal will be less uncomfortable and easier to handle if you heed these energizing suggestions:

❖ Keep your blood sugar, and thus your energy level, up. Eat frequent small meals that are rich in protein and complex-carbohydrate foods. And be sure to take your pregnancy vitamin-mineral supplement.

❖ Get some outdoor exercise every day.

❖ Be sure to get enough sleep—

which will probably be easier without caffeine.

If you decide that a completely caffeine-free life isn't for you, don't despair. Based on the evidence, a cup or two of caffeinated beverage daily should pose no problem.

SUGAR SUBSTITUTES

"I'm trying not to gain too much weight. Can I use sugar substitutes?"

It usually comes as an unpleasant surprise to hopeful dieters, but the use of sugar substitutes rarely helps control weight. Maybe it's because the person who uses a substitute in her tea figures she's saved enough calories to have a few cookies with it. Even if sugar substitutes could guarantee weight control, however, caution would be recommended concerning their use by expectant mothers.

Unfortunately, not much human research has been done on saccharin use in pregnancy. Animal studies, however, show an increase in cancer in the offspring when pregnant mothers ingest the chemical. Added to evidence that the sweetener crosses the placenta in humans and is eliminated very slowly from fetal tissues, these studies suggest that it is sensible not to use saccharin while preparing for pregnancy, around the time of conception, or during pregnancy itself. Don't worry, however, about saccharin you've had before finding out that you're pregnant, since the risks, if any, are certainly extremely slight.

On the other hand, studies have shown no harmful effects from the use of typical amounts of the sweetener aspartame (Equal, NutraSweet) by most women during pregnancy.[5] Aspartame is composed of two common amino acids (phenylalanine and aspartic acid) plus methanol, and

most doctors will okay *moderate* use of this sweetener for pregnant women. But because so many products sweetened with aspartame are nutritionally unworthy of a Best-Odds dieter—they're often overloaded with artificial additives and underloaded with nutrients—pregnant women should be selective in choosing among them. Adding a packet of Equal to your homemade ice cream or hot chocolate or using NutraSweet-sweetened yogurt should be fine. Filling up on diet sodas in place of more nourishing fare wouldn't be.

During pregnancy, the best sweeteners to rely on are natural and nutritious fruits and fruit juices. In the past few years, products sweetened entirely with fruit and fruit juice concentrates have proliferated in health food stores and supermarkets. Besides the Best-Odds treats you can bake (see the recipes on page 96 and in *What to Eat When You're Expecting,* or modify your own favorites), there are dozens that you can buy, including jams and jellies, cookies and muffins, ice creams and sorbets, candy bars and granola bars—even pop-up toaster pastries and sparkling natural "sodas." And unlike most products sweetened with sugar or sugar substitutes, the majority are nourishing, combining whole-grain flours with a host of other wholesome ingredients. Avoid those that, like most sugar-sweetened products, are made with refined flours, "bad" fats, or a long list of chemicals.

5. Women with PKU (phenylketonuria), however, must limit their intake of phenylalanine and are generally advised not to use aspartame. The suggestion has been made that some women—estimates vary from 1 in 10 to 1 in 50—may not metabolize phenylalanine properly, yet exhibit no symptoms of PKU. The theory that these women may damage their babies' brains by ingesting large amounts of aspartame remains unproven.

Your Pregnancy Lifestyle

Whereas most of your lifestyle habits used to affect only your body, many now have the potential of affecting your baby's body too. Old habits may now be bad habits, ones you'd like to break in a hurry.

Fortunately, there are some strategies that can help.

Eliminate Temptation. That means keeping everything that you shouldn't have out of sight. No wine in the fridge; no liquor on top of the bar. No cake mixes in the kitchen cupboard; no white bread in the bread box.

Stock Up on Substitutes. Sparkling cider in your wineglass at dinner, a Mock Strawberry Daiquiri (page 98) at cocktail time (unless imitations make you yearn for the real thing). Fruit-sweetened cookies and cakes in the cupboard; delicious whole-grain breads and muffins in the freezer.

Use Cues. One of the major obstacles to changing habits is forgetting what your goals are; they can easily slip from your mind when temptation is near. So tape pictures of babies (cute, healthy-looking babies) on the refrigerator, inside kitchen cupboards, on the outside of the liquor cabinet, on your desk at work. If skipping breakfast is your vice, put a sign inside your front door that asks, "Have you fed your baby breakfast today?"

Forgive Yourself. If you slip up and eat something that's less than good for your baby, or even if you have a glass of wine or a beer, don't throw in the towel and go back to your old ways. Get right back on the healthy-living wagon. Try to analyze what it was that caused you to fall off, and try to avoid such situations for the duration.

Identify, Then Squelch, Feelings That Weaken Your Resolve. Many people find it difficult to stay on a diet, avoid alcohol, tobacco, or drugs, or shun other negative habits in the face of hunger, anger, boredom, fatigue, or loneliness. So get a jump on these saboteurs. Eat frequent small meals to keep hunger in check. Diffuse feelings of annoyance or resentment immediately, before they get the best of you. Get plenty of rest—when your body says "slow down," listen. And if you feel isolated or bored a good deal of the time, join a prenatal group, do some volunteer work, or take some stimulating courses. Make sure your spouse knows that you're craving extra attention—and the important reasons why you need it now more than ever.

Rely on Relaxation. It's often tension that makes us susceptible to forgetting our good intentions, so take spare moments during the day to do relaxation exercises (see page 114).

Learn to Say No... to that second cup of coffee, that social cigarette, that glass of bubbly being passed your way, one too many fudge brownies. Be polite but firm: "You know I love your brownies, Grandma, but my baby's too young for them" or "Thanks, but I'll toast your birthday with orange juice—my baby's underage."

Enlist an Ally. Your husband is the most logical one, but it can also be a friend at work, a sister, or someone else you spend a lot of time with. Your ally should be willing to stick to the rules with you when you're together; this will help strengthen your resolve and remove a good deal of temptation.

If You Can't Do It Alone, Get Help. Some habits are harder to break than others. If you're having difficulty kicking a potentially dangerous habit, whether it's smoking, drinking, or taking drugs, then talk to your practitioner or seek other professional help.

THE FAMILY CAT

"I have two cats at home. I've heard that cats carry a disease that can harm a fetus. Do I have to get rid of my pets?"

Probably not. Since you've lived with cats for a while, the odds are pretty good that you've already contracted the disease, toxoplasmosis (see page 313), and developed an immunity to it. It's estimated that about half of the American population has been infected (the estimates in some countries—France, for example—are as high as 90%), and the rates of infection are much higher among people who have cats or who frequently eat raw meat or drink unpasteurized milk (both of which can also harbor and transmit the infection). If you weren't tested prenatally to see if you were immune, it's not likely you will be tested now—unless you show symptoms of the disease (although some doctors will run regular tests on pregnant women who live with a lot of cats).

If you were tested prenatally and were not immune, or if you're not sure whether you are or not, you should take the following precautions to avoid infection:

❖ Have your cats tested by a veterinarian to see if they have an active infection. If one or both of them does, board them at a kennel or ask a friend to care for them for at least six weeks—the period during which the infection is transmissible. If they are free of infection, keep them that way by not allowing them to eat raw meat, roam outdoors, hunt mice or birds (which can transmit toxoplasmosis to cats), or fraternize with other cats. Have someone else handle the litter box. If you must do it yourself, use

gloves when handling the litter box and wash your hands when you've finished. The litter should be changed daily since the oocytes that transmit the disease become more infectious with time.

❖ Wear gloves when gardening. Don't garden in soil, or let your children play in sand, in which cats may have deposited feces. Wash fruits and vegetables, especially those grown in home gardens, with dish detergent (rinsing very thoroughly), and/or peel or cook them.

❖ Don't eat raw or undercooked meat or unpasteurized milk; a thermometer inserted in the center of the meat when it comes from the oven should register at least 140°F. In restaurants, order meat well done.

Some doctors are urging routine testing before conception or in very early pregnancy for all women, so that those who test positive can relax, knowing they are immune, and those who test negative can take the necessary precautions to prevent infection. Other doctors believe the costs of such testing may outweigh the benefits it may provide.

HOT TUBS AND SAUNAS

"We have a hot tub. Is it safe for me to use it while I'm pregnant?"

You won't have to switch to cold showers, but it's probably a good idea to refrain from long stays in the hot tub. Anything that raises the body temperature over 102°F (38.9°C) and keeps it there for a while—whether it's a dip in a hot tub or an extremely hot bath, too long a session in the sauna or steam room, an overzealous workout in hot weather, or a virus—is potentially hazardous to the developing embryo or fetus, particularly in the early months. Some studies have shown that a hot tub doesn't raise a woman's temperature to dangerous levels immediately—it takes at least 10 minutes (longer if the shoulders and arms are not submerged or if the water is 102°F or less)—but because individual responses and circumstances vary, play it safe by keeping your belly out of the hot tub. But feel free to soak your feet.

If you've already had some brief sojourns in the hot tub, there is probably no cause for alarm. Studies show that most women spontaneously get out of a hot tub before their body temperatures reach 102°F, because they've become uncomfortable. It's likely you did too. If you are concerned, however, speak to your doctor about the possibility of having an ultrasound exam or other prenatal test to help put your mind at ease.

Lengthy stays in the sauna may also be unwise, though the evidence is not clear. The weekly sauna is customary in Finland, even for pregnant women, and yet the kind of central nervous system defects believed to be caused by hyperthermia (a dangerous rise in body temperature) aren't common in babies there. Still, most U.S. experts recommend avoiding the sauna.

MICROWAVE EXPOSURE

"I've read that exposure to microwave ovens is dangerous to a developing fetus. Should I unplug ours until after the baby's born?"

A microwave oven can be a working mother-to-be's best friend, helping to make nutritious eating-on-the-run possible. But like so many of our modern miracles, there's talk that it may also be a modern menace. Whether or not we can be zapped by exposure to microwaves is still very controversial. Much more research needs to be done before the answer is definitively known. It is believed, however, that two types of human tissue—the developing fetus and the eye—are particularly vulnerable to the effects of microwaves because they have a poor capacity to dissipate the heat the waves generate. However, rather than unplugging your microwave oven, you should take some precautions.

First of all, be sure your oven doesn't leak. Don't operate it if seals around the door are damaged, if the oven doesn't close properly, or if something is caught in the door. Since inexpensive home devices for measuring radiation are unreliable, don't attempt to test for leaks yourself. Consult an appliance service center, the city or state consumer protection office, or your local health department. They may be able to do the testing for you, or recommend someone who can. Second, don't stand in front of the oven when it is in operation. Finally, follow the manufacturer's directions to the letter.

ELECTRIC BLANKETS AND HEATING PADS

'We use an electric blanket all winter long. Is this safe for the baby we're expecting?'

Cuddle up to your sweetie instead, or if his toes are as cold as yours, invest in a down comforter, push up the thermostat, or heat the bed with the blanket and then turn it off before you get in. Electric blankets can raise body temperature excessively, and although their use hasn't been clearly associated with fetal damage, the theory is there. Furthermore, although studies have been contradictory, some researchers have suggested that there is also some potential risk from the electromagnetic field created by electric blankets. So it would be prudent to try alternative routes to warmth. Don't, however, worry about nights you've already spent beneath an electric blanket—the chance that your baby was harmed is extremely remote, even in theory.

Be cautious, too, when using a heating pad. If treatment with one has been recommended by the doctor, wrap it in a towel to reduce the heat it passes along, limit applications to 15 minutes, and don't sleep with it.

Electrically heated water beds have also been linked to pregnancy problems. Those who sleep in them seem to be at increased risk of miscarrying. Scientists suggest this may be because of the electromagnetic field that these beds emit. Though the increased risk is probably very small, if you've been sleeping in a heated water bed, it makes sense to switch to another type of bed or to sleep on the sofa until your baby arrives.

X-RAYS

"I had an x-ray series at the dentist before I found out I was pregnant. Could this have hurt my baby?"

D on't worry. First of all, dental x-rays are directed far away from your uterus. Second, a lead apron shields your uterus and your baby effectively from any radiation.

Determining the safety of other types of x-rays during pregnancy is more complicated, but it is clear that diagnostic x-rays rarely pose a threat to the embryo or fetus. Three factors affect whether or not radiation from x-rays might be harmful:

❖ **The Amount of Radiation.** Severe damage to the embryo or fetus occurs only at very high doses (50 to 250 rads). No damage appears to occur at doses lower than 10 rads. Since modern x-ray equipment rarely delivers more than 5 rads during a typical diagnostic exam, such exams should not present a problem in pregnancy.

❖ **When the Exposure Occurs.** Even at high doses, there appears to be no teratogenic risk to the embryo before implantation (the sixth to eighth day postconception). There is a somewhat greater risk of damage during the period of early development of a baby's organs (the third and fourth weeks after conception), and some continued risk of damage to the central nervous system throughout pregnancy. But again, only at high doses.

❖ **Whether There Is Actual Exposure of the Uterus.** Today's x-ray equipment is able to precisely pinpoint the area that needs to be viewed, which protects the rest of the body from radiation exposure. Most x-rays can be done with the mother's abdomen and pelvis, and thus the uterus, shielded by a lead apron. But even an abdominal x-ray is unlikely to be hazardous, since it practically never delivers more than 10 rads.

Of course it still isn't wise to take unnecessary risks, no matter how small, so it's usually recommended that elective x-rays be postponed until after delivery. Necessary risks are another matter. Since the likelihood of damage to the fetus from x-ray exposure is slight, the health of the expectant mother shouldn't be endangered by putting off an x-ray that is genuinely needed. And the already minimal hazards of an x-ray during pregnancy can be minimized still further by observing the following guidelines:

❖ Always inform the doctor ordering the x-ray and the technician performing it that you are pregnant.

❖ Never have an x-ray, even a dental x-ray, during pregnancy if the benefit does not outweigh the risk. (Read Weighing Risk vs. Benefit, page 77.)

❖ Do not have an x-ray if a safer diagnostic procedure can be used instead.

❖ If an x-ray is necessary, be certain that it is taken in a licensed or regularly inspected facility. Equipment should be up-to-date, in good condition, and operated by well-trained, conscientious technicians under the supervision of a full-time radiologist. The x-ray equipment should, when possible, be directed so that only the minimum area necessary is exposed to radiation; the uterus should be shielded with a lead apron.

❖ Follow the technician's directions precisely, being especially careful not to move during the shot, so that retakes won't be needed.

❖ Most important, if you've had an x-ray, or need an x-ray, don't waste your time worrying about the possible consequences. Your baby is in more danger when you forget to buckle your seat belt.

HOUSEHOLD HAZARDS

"The more I read, the more I'm convinced that the only way to protect my baby in this day and age is to spend the next nine months locked up in a sterile room. Even my home isn't safe."

The threats you and your baby face from the increasing number of environmental hazards, including those in your own backyard, quickly pale when compared to those faced by your great-grandmothers, when modern obstetrical medicine was in its infancy. All of today's environmental perils combined (alcohol, tobacco, and other drugs excepted) are far less of a threat to you and your baby than one untrained midwife with unwashed hands was to your ancestresses. So in spite of all the trumpeting about the perils around us, we repeat: Pregnancy and childbirth have never been so safe.

But while you won't have to trade in your home for a sterile room, a little caution is certainly warranted when dealing with hazards around the house:

Household Cleaning Products. Since many cleaning products have been in common use for the better part of the century and no correlation has ever been noted between clean homes and birth defects, it's unlikely that disinfecting your toilet bowl or polishing your dining-room table will in any way compromise the well-being of your baby. In fact, much the opposite is probably true: The elimination of bacteria and other germs by chlorine, ammonia, and other cleaning agents can protect your baby by preventing infection.

No studies have proven that the occasional incidental inhalation of ordinary household cleansers has any detrimental effect on the developing fetus; on the other hand, no studies have proven frequent inhalation completely safe. If you've already been "exposed" to cleaning products, there's no reason for concern. But for the rest of your pregnancy, clean with prudence. Let your nose, and the following tips, be your guide in screening out potentially hazardous chemicals:

❖ If the product has a strong odor or

fumes, don't breathe it in directly. Use it in an area with plenty of ventilation, or don't use it at all.

❖ Use pump sprays instead of aerosols.

❖ Never (even when you're not pregnant) mix ammonia with chlorine-based products; the combination produces deadly fumes.

❖ Try to avoid using products such as oven cleaners and dry-cleaning fluids whose labels are plastered with warnings about toxicity.

❖ Wear rubber gloves when you're cleaning. Not only will they spare your hands a lot of wear and tear, they'll prevent the absorption through the skin of potentially toxic chemicals.

Lead. Not that expectant mothers need something else to worry about, but in recent years it's been discovered that lead—long known to reduce the IQ of children who ingest it from crumbling paint—can also affect pregnant women and their fetuses. Heavy exposure to the mineral can put a woman at increased risk of developing pregnancy-induced hypertension, and even of pregnancy loss. It puts her baby at risk for a variety of problems, ranging from serious behavioral and neurological problems to relatively minor birth defects. The risks multiply when a baby is exposed to lead in the uterus and then continues to be exposed after birth.

Fortunately, it's fairly easy to avoid lead exposure, along with all the problems it can cause. Here's how: Since drinking water is a common source of lead, be sure that yours is lead-free (see below). If your home dates back to 1955 or earlier and layers of paint are to be removed for any reason, stay away from the house while the work is being done. Still another common

source of lead is food or drink contaminated by lead leached from earthenware, pottery, or china. If you have pitchers or dishes that are home-crafted, imported, antique, just plain old (the FDA did not set limits on lead in dishes until 1971), or of otherwise questionable safety, don't use them for serving or storing, particularly of acidic food or beverages (citrus, vinegar, tomatoes, wine, soft drinks).

Tap Water. Water ranks second only to oxygen on the list of substances essential to life. Humans can survive for at least a week without food (though starvation isn't medically recommended), but for only a few days without water. In other words, you've got more to worry about if you *don't* drink the water than if you do.

It's true that water once posed a serious threat to the lives it sustained, carrying deadly typhoid and other diseases. But modern water treatment has eliminated such threats, at least in developed areas of the world. Though there are some who suspect that a new threat to the unborn now exists in the very chemicals that are used to purify water, there is no conclusive evidence that this is true. Any possible hazard is eliminated in systems that use filters instead of chemicals in the water purification process.

Most tap water in the United States is safe and drinkable. But there are exceptions. Some water is contaminated with lead as it passes through old lead pipes or through newer pipes that were soldered with lead. And in a few areas, seepage of sewer wastes and chemicals from factories, toxic waste sites, dumping grounds, underground storage tanks, and farms has also led to potentially hazardous contamination. Water that comes from an underground well is at least as subject to such contamination as water from rivers, lakes, and streams. To be sure that when you fill a glass of water you will be drinking to your—and your baby's—health, do the following:

❖ Check with your local Environmental Protection Agency (EPA) or health department about the purity and safety of community drinking water. If you lack confidence in the answers, you can also consult a local environmental group (contact the Environmental Defense Fund for a referral). If there is a possibility that the quality of your water (because of pipe deterioration, because your home borders on a waste disposal area, or because of odd taste or color) might differ from the rest of the community's, arrange to have it tested (your local EPA or health department can tell you where).

❖ If your tap water looks suspicious or has an "off" taste, invest in a carbon filter for your kitchen sink. (It will last longer if it is used only for cooking and drinking water and not for the dishwasher and other purposes.) Or use bottled water for drinking and cooking.

Be aware, however, that no water that is bottled and advertised as "pure" is automatically free of impurities. Some bottled waters are as contaminated as contaminated tap water, and most do not contain fluorides, which could be important for your bones and teeth, and later for your baby's.

❖ If you suspect lead in your water, or if testing reveals high levels, changing the plumbing would be the ideal solution, but this is not always feasible. To reduce the levels of lead in the water you drink, use only cold water for drinking and cooking (hot leaches more lead from the pipes), and run the cold-water tap for about five minutes in the morning (as well as any time the water has been off for six hours or more) before using it. You can tell that fresh water from the street pipes has reached your faucet when the water has gone from cold to warmer to cold again.

❖ If your water smells and/or tastes like chlorine, boiling it or letting it stand for 24 hours will evaporate much of the chemical.

Insecticides. Though some insects, such as gypsy moths, pose a considerable threat to trees and plants, and others, such as roaches and ants, to your esthetic sensibilities, they rarely pose a health risk to human beings—even pregnant ones. And it's generally safer to live with them than to eliminate them through the use of chemical insecticides, some of which have been linked to birth defects.

Of course, your neighbors and/or your super (if they don't happen to be pregnant or have small children) may not agree. If your neighborhood is currently being sprayed, avoid being outdoors as much as possible until the chemical odors have dissipated—about two to three days. When indoors, keep the windows closed. If your super is spraying apartments for roaches or other insects, ask him to skip yours if possible. If not, be sure that all closets and kitchen cabinets are tightly closed to prevent contamination of their contents, and that all food preparation surfaces are covered. Stay out of the apartment for a day or two if that's possible, and ventilate with open windows for as long as practical. The chemicals are potentially dangerous only as long as the fumes linger. Once the spray has settled, have someone else scrub all the food preparation surfaces in or near the sprayed area.

Whenever possible, try to take the natural approach to pest control. Pull weeds instead of spraying them. Have someone remove gypsy moth larvae or other insect pests manually from trees and plants, then drop them in a jar of kerosene. Some pests can be eliminated from garden and house plants by spraying with a forceful stream from the garden hose or with a biodegradable insecticidal soap mixture, though the procedure may need to be repeated several times to be effective. Investing in an infantry of ladybugs or other beneficial predators (available from some garden supply houses) can also wipe out some unfriendly pests.

Inside the house, use "motel" or Combat-type traps, strategically placed in heavy bug traffic areas, to get rid of roaches and ants; use cedar blocks instead of mothballs in clothes closets; and use other nontoxic types of pest control. If you have young children or pets, avoid boric acid, which can be toxic when ingested. For more information on natural pest control, contact your regional Cooperative Extension Service or a local environmental group.

If you have been accidentally exposed to insecticides or herbicides, don't be alarmed. Brief, indirect exposure isn't likely to have done any harm to your baby. What does increase the risk is frequent, long-term exposure, the kind that working daily around such chemicals (as in a factory or heavily sprayed field) would involve.

Paint Fumes. In the entire animal kingdom, the period before birth (or egg laying) is passed in hectic preparation for the arrival of the new offspring. Birds feather their nests, squirrels line their tree-trunk homes with leaves and twigs, and human mothers and fathers sift madly through volumes of wallpaper and fabric samples.

And almost invariably, painting the baby's room is involved—which, in the days of arsenic- or lead-based paints, might have posed some threat to the health of the unborn. For a long while it was believed modern latex paints were much safer, but it was recently reported that they contain unsafe amounts of mercury. Federal regulations now require that paints be reformulated so they don't contain mercury. But because you don't know what hazard may turn up in paint next, it's a good idea to consider painting an inappropriate avocation for an expectant mother—even one who's trying desperately to keep busy in those last weeks of waiting. In addition, balancing on ladder tops is precarious, to say the least, and paint odors can bring on an attack of nausea. Try, instead, to get the expectant father, or someone else, to handle this aspect of the preparations.

While the painting is being done, try to arrange to be out of the house. Whether you're there or not, be sure to keep windows open for ventilation (for this reason human nest renovations are best accomplished, as they are for much of the animal kingdom, during the mild days of spring.) Avoid

Let Your House Breathe

Though making your house as airtight as possible will cut your fuel bills, it will also increase the risk of indoor air pollution. So don't caulk every crack and weatherstrip every door. Allow some fresh air to leak in and some indoor air to leak out. Weather permitting, keep some windows open.

The Green Solution

There is no way to totally eliminate indoor air pollution. Furniture, paints, carpets, paneling, all can give off invisible fumes and pollute the air you breathe at home. Though there's no evidence that at typical levels such pollution is harmful to you or your baby, you may be more comfortable if you know you are doing something to reduce it. You can accomplish this very easily and effectively by filling your home with house plants. Plants have the ability to absorb noxious fumes in the air while adding oxygen, and of course beauty, to the indoor environment.

entirely exposure to paint removers, which are highly toxic, and steer clear of the paint removing process (whether chemicals or sanders are used), particularly if the paint that's being removed might be mercury- or lead-based.

AIR POLLUTION

"It seems it isn't even safe to breathe when you're pregnant. Will city air pollution hurt my baby?"

Living in a bus terminal or sleeping nightly in a tollbooth on a congested highway might, of course, expose your fetus to excessive pollutants while depriving it of essential oxygen. Ordinary breathing in the big city, however, isn't as risky as you might think, particularly when you consider the alternative. Millions of women live and breathe in major cities across the nation and give birth to millions of healthy babies. Even in the 1960s, when pollution was at its worst levels in such smoggy places as Los Angeles and New York, no damage to the unborn was documented.

Day-to-day breathing, then, will have no detrimental effect on your baby. Even enough carbon monoxide to cause illness in the mother appears not to have deleterious effects on the fetus early in pregnancy (although carbon monoxide poisoning later in pregnancy might). It's common sense, however, to avoid extraordinarily high doses of most air pollutants. Here's how:

❖ Avoid smoke-filled rooms for extended, repeated periods. Keep in mind that cigars and pipes, because they aren't inhaled, release even more smoke into the air than cigarettes do. Ask family, guests in your home, and co-workers not to smoke in your presence.

❖ Have the exhaust system on your car checked to be sure there is no leakage of noxious fumes and that the exhaust pipe isn't rusting away. Never start your car in the garage with the garage door closed; keep the tailgate on a station wagon closed when the engine is running; avoid waiting in gas lines with other cars spewing out carbon monoxide; keep your car's air vent closed when driving in heavy traffic.

❖ If a pollution alert is called in your city, stay indoors as much as you can, with the windows closed and the air conditioner, if you have one, running. Follow any other instructions given by the city for residents who are at special risk.

❖ Don't run, walk, or bicycle along congested highways, or exercise outdoors when there's a pollution alert, since you breathe in more air—and pollution—when you're active.

❖ Make sure gas stoves, fireplaces, and wood-burning stoves in your home are vented properly. If they aren't, they can fill the air with carbon monoxide and other possibly hazardous gases.

❖ Keep the air around you cleaner with greenery. Living plants improve air quality in and around your home.

❖ If you *do* work in a bus terminal or in a tollbooth on a busy highway, consider asking for a temporary transfer to a desk job to eliminate even the hypothetical risk that the pollution might pose to your baby.

OCCUPATIONAL HAZARDS

"You hear a lot about dangers on the job, but how do you know if your workplace is safe?"

The hazards of the workplace, and the threats they may pose to the reproductive capabilities of both male and female workers and to the well-being of their unborn children, have only just begun to be explored and identified. Conclusive answers have been elusive, as they are whenever cause-and-effect connections between environmental factors and poor pregnancy outcomes are sought. First of all, it's hard to separate out all the various possible contributing risk factors in a woman's life, or to prove that an unfavorable outcome wasn't caused by a genetic accident. Second, though animal studies often yield interesting results, there's no way to ascertain whether the results apply to humans, since experiments on humans aren't, of course, feasible.

Therefore, effects on humans can be determined only through epidemiological studies. These studies can be done in two ways: Large groups of women who are exposed to certain substances can be looked at to see if they show an increase in one or more types of poor pregnancy outcome (miscarriages, birth defects, etc.). Or small groups of women who have poor outcomes can be studied to see if there is a common risk factor shared by all of them. Either way, such studies give us clues but not definitive answers.

From what we presently know, it is clear that some workplaces do present hazards for the pregnant woman (e.g., chemical factories, operating rooms, x-ray departments). Other workplaces so far have fallen into gray areas because not enough research has been done to establish their safety—or lack of it. In the majority of workplaces, much of the concern about potential risks on the job is unwarranted.

The following is a brief rundown on what's known (and what's not) about the safety of certain jobs during pregnancy:

Office Work. Far and away the most controversial potential occupational hazard sits on the desks of over 10 million American women of childbearing age: the video display terminal. VDTs have become the intensely scrutinized focus of media and public attention since the early 1980s, when reports began to link them with pregnancy problems. Several studies have been done since then, and very little solid incriminating evidence has been uncovered. No study has been able to prove a definite link between the low-level radiation (actually lower than that of sunshine) emitted by VDTs and miscarriages, though the link had been suggested. And the most recent government study (sponsored by NIOSH) has shown no greater miscarriage rate among women who use

VDTs than those who don't. One study did show an increase in miscarriages among clerical workers (but not executives) who worked 20 or more hours in front of a VDT, but experts suggest that other factors might have been responsible. Isolated reports of birth defects in babies of VDT users have not been consistent with the kinds of defects that would be expected from radiation exposure; researchers therefore considered it unlikely that the defects are related to VDT use.

Unquestionably, more large-scale study needs to be done—and it's very possible that when it is, VDTs will be vindicated. In the meantime, panic is certainly not justified, nor, according to researchers, is a change of career, even if you spend the better part of your work week in front of a terminal. If all the reassurances in the world won't make you comfortable sitting at your VDT, however, and you feel as though you would like to take some concrete steps to minimize any possible risks, consider the following:

❖ No pregnancy-related problems have been reported among pregnant women who used a VDT for 20 hours a week or less. A temporary decrease in hours spent in front of the screen to under this number would seem to wipe out even a theoretical risk.

❖ If the radiation is responsible for any negative effects, some theorize, then it would be more dangerous to sit *behind* someone else's terminal (more radiation is emitted from the back of a unit) than in front of your own. If your desk is in a less than ideal position relative to other VDTs, see if you can change its location or change desks temporarily, or if barriers can be erected between units.

❖ Some experts have suggested that

wearing a protective apron or using a grounded electrically conductive filter over the screen may protect against nonionizing radiation; others have termed these precautions ineffective. Discuss this option with your practitioner.

Though there isn't any hard evidence that working with a VDT can cause miscarriage, there is evidence that it can cause a multitude of physical discomforts, including neck, eye, wrist, arm, and back strain, dizziness, and headaches, all of which can compound the normal discomforts of pregnancy. To reduce these symptoms, try the following:

❖ Take frequent breaks from the sitting position during the day—even a brisk walk to the rest room or to deliver a memo will help.

❖ Do stretching and/or relaxation exercises (see page 194) periodically while sitting at the terminal.

❖ Use a height-adjustable chair with a backrest that supports your lower back. And be sure the keyboard and monitor are at comfortable heights.

❖ Make sure that your eyeglasses are appropriate for use at a VDT.

Health Care Work. Ever since the first doctor cared for the first patient, health care workers (physicians, dentists, veterinarians, nurses, laboratory and x-ray technicians) have taken risks with their own lives in order to save or improve the quality of the lives of others. And while some such risks are an inevitable part of the job, it makes sense for the health care worker, particularly the pregnant one, to protect herself from as many as possible. Potential risks include exposure to waste anesthesia gases (either through leakage in the operating room or the exhaled breath of recovery room patients), to chemicals (such as ethylene

Getting all the Facts

By law, you have the right to know what chemicals you are exposed to on the job; your employer is obliged to tell you. Information on workplace hazards can also be obtained by contacting the National Institute of Occupational Safety and Health, Clearing House for Occupational Safety and Health Information, 4676 Columbia Parkway, Cincinnati, OH 45226; or the Occupational Safety and Health Administration, 200 Constitution Avenue NW, Washington, DC 20210. NIOSH also makes available a booklet titled *Technical Guidelines for Protecting the Safety and Health of Hospital Workers*. Information about the safety of machinery or other equipment that you operate on the job can often be secured by writing directly to the manufacturer's corporate medical director.

If your job does expose you to hazards, either ask to be transferred temporarily to a safer post or, finances permitting, begin your maternity leave early.

---

oxide and formaldehyde) used for sterilization of equipment, to ionizing radiation (such as that used in diagnosis or treatment of disease),[6] to anti-cancer drugs, and to infections, such as hepatitis B and AIDS. Depending upon the particular risk you are exposed to, you might want to either take safety precautions as recommended by the National Institute of Occupational Safety and Health (NIOSH; see box above) or switch to safer work for the time being.

Manufacturing Work. How safe conditions are in a factory depends on what's being made in it and, to a certain extent, on how principled the people who run it are. The Occupational Safety and Health Administration (OSHA) lists a number of substances that a pregnant woman should avoid on the job. They include such chemicals as alkylating agents, arsenic, benzene, carbon monoxide, chlorinated hydrocarbons, dimethyl sulfoxide, organic mercury compounds, lead, lithium, aluminum, arsenic, ethylene oxide, dioxin, and polychlorinated biphenyls. Where proper safety protocols are implemented, exposure to such toxins can be avoided. Your union or other labor organization may be able to help you determine if you are protected. You can also get useful information from OSHA (see box above).

In-Flight Work. It has recently been suggested that flight attendants and airline pilots (possibly along with very frequent flyers) may run the risk of excessive exposure to radiation from the sun if their flights often bring them to very high altitudes. Radiation is more intense nearer the poles and less so near the equator, so flights across the southern United States pose less potential risk than those across the northern states. Though at this

---

6. Most technicians working with low-dose diagnostic x-ray will not be exposed to dangerous levels of radiation. It is recommended, however, that women of childbearing age working with higher-dose radiation wear a special device that keeps track of daily exposure, to ensure that cumulative annual exposure does not exceed safe levels.

time the risk appears to be very small, those who ordinarily spend a lot of time flying long distances, particularly at closer proximity to the poles, might want to consider a switch during pregnancy to shorter routes that fly at lower altitudes, or to ground work. If you're concerned about the flying you did before you found out you were pregnant, discuss this with your practitioner—you're more than likely to find reassurance.

Physically Strenuous Work. Work that involves heavy lifting, physical exertion, long hours, rotating shifts, or continuous standing may somewhat increase a woman's risk for early and late miscarriage as well as preterm deliveries and stillbirth. If you have such a job, you should request a transfer to a less strenuous position until after delivery and postpartum recovery. (See page 204 for recommendations on how long it is safe for you to stay at various strenuous jobs during your pregnancy.)

Other Work. Teachers and social workers who deal with young children may come into contact with potentially dangerous infections, such as rubella. Animal handlers, meat cutters, and meat inspectors may be exposed to toxoplasmosis (but may well have developed immunity already, in which case their babies would not be at risk), and laundry workers to a variety of infections. If you work where infection is a risk, be sure you're immunized as needed and take appropriate precautions, such as using gloves, masks, and so on. (See individual infections.)

Artists, photographers, chemists, cosmeticians, dry cleaners, agricultural and horticultural workers, and others may be exposed to a variety of possibly hazardous chemicals in the course of their work. If you work with any suspect substances, you should take appropriate precautions, which in some cases may mean avoiding that part of your work that involves the use of chemicals. Don't be overly concerned about exposure that's already occurred, since in most cases exposure to toxins that isn't massive enough to cause illness in the mother rarely results in damage to the fetus.

Quiet Please

Noise is probably the most prevalent of all occupational hazards, and has long been known to cause hearing loss in those exposed to it on a regular basis. But it isn't known how it affects the unborn baby—if at all. Noise has been shown to increase the risk of miscarriage in animals, but it isn't clear that it also does so in humans. Studies to try to determine whether excessive exposure to loud noise can cause birth defects have been contradictory, and there just isn't enough research to determine whether vibration, which often accompanies noise, is harmful. Until more is known, expectant mothers who work in an extremely noisy environment or are exposed to vibration and want to play it safe can consider asking about a temporary transfer.

WHAT IT'S IMPORTANT TO KNOW:
PLAYING BABY ROULETTE

When a gambler playing roulette puts down a bet on his lucky number, the odds are very high against the wheel coming to a stop there. It's the same when a pregnant woman plays baby roulette (intentionally or inadvertently), exposing her baby to teratogens, substances potentially harmful to the fetus. Almost all of the time the baby roulette wheel will pass innocuously by, and the baby won't be affected.

Although the gambler will call it luck, where the roulette wheel stops depends on the weight of the wheel, the friction it encounters, and the force with which it is spun. And though baby roulette may also appear to be a game of chance, its outcome, too, is actually dependent on a variety of factors:

How Strong Is the Teratogen? A very few drugs are powerful teratogens. For example, thalidomide, a drug used in the early 1960s, caused severe deformities in all fetuses who were exposed in utero at a particular time in their development (1 in 5 of all babies exposed at any time prenatally), and the acne medicine Accutane, a more recently recognized teratogen, caused defects in almost 1 in 5 exposures. At the other extreme are drugs such as the hormone Provera—a progestin—that are believed to cause defects only rarely (an estimated 1 in 1,000 exposed fetuses for Provera). Most drugs fall somewhere in between, and fortunately, few are as potent as thalidomide and Accutane (and Accutane-like compounds).

Often it's very difficult to tell whether a drug is teratogenic at all, even when its use appears to be re-lated to the occurrence of certain birth defects. Say, for example, a defect shows up in babies whose mothers took a particular antibiotic for infection with high fever when they were pregnant; the cause of the defect could turn out to be the fever or the infection, not the medication. Or, as some surmise may be the case with Provera, which has been used to prevent miscarriage, the malformations associated with its use may have nothing to do with the drug, but may show up only because the drug averted the miscarriage of an embryo that was blighted to begin with.

Is the Fetus Genetically Susceptible to the Teratogen? Just as not everybody exposed to cold germs succumbs, not every fetus who is exposed to a teratogen is affected by it.

When Was the Fetus Exposed to the Teratogen? The period of gestation during which most teratogens are capable of doing harm is very brief. For example, thalidomide caused no damage at all when taken after the 52nd day. Likewise, the rubella virus causes damage in less than 1% of fetuses if exposure takes place after the third month.

During the six to eight days after conception (before a woman has even missed her period), the fertilized egg, or conceptus, which expands into a ball of cells and travels down the fallopian tubes to the uterus, is largely insensitive to assault from what passes through its mother's system, and rarely suffers malformation. In fact, if it does sustain a minor injury, it has the ability to repair itself. The only risk at this point is that the conceptus will fail to survive because of a genetic mistake or that it will be destroyed by certain external factors, such as a very powerful dose of radiation.

The period during which the organs are being formed—from implantation of the conceptus in the uterus around days six to eight through the end of the first trimester—is the interval when the risk of malformation is greatest. After the third month, the risk of this kind of injury is greatly reduced; any damage that does occur usually affects the rate of growth of the fetus or its central nervous system.

How Much Exposure Was There? Most teratogenic effects are dose-related. One brief diagnostic x-ray will be unlikely to cause a problem. A series of heavy-dose radiation treatments could. Smoking lightly for the first few months is not likely to harm a fetus; heavy smoking for the entire pregnancy increases certain risks very significantly.

What Is the Mother's General Nutritional Status? Animal experiments show that defects apparently caused by a drug were, in some cases, actually caused by poor nutrition; the drug only reduced appetite, and thus water and food intake. Just as you will resist a cold virus more effectively if you are well nourished and not run-down, so will your fetus resist teratogens better if he or she is well nourished— through you, of course.

Was the Mother Affected by the Exposure? It's reassuring to know that chemical exposure that isn't toxic enough to cause symptoms in the mother usually is not toxic enough to cause problems in the fetus.

Are Several Factors Combining to Increase Risk? The trio of poor diet, smoking, and alcohol abuse, the duet of smoking and tranquilizers, and other "losing combinations" can greatly increase risk.

Is Some Unknown Protective Factor in Play? Even when all factors appear identical, not all fetuses are affected in the same way. In experiments with mouse fetuses of identical genetic strains who were exposed to the same teratogens at identical stages in development and at identical dosages, only 1 in 9 was born malformed. No one knows exactly why, though perhaps someday medical science will come up with the solution to this mystery.

WEIGHING RISK VS. BENEFIT

Should today's pregnant woman fear for her baby's life and well-being because he or she is developing in a world filled with environmental threats? Absolutely not—and for several reasons. First of all, drugs and other environmental factors account for less than 1% of all birth defects— and birth defects affect only 3% to 4% of all newborns. The general risk is extremely slight, even if you have already been exposed to a specific teratogen. Second, if you haven't, knowing what the risks are can help you to avoid them, improving your baby's odds still more. Third, in spite of the dire warnings making headlines and highlighting news programs daily, never have the chances of having a healthy, normal baby been better.

Of course, no decision is totally without risk. But when making choices, we need to learn to weigh risks against benefits. This is never more important than during pregnancy, when each decision potentially affects the safety and well-being of not one but two lives. When you're faced with the decision of whether or not to smoke, to have a before-dinner cocktail, to nibble on a chocolate bar instead of an apple while watching TV, you should weigh risk against benefit. Are the benefits, if any, you are going to derive from smoking, drinking, or junk-food snacking worth the risks to your baby?

Well, most of the time your answer will probably be no. But once in a while you may decide that a little risk will be worth it. One small glass of wine, for example, to toast your anniversary: the risk to your baby is practically nil, and the benefit (a more festive anniversary) is really important. Or a big chunk of sugar- and butter-rich cake for your birthday—a lot of empty calories, true. But they won't really deprive baby of necessary nutrients over the long run, and after all, it *is* your birthday.

Some risk vs. benefit decisions are easy. For instance, regular heavy alcohol consumption throughout pregnancy can handicap your child for life (see page 52). Giving up the pleasure you derive from drinking may take considerable effort, but the risks if you don't are clear.

Or say you have the flu and you are running a fever that's high enough to pose a threat to your baby. Your doctor won't hesitate to prescribe a safe medication to bring down the fever. In this case, the benefit of using the drug far outweighs its possible harm. On the other hand, if your temperature is only slightly elevated, it poses no threat to your baby and will actually help your body fight the flu virus. So before resorting to medication, your doctor will feel secure in giving your body a chance to cure itself, on the grounds that the possible risk of taking the drug outweighs its potential benefits.

Other decisions are not so clear-cut. What if you have a terrible cold with sinus headaches that have been keeping you up at night? Should you take a cold tablet to help you get some rest? Or should you suffer through sleepless nights, which won't do you or the baby any good? The best way to approach such decisions is:

❖ Determine if there are alternative lower-risk ways of obtaining the benefits you are seeking—perhaps through non-drug approaches (see Appendix). Try them. If they don't work, continue to evaluate your original option—in this case, cold tablets.

❖ Ask your physician about risks and benefits. It's important to remember that not all drugs are known to cause birth defects, and that many have been used safely in pregnancy. New studies are turning up more information on drug safety, or lack of it, daily. Your practitioner has access to this information.

❖ Do some research on your own. For the latest information on the safety of a particular drug during pregnancy, check with the Federal Drug Administration or the March of Dimes. (See Appendix.)

❖ Determine if there are ways of increasing the benefits and/or decreasing the risks (taking the safest, most effective pain reliever in the smallest effective doses for the shortest possible time), and try to ensure that if you do take the risk, you will receive the benefit (take your cold tablet before you go to bed, when you are most likely to get that needed rest).

❖ In consultation with your practitioner and, if necessary, a genetic counselor or maternal-fetal subspecialist, review all the information you've gathered—weighing risks against benefits—and make your decision.

During pregnancy you will be challenged to make intelligent decisions in dozens of situations, weighing risk against benefit. Almost every decision you make will impact on your chance of having a healthy baby. But an occasional wrong choice isn't likely to be catastrophic—it will change the odds only very slightly. If you've already made a few not-so-terrific choices and there's no way to undo them, forget them. Just try to make better decisions for the rest of your pregnancy. And remember, the odds are very much in your baby's favor!

4
The Best-Odds Diet

There's a tiny new being developing inside you. The odds are already fairly good that he or she will be born healthy. But you have the chance to improve those odds significantly—to come as close as possible to guaranteeing your baby not just good health, but excellent health—with every bite of food you put in your mouth.

That's not just idle theory. A study done at the Harvard School of Public Health dramatically illustrates how closely the state of a baby's health at birth is tied to its mother's diet during pregnancy. Of the women in the study whose diets were good to excellent, fully 95% had babies in good or excellent health. On the other hand, only 8% of women whose diets were really awful (composed largely of junk foods) had babies in good or excellent health, and 65% of them had infants who were stillborn, premature, functionally immature, or who had congenital defects.

Of course, the diets of most of the women in the study (like those of most pregnant women) were neither excellent nor extremely poor. They were average, and so was the health of their children. Eighty-eight percent had babies in good or fair health. But only 6% had infants in really excellent health—which is, after all, what most of us want for our children.

Other studies, too, have shown that the effects of diet can be far-reaching. What a pregnant woman eats or doesn't eat can have an effect on her baby's developing organs. For example, lack of protein and calories in the last trimester can interfere with brain development, and a lack of folic acid, it is believed, may be linked to spinal tube defects. What she eats can also affect her baby's general growth (eating too little or the wrong kinds of food can retard growth in the uterus).

Research also shows that her eating habits can have an effect on the course of her pregnancy (some complications, such as anemia and pre-eclampsia, are more common among poorly nourished women); her comfort (fatigue, morning sickness, constipation, leg cramps, and a host of other pregnancy symptoms can be minimized or avoided altogether with good diet); her labor and delivery (in general, women on excellent diets are less likely than women on poor diets to deliver too early; specifically, deficiency in zinc has been linked to an increased risk of premature labor); her emotional state (good diet can help to moderate mood swings); and her postpartum recovery (a well-nourished body can bounce back faster and more easily, and weight that's been gained at a sensible rate and on nutritious foods can be shed more quickly).

If your eating habits aren't that disciplined or virtuous to begin with, following the Best-Odds Diet will probably present you with quite a challenge. But when you consider the result of your extra efforts—better odds that your baby will be born in excellent health and better odds that you'll recover faster from pregnancy and delivery—we think you'll agree that it's a challenge worth accepting.

NINE BASIC PRINCIPLES FOR NINE MONTHS OF HEALTHY EATING

Every Bite Counts. You've got only nine months of meals and snacks with which to give your baby the best possible start in life. Make every one of them count. Before you close your mouth on a forkful of food, consider, "Is this the best bite I can give my baby?" If it will benefit your baby, chew away. If it'll only benefit your sweet tooth or appease your appetite, put your fork down.

All Calories Are Not Created Equal. For example, the 150 calories in a doughnut are not equal to the 150 calories in a whole-grain, juice-sweetened bran muffin. Nor are the 100 calories in ten potato chips equal to the 100 in a baked potato served in its skin (or in a batch of Best-Odds Fries; see page 93). So choose your calories with care, selecting quality over quantity. Your baby will benefit a lot more from 2,000 nutrient-rich calories daily than from 4,000 mostly empty ones.

Starve Yourself, Starve Your Baby. Just as you wouldn't consider starving your baby after it's born, you shouldn't consider starving it in utero. The fetus can't thrive living off your flesh, no matter how ample. It needs regular nourishment at regular intervals. Never, never skip a meal.[1] Even if you're not hungry, the baby is. If persistent heartburn or a constant bloated feeling is spoiling your appetite, spread your daily requirements out over six small meals instead of three large ones.

Efficiency Is Effective. Fill your daily nutritional requirements in the most efficient way possible within your caloric needs. Eating 6 tablespoons of peanut butter (if you can get it down) at 600 calories, or about 25% of your daily allotment, is a considerably less efficient way of getting 25 grams of protein than eating 3½ ounces of water-packed tuna at 125 calories. And eating a cup and a half of ice cream (about 450 calories) is a far less efficient way of getting 300 milligrams of calcium than drinking a glass of skim milk (90 calories) or eating a cup of nonfat yogurt (100 calories). Fat, because it has more than twice as many calories per gram as either proteins or carbohydrates, is a particularly inefficient source of calories. Choose lean meats over fatty ones, low-fat milk and dairy products over full-fat, broiled foods over fried; spread butter lightly; sauté in a teaspoon of fat, not a quarter of a cup.

Efficiency is important, too, if you're having trouble gaining enough weight. To start tipping the scale toward a healthier weight gain, choose foods that are dense in nutrients and calories—avocados, nuts, and dried fruits, for instance—that can fill you and your baby out without filling you up too much. And avoid such calorie bargains as popcorn and large salads, which will do just the opposite.

---

1. Never fast during pregnancy, either. An Israeli study shows a jump in deliveries just after Yom Kippur, the Day of Atonement, suggesting that fasting late in pregnancy could trigger an early delivery.

Whether you are trying to gain less or gain more, or just trying to squeeze your Daily Dozen into a queasy, upset, or too-full tummy, whenever possible opt for foods that efficiently fulfill two or more requirements with one serving—for example, broccoli (Vitamin C, Green Leafy, and Calcium); yogurt or canned salmon (Protein and Calcium); dried apricots (Yellow Fruits and Iron). (The Daily Dozen requirements are described beginning on page 83.)

Carbohydrates Are a Complex Issue. Some women concerned about gaining too much weight during pregnancy mistakenly drop carbohydrates from their diets like so many hot potatoes. True, refined and/or simple carbohydrates (like white bread, white rice, refined cereals, cakes, cookies, pretzels, sugars, syrups) are nutritionally weak—supplying little but calories. But unrefined and/or complex carbohydrates (whole-grain breads and cereals, brown rice, vegetables, dried beans and peas, and, of course, hot potatoes—especially in their skins) and fresh fruit supply essential B vitamins, trace minerals, protein, and important fiber. Good not only for your baby, but for you. They'll help keep nausea and constipation in check, and because they are filling and fiber-rich but not fattening (as long as they're not bathed in buttery sauces or slathered with rich toppings), they'll help keep your weight gain in check, too. Recent research suggests yet another bonus for complex carbohydrate eaters: consuming plenty of fiber may reduce the risk of developing gestational diabetes.

Sweet Nothings: Nothing But Trouble. No calorie is as empty, and therefore as wasted, as a calorie of sugar. In addition, researchers are finding that sugar may be not only void of value, but harmful. Research suggests that, in addition to causing tooth decay, it may be implicated in diabetes, heart disease, depression, and in some cases of hyperactivity. Perhaps the worst thing about sugar is that it is most often found in foods that are on the whole nutritionally bankrupt: sweets and baked goods made with bleached white flour and excessive quantities of unhealthy fats. Sugar substitutes (even aspartame, which is believed to be safe for use in pregnancy; see page 62) are a questionable replacement for all the sugar the average pregnant woman is used to consuming, partly because these sweeteners, too, are often found in less-than-best foods.

For delicious *and* nutritious sweetness, substitute fruit and fruit juice concentrates (undiluted frozen juices) for sugar. They are about as sweet as sugar but contain more vitamins and trace minerals. Products sweetened with them are almost invariably made with whole grains and healthy fats and without questionable chemical additives. Make your own at home, using recipes such as those found in this chapter, or choose from the increasingly abundant selection available in health food stores and supermarkets. But read labels to be sure that the fruit sweeteners have not simply replaced the sugar in what is otherwise a poor food choice.

The Best-Odds Diet recommends limiting refined sugars (brown, white, turbinado, honey, maple syrup, corn syrup, fructose, and so on) during pregnancy to an occasional special-occasion fling. Every sugar calorie can better come from foods that yield a higher nutritional return for your baby.

Good Foods Remember Where They Came From. If your green beans haven't seen their native fields for months (having been boiled, processed, preserved, and canned since harvesting), they probably don't have much of their natural goodness left to offer you or your baby. Choose fresh vegetables and fruits when they're in season, or fresh-frozen when fresh are unavailable or you don't have time to prepare them (they're as nutritious as fresh because they're frozen immediately after harvesting). Try to eat some raw vegetables and/or fruit every day. When cooking vegetables, steam or stir-fry them lightly, so they'll retain their vitamins and minerals. Poach fruits in juice with no sugar added. Avoid prepared foods that have picked up a lot of chemicals, sugar, and salt on the assembly line; they're frequently low in nutrition. Choose a fresh chicken breast over processed chicken roll; a casserole made from fresh ingredients rather than a dehydrated mix of overprocessed ingredients and chemicals; fresh oatmeal made from rolled oats (you can flavor it with cinnamon and chopped dried fruit) rather than the sugared instant varieties.

Healthful Eating Should Be a Family Affair. If there are subversive elements at home, urging you to bake chocolate chip cookies or to add potato chips to your shopping list, it's a sure bet that the Best-Odds Diet won't stand a chance. So make other family members your allies by putting the whole household on the diet with you. Bake naturally sweet Fruity Oatmeal Cookies (page 96) instead of chocolate chip; bring home whole-wheat pretzels or toasted sunflower seeds instead of potato chips. In addition to a healthier baby and a relatively slimmer you, there will be the postpartum bonus of a fitter, trimmer husband and older children (if you have them) with better eating habits. Continue the Best-Odds Diet for the whole family after delivery and you will be giving each member—particularly that important newest member—the best odds for a longer and healthier life.

Bad Habits Can Sabotage a Good Diet. The best prenatal diet in the world is easily undermined if the expectant mother fails to heed the advice to eliminate alcohol, tobacco, and other unsafe drugs from her life. Read about these saboteurs in Chapter 3, and if you haven't done so already, change your habits accordingly.

THE BEST-ODDS DAILY DOZEN

Calories. The old adage that a pregnant woman is eating for two is true. But it's important to remember that one of the two is a tiny developing fetus whose caloric needs are significantly lower than yours—a mere 300 a day, more or less. So, if you're of average weight, you need only about 300 calories more than was necessary to maintain your prepregnancy weight.[2] During the first trimester you may need fewer than 300 extra calories daily, unless you're trying to compensate for starting out underweight. As your metabolism speeds up later in pregnancy, you may need somewhat more than 300 extra calories daily. In spite of the numerous pregnancy diets you may see that seem to recommend you eat enough food to feed a family of four, consuming calories beyond what your baby needs for growth and what you need for baby-making is not only unnecessary but unwise. Eating fewer calories, on the other hand, is

---

2. To determine roughly how many calories you need to maintain your prepregnancy weight, multiply that weight by 12 if you're sedentary, 15 if you're moderately active, and up to 22 if you're very active. Because the rate at which calories are burned varies from person to person even during pregnancy, calorie requirements vary too, so the figure you arrive at is just an estimate.

not only unwise but potentially dangerous; women who don't take in sufficient calories during pregnancy—particularly in the second and third trimesters—can seriously hamper the development of their babies.

There are four exceptions to this basic formula. In each of these cases the expectant mother should discuss her caloric needs with her practitioner: the overweight woman, who, with proper nutritional guidance, can possibly do with fewer calories; the seriously underweight woman, who certainly needs more; the adolescent, who is still growing herself and has special nutritional needs; and the woman carrying multiple fetuses, who will have to add 300 calories for each of them.

Having to eat 300 extra calories a day sounds like a food lover's fantasy, but sad to say, it isn't. By the time you've guzzled your four glasses of milk (total of 380 calories for skim) or the equivalent in calcium-rich foods and taken your required extra servings of protein, you've exceeded your allowance. Which means that instead of adding tantalizing frills, you'll probably have to cut out those you're accustomed to in order to nourish your baby adequately and keep your weight gain reasonable. To make sure you get the maximum nutritional punch out of your calories, become a dietary efficiency expert (see page 81).

But while calories count during pregnancy, they don't have to be counted. Instead of concerning yourself with complicated computations at every meal, step on a reliable scale once a week to check your progress. Weigh yourself at the same time of day, naked or wearing the same clothing (or clothing that weighs about the same), so that your calculations won't be thrown off by a heavy meal one week or a heavy sweater the next. If your weight gain is going according to schedule (an average of about 1 pound a week in the second and third trimesters; see page 147), you're getting the right number of calories. If it's less than that, you're getting too few; if it's more than that, you're getting too many. Maintain or adjust your food energy intake as necessary, but be certain you never cut out required nutrients along with calories. And continue to weigh yourself weekly to make sure you stay on track.

Protein: four servings daily. Protein is composed of substances called amino acids, which are the building blocks of human cells; they are particularly important in building the cells of a new baby. Research has shown that inadequate protein intake in expectant mothers, like inadequate calorie intake, can result in babies being smaller than normal at birth. Therefore, the pregnant woman should aim to have at least 60 to 75 grams of protein every day. It's possible that 100 grams, the amount often recommended in high-risk pregnancies, may be a better goal since the increased intake may help prevent a pregnancy from becoming high risk in the first place.[3] Though a goal of 100 grams of protein may seem like a lot, most Americans consume that much or more per day. To get your 100 grams, all you have to do is eat a total of four servings of Protein Foods from the Best-Odds Food Selection Groups (see page 89). When tallying your protein servings, don't forget to count the protein found in many high-calcium foods: a glass of milk and an ounce of cheese each provide a third of a protein serving; a cup of yogurt equals

---

3. Women who are not taking in an adequate amount of calories (perhaps because of nausea and vomiting) need a greater protein intake so that there is enough both for energy and for baby-building purposes. They should be sure to get at least four servings daily.

half a serving; 4 ounces of canned salmon, a whole serving.

If at the end of the day you come up a half or even a whole serving short, you can meet your quota quickly with a high-protein bedtime snack. For example, try egg salad (half a protein serving when made with 1 egg and 2 egg whites) with whole-wheat crackers; a Double-the-Milk Shake (two-thirds of a protein serving; see page 95); or ¾ cup of low-fat cottage cheese (a full protein serving) garnished either with fresh fruit, raisins, and cinnamon or chopped tomato and basil. *Do not,* however, use liquid or powdered high-protein supplements to help fill your protein requirement—they could be harmful.

Vitamin C Foods: two servings daily.
You and baby both need vitamin C for tissue repair, wound healing, and various other metabolic (nutrient-utilizing) processes. Your baby also needs it for proper growth and for the development of strong bones and teeth. Vitamin C is a nutrient the body can't store, so a fresh supply is needed every day. Vitamin C–rich foods are best eaten fresh and uncooked, as exposure to light, heat, and air destroys the vitamin over time. As you can see from the list of Vitamin C Foods on page 90, the old standby orange juice is far from the only, or even the best, source of this essential vitamin.

Calcium Foods: four servings daily.
Back in elementary school you probably learned that growing children need plenty of calcium for strong bones and teeth. Well, so do growing fetuses on their way to becoming growing children. Calcium is also vital for muscle, heart, and nerve development, blood clotting, and enzyme activity. But it's not only your baby who stands to lose when you don't get enough calcium. If incoming supplies are inadequate, your baby-making fac-

tory will draw upon the calcium in your own bones to help meet its quota, setting you up for osteoporosis later in life. Still another reason to drink your milk (or take your calcium in other forms) is the recent research indicating that a high calcium intake may help prevent pregnancy-induced hypertension (preeclampsia).

So be diligent about getting your four servings of calcium-rich foods a day. And don't worry if the idea of four glasses of milk doesn't appeal to you. Calcium doesn't have to be served in glasses at all. It can be served up as a cup of yogurt, a piece of cheese, or a large portion of cottage cheese. It can be disguised in soups, casseroles, breads, cereals, desserts; this is especially easy when it's in the form of nonfat dry milk or evaporated skim milk (⅓ cup and ½ cup, respectively, measure up to a full glass of liquid milk, or one Calcium serving). And if you do opt for the glass, you can double the calcium power in each one by stirring in ⅓ cup of nonfat dry milk (see Double-the-Milk Shake, page 95). For those who can't tolerate or don't eat milk products at all, calcium can also come in nondairy form. The Calcium-Rich Foods listing on page 90 provides a variety of nondairy equivalents.

For those who cannot be sure of getting enough calcium from their diets (such as vegetarians or the lactose-intolerant), a calcium supplement may be recommended.

Green Leafy and Yellow Vegetables and Yellow Fruits: three servings daily, or more. These bunny-set favorites supply the vitamin A, in the form of beta-carotene, that is vital for cell growth (your baby's cells are multiplying at a fantastic rate), healthy skin, bones, and eyes, and may even reduce the risk of some types of cancer. The green leafies and yellows also deliver doses of essential vitamins (vitamin E, riboflavin, folic acid, B₆), numerous minerals (many green leafies provide a good deal of calcium as well as trace minerals), and constipation-fighting fiber. A bountiful selection of nature's most efficient sources of vitamin A can be found in the Green Leafy and Yellow Vegetables and Yellow Fruits list on page 91. Those with an anti-vegetable bent may be surprised to discover that carrots and spinach are not the only sources of vitamin A and, in fact, that the vitamin comes packaged in some of nature's most tempting sweet offerings—dried apricots, yellow peaches, cantaloupe, and mangoes, for example. And those who like to drink their vegetables may be happy to know that they can occasionally count a glass of vegetable juice cocktail toward their Green Leafy and Yellow allowance.

Other Fruits and Vegetables: two servings daily, or more. In addition to produce rich in beta-carotene-vitamin A and vitamin C, you need at least two other types of fruit or vegetable daily—for extra fiber, vitamins, and minerals. Many of these are rich in potassium and/or magnesium, both of which are important to good pregnancy health, and in boron, the importance of which is only beginning to be understood. A variety of these fruits and vegetables are suggested on page 91.

Whole Grains and Legumes: five servings daily, or more. Whole grains (whole wheat, oats, rye, barley, corn, rice, millet, triticale, soy, and so on) and legumes (dried peas and beans) are packed with nutrients, particularly the B vitamins that are needed for just about every part of your developing baby's body. These concentrated complex carbohydrates are also rich in trace minerals, such as zinc, selenium, and magnesium, which have been shown to be very signifi-

cant in pregnancy. Starchy foods may also help reduce morning sickness.

Though these staff-of-life foods have many nutrients in common, each has its own strengths. To get the maximum benefit, include a variety of complex carbohydrates in your diet. Be adventurous: Bread your fish with oat bran seasoned with herbs and Parmesan cheese. Add triticale to your rice pilaf. Use rolled barley in your favorite oatmeal cookie recipe. Substitute navy beans for limas in your soup.

Don't count refined grains (breads or cereals made with white flour, for example) as meeting this requirement on a regular basis. Even if they are "enriched," they are still lacking in the fiber and in more than a dozen vitamins and trace minerals that are found in the originals.

Iron-Rich Foods: some daily. Since large amounts of iron are essential for the developing blood supply of the fetus and for your own expanding blood supply, you'll need more during these nine months than at any other time in your life. Get as much of your iron as you can from your diet (see the list on page 92). Eating foods rich in vitamin C at the same sitting as iron-rich foods will increase the absorption of the mineral by the body.

Because it's often difficult to fill the pregnancy iron requirement through diet alone, it is recommended that, from about the 12th week on, pregnant women take a daily supplement of 30 milligrams of ferrous iron. To enhance the absorption of the iron in the supplement, it should be taken between meals with a fruit juice rich in vitamin C or with water (but not with milk, tea, or coffee). If a pregnant woman's iron stores are low, 60 to 120 milligrams may be prescribed by her practitioner.

High-Fat Foods: four full or eight half servings, or an equivalent combina-

tion daily. According to generally accepted nutritional guidelines, no more than 30% of an adult's calories should come from fat (in the average American diet, 40% of calories come from fat). The same guidelines apply to pregnant adults. That means that if you weigh about 125 pounds and need about 2,100 calories a day (see page 83 and the Appendix if you weigh more or less), no more than 630 of these should come from fat. Since it takes only 70 grams of fat (as much as you would find in a hefty slice of quiche) to reach 630 calories, this requirement is definitely the easiest to fill—and the easiest to overfill. And though there's no harm in having a couple of extra Green Leafies or Vitamin C foods, or even additional Whole Grains or Calcium foods, excess fat servings could spell excess pounds. Still, while keeping fat intake moderate is a good idea, eliminating all fat from your diet is a potentially dangerous one. Fat is vital to your developing baby; the essential fatty acids it provides are just that—essential.

Keep careful track of the high-fat foods you eat each day; fill your quota but stop before you exceed it. Don't forget that the fat used in cooking and preparing foods counts, too. If you've fried your eggs in ½ tablespoon of margarine (½ a serving) and mashed your tuna with a tablespoon of mayonnaise (1 serving), include these amounts in your daily tally.

If you're not gaining enough weight, and increasing your intake of other nutritious foods is not effective, try adding one extra fat serving each day (but no more); the concentrated calories it provides may help you hit your optimum weight gain stride.

For information on cholesterol in pregnancy, see page 126.

Salty Foods: in moderation. At one time, the medical establishment pre-scribed limiting salt (sodium chloride) during pregnancy because it contributed to water retention and bloating. Now it is believed that some increase in body fluids in pregnancy is necessary and normal, and that a moderate amount of sodium is needed to maintain adequate fluid levels. Still, very large quantities of salt and very salty foods (such as pickles, soy sauce, and potato chips) aren't good for anyone, pregnant or not. High sodium intake is closely linked to high blood pressure, a condition that can cause a variety of potentially dangerous complications in pregnancy, labor, and delivery. Though iodine deficiency is not a problem in the United States, you may want to use iodized salt to be sure that you meet the increased need for iodine in pregnancy. As a general rule, rather than adding salt during cooking, salt your food to taste at the table.

Fluids: at least eight 8-ounce glasses daily. You're not only eating for two, you're drinking for two. If you've always been one of those people who goes through the day with barely a sip of anything, now's the time to change that habit. As body fluids increase during pregnancy, so does your need for fluid intake. Your fetus, too, needs fluids. Most of its body, like yours, is composed of water. Extra fluids also help keep your skin soft, lessen the likelihood of constipation, rid your body of toxins and waste products, and reduce excessive swelling and the risk of urinary tract infection. Be sure to get at least 8 cups (2 quarts) a day—more if you're retaining a lot of fluid (paradoxically, a plentiful fluid intake can flush excess fluids from your body). Of course, all your water doesn't have to come from the tap. You can count milk (which is two-thirds water), fruit and vegetable juices, naturally decaffeinated coffee and teas, soup, and plain soda water. Be sure, however, that all your fluids aren't caloric, or you may end up with too many calories each day.

Using 12-ounce glasses or mugs each time you take a drink will give you 1½ cups of fluid at a shot and mean fewer refills. Spread your fluid intake out over the day, and don't try to drink more than two glassfuls at a sitting—which could dilute your blood excessively, causing a chemical imbalance.

Nutritional Supplements: a pregnancy formula taken daily. Vitamin supplements have always generated controversy in the scientific community. The controversy surrounding prenatal vitamin supplements has now intensified with a statement from the National Academy of Sciences, which concluded that there is currently insufficient evidence to encourage routine use of supplements (except for 30

What's in a Pill?

There are no standards set either by the FDA or by the American College of Obstetricians and Gynecology specifying exactly what must be in a pill for it to be called a prenatal supplement. So selecting the right formula can be complicated. Often a practitioner will prescribe a supplement, and in general prescribed formulas are superior to those bought over the counter.

If you are selecting a vitamin/ mineral supplement yourself, look for a formula that contains:

❖ No more than 8,000 IU of vitamin A; 4,000 or 5,000 IU would probably be better.

❖ 800 to 1,000 mcg (1 mg) of folic acid.

❖ The pregnancy RDA for vitamins D and C. Some formulas contain slightly more or less than the RDA, and that's okay. But avoid those that contain much more than that unless prescribed by your doctor.

❖ The pregnancy RDA, or slightly more or less, of niacin (or niacinamide or B_3), pantothenic acid (B_5; absent in many supplements), iron, iodine, zinc, and copper.*

❖ The pregnancy RDA for vitamin E.

❖ At least the pregnancy RDA for thiamine (B_1), riboflavin (B_2), pyridoxine (B_6), and cyanocobalamin (B_{12}). Many formulas contain from 1½ to 3 times the RDA for these vitamins; there are no known harmful effects from such doses.

❖ No more than 250 mg of elemental calcium or 25 mg of magnesium, if the formula also contains iron, since large amounts of either of these minerals can interfere to some extent with iron absorption. (If the doctor has prescribed larger doses of calcium and/or magnesium, take them at least two hours before or after any supplement containing iron.)

❖ Trace minerals, such as chromium, manganese, molybdenum, and the vitamin biotin; these offer added insurance, but they are included in few supplements.

---

*Copper is necessary in any supplement containing zinc, since zinc can interfere with the body's absorption of copper from the diet, increasing the need for this mineral. Zinc and copper are both necessary in a supplement containing iron, since the iron may interfere with their absorption.

milligrams of iron) for all pregnant women. The Academy urged more research to see if supplementation with certain vitamins and minerals could indeed be valuable for everyone. But for the present, they recommend that physicians carefully evaluate the diet of each patient and prescribe supplements only when they determine that the diet is lacking—with routine supplementation limited to those at nutritional high risk, including vegetarians, women carrying more than one fetus, heavy smokers, and alcohol and drug abusers.

The theory that a healthy pregnant woman can get virtually all of her nutritional requirements at the kitchen table is a common one. And, indeed, she could—if she lived in a laboratory where her food was prepared to ensure retention of vitamins and minerals and measured to ensure an adequate daily intake, if she never ate on the run or felt too sick to eat, if she always knew for sure that she was carrying only one baby and that her pregnancy wouldn't turn out to be high-risk. But in the real world, a nutritional supplement provides extra health insurance—and women who like to play it safe may feel safer with such insurance.

Still, a supplement is just a *supplement.* No pill, no matter how complete, can replace a good diet. It's very important that most of your vitamins and minerals come from foods, because that is the way nutrients can be most effectively utilized. Fresh foods (not processed) contain not only nutrients that we know about, and that can be synthesized in a pill, but probably a great many others that are as yet undiscovered. Thirty years ago, a prenatal supplement didn't contain zinc and the other trace minerals we now know to be necessary to good health. But whole-wheat bread has always contained it. Likewise, food supplies fiber and water (fruits and vegetables are loaded with both) and important calories and protein—none of which come packaged in a pill. (Incidentally, beware of those pills claiming to be equivalent to daily vegetable requirements—those claims are totally fraudulent.)

And don't think that because a little is good, a lot is better. Vitamins and minerals at high doses act as drugs in the body and should be treated as drugs, especially by expectant moms; a few, such as vitamins A and D, are toxic at levels not much beyond the RDA (recommended daily allowance).[4] Any supplementation beyond the RDA should be taken only under medical supervision, when benefits outweigh risks.

THE BEST-ODDS DIET FOOD SELECTION GROUPS

Many foods fill more than one nutritional requirement, so Food Selection Groups may overlap. The same three glasses of milk, for example, will give you three Calcium and one Protein serving.

PROTEIN FOODS

Every day have four of the following, or a combination equivalent to four servings. Servings contain between 18 and 25 grams of protein, and you should consume 75 to 100 grams a day.

3 8-ounce glasses of skim or low-fat milk or low-fat buttermilk

---

4. Getting more than the RDA of such vitamins from your daily diet, however, is not considered dangerous.

¾ cup low-fat cottage cheese
1¾ cups low-fat yogurt
1¾ ounces (½ cup) Parmesan cheese
2½ ounces Edam cheese
3 ounces Swiss or Cheddar cheese or low-fat cheese
5 large egg whites
2 large whole eggs, plus 2 egg whites
3½ ounces tuna
2½ ounces white meat chicken or turkey, without skin
3½ ounces fish or shrimp
5 ounces clams, crab, or lobster meat
3 ounces lean beef, lamb, or pork, or dark meat chicken
3 ounces veal
4 ounces fatty beef or lamb
3 ounces liver (use infrequently)
5 or 6 ounces tofu (bean curd)
Texturized vegetable protein[5]
1 serving of a complete protein combination (see box, page 97)

HIGH-PROTEIN SNACKS

Nuts and seeds
Whole-grain baked goods
Soy baked goods
Yogurt
Hard cheese
Hard-cooked eggs
Wheat germ

VITAMIN C FOODS

Have at least two Vitamin C foods, or a combination equal to two, every day. Your body can't store this vitamin, so don't skip a day.

½ grapefruit

½ cup grapefruit juice
2 small oranges
½ cup orange juice
2 tablespoons orange juice concentrate
½ medium mango
½ cup cubed papaya
¼ small cantaloupe
½ cup strawberries
1⅓ cup blackberries or raspberries
1½ large tomatoes
1 cup tomato juice
¾ cups vegetable juice (V-8)
1½ cups shredded raw cabbage or coleslaw
½ small red or green pepper
⅔ cup cooked broccoli
¾ cup cooked cauliflower
¾ cup cooked fresh kale
1 cup collard greens, frozen chopped
¾ cup cooked kohlrabi
3 cups raw spinach

CALCIUM-RICH FOODS

Take four servings of these foods daily, or any combination that is equivalent to four servings. You need 1,280 to 1,300 milligrams of calcium daily. Each serving contains about 300 milligrams of calcium.

8 ounces skim or low-fat milk or low-fat buttermilk
½ cup evaporated skim or low-fat milk
1¾ cups low-fat cottage cheese
1½ ounces Cheddar or American cheese
1¼ ounces Swiss cheese
1 cup low-fat or nonfat yogurt
⅓ cup nonfat dry milk
6 ounces calcium-added milk[6]

---

5. Recipes vary; some have a high protein/calorie ratio, others low, so read nutrition labels, remembering that 20 to 25 grams of protein equals 1 Protein serving.

6. Calcium-added milk may also be available in lactose-reduced form, which is often tolerated by those who can't otherwise tolerate dairy products.

6 ounces calcium-added orange juice
4 ounces canned salmon with bones
3 ounces canned sardines with bones
3½ ounces canned Pacific mackerel
   with bones
2 to 3 tablespoons ground sesame
   seeds
Soy milk and soy protein[7]
1 cup collard greens
1½ cups cooked kale
1½ cups cooked mustard or turnip
   greens
1¾ cups broccoli
2½ tablespoons blackstrap molasses
2 corn tortillas
10 dried figs
3 cups cooked dried beans (Great
   Northern, navy, pinto)

CALCIUM-RICH SNACKS

Almonds, filberts, peanuts
Dried fruit
Baked goods made with sesame seeds,
   soy flour, or carob

GREEN LEAFY AND YELLOW VEGETABLES AND YELLOW FRUITS

You need three or more servings a day, one of which should be raw. Try to choose some yellow and some green daily.

⅛ cantaloupe (about 5 inches long)
2 large fresh or dried apricots
½ medium mango
1 large nectarine or yellow peach

---

1 cup cubed papaya
½ medium persimmon
1 tablespoon canned unsweetened
   pumpkin
⅓ cup cooked beet greens
¾ cup cooked broccoli or turnip
   greens
½ raw carrot, or ⅓ cup cooked
½ cup cooked collard greens
1½ cups endive or escarole
⅓ cup cooked kale or mustard greens
8 to 10 large leaves dark green leafy
   lettuce
½ cup raw spinach, or ¼ cup cooked
¼ cup cooked winter squash
¼ small sweet potato or yam
⅓ cup cooked Swiss chard

OTHER FRUITS AND VEGETABLES

Have at least two of the following daily.

1 apple or ½ cup unsweetened applesauce
6 to 7 asparagus spears
1 small banana
1 cup bean sprouts
¾ cup green beans
⅔ cup blueberries or lingonberries
⅔ cup Brussels sprouts
⅔ cup pitted fresh cherries
⅔ cup grapes
1 cup fresh mushrooms
1 medium white peach
9 pods okra
½ cup parsley
1 medium pear
1 medium slice fresh or unsweetened
   canned pineapple
1 medium potato
⅔ cup zucchini

WHOLE GRAINS AND LEGUMES

Have four or five, or more, of the following every day:

1 slice whole-wheat, whole-rye, other whole-grain or soy bread
½ cup cooked brown rice
½ cup cooked wild rice
½ cup cooked whole-grain cereal (oatmeal, Wheatena, Ralston)
1 ounce whole-grain ready-to-eat cereal with no added sugar (shredded wheat, Nutri-Grain, health food brands)
2 tablespoons wheat germ
½ cup cooked millet, bulgur, triticale, or kasha (buckwheat groats)
½ cup cooked whole-grain, soy, or high-protein-type pasta
2 × 2 × 1-inch cornbread (made with nondegerminated meal)
½ cup cooked beans or peas
1 corn or whole-wheat tortilla

IRON-RICH FOODS

S mall amounts of iron are found in most of the fruits, vegetables, grains, and meats you eat every day. But try to have some of the following higher-iron-content foods daily, along with your supplement.

Duck
Beef
Liver and other organ meats (choose infrequently)
Oysters (cooked; don't eat raw)
Sardines
Collards, kale, and turnip greens
Jerusalem artichokes
Pumpkin
Potatoes in their skin
Spinach
Spirulina (seaweed)
Legumes (green peas, chick-peas, lentils, kidney and lima beans, for example)
Soybeans and soy products
Carob flour and carob powder
Blackstrap molasses
Dried fruits

HIGH-FAT FOODS

H ave four full or eight half servings, or a combination, daily, if you weigh about 125 pounds (see Appendix if you weigh more or less). Do not exceed this quantity unless you are gaining weight too slowly (see page 147); do not reduce this quantity unless you are gaining weight too quickly. On most days, no more than two servings should come from pure fats, such as butter, margarine, or oil.

Half Servings

1 ounce cheese (Swiss, Cheddar, provolone, mozzarella, blue, Camembert)
1 ½ ounces skim-milk mozzarella
2 tablespoons grated Parmesan cheese
1 ½ tablespoons light cream
1 tablespoon heavy, or whipping, cream
2 tablespoons whipped cream
2 rounded tablespoons sour cream
1 tablespoon cream cheese
1 cup whole milk
1 ½ cups 2% milk
⅔ cup whole evaporated milk
½ cup regular ice cream
1 cup whole-milk yogurt
1 tablespoon "light" margarine
1 tablespoon peanut butter
½ cup white sauce
⅓ cup hollandaise sauce
1 egg or 1 egg yolk
¼ small avocado
2 servings Best-Odds cake, cookies, or muffins
6 ounces tofu
7 ounces light-meat turkey or chicken, no skin
3 ½ ounces dark-meat turkey or chicken, no skin
4 ounces fresh or canned salmon
3 ounces canned tuna in oil

Full Servings[8]

1 tablespoon vegetable oil
1 tablespoon regular margarine or butter

1 tablespoon regular mayonnaise
2 tablespoons regular salad dressing[9]
3 to 6 ounces lean meat (varies with cut)
¾ cup tuna salad

BEST-ODDS RECIPES

H ere are some recipes to pacify your sweet or snacking tooth and to give you a few cocktail or breakfast ideas. For more, see *What to Eat When You're Expecting.*

CREAM OF TOMATO SOUP

Makes 3 servings

> **1 tablespoon margarine or butter**
> **2 tablespoons whole-wheat flour**
> **1 ¾ cups evaporated skim milk**
> **3 cups tomato or vegetable juice**
> **¼ cup tomato paste**
> **Salt and pepper to taste**
> **Fresh or dried oregano and basil to taste (optional)**

Optional Garnishes
> **6 tablespoons cottage cheese (½ Protein serving)** *or*
> **2 tablespoons grated Parmesan cheese (¼ Protein serving; ½ Calcium serv-**

ing) *or* **1 tablespoon wheat germ (½ Whole Grains serving)**

1. In a saucepan, melt the margarine over low heat. Add the flour, and blend over very low heat for 2 minutes. Gradually blend in the milk and continue cooking over low heat, stirring occasionally, until thickened.

2. Stir in the juice, tomato paste, and seasonings until smooth. Continue cooking over low heat, stirring frequently, for 5 minutes.

3. Serve soup warm, topped with cottage cheese, Parmesan cheese, or wheat germ if desired.

1 serving = 1 + Calcium serving; 1 Vitamin C serving; 1 Green Leafy serving if vegetable juice is used.

BEST-ODDS FRIES

Makes 2 servings

> **1 ½ teaspoons vegetable oil**
> **2 large baking potatoes**
> **2 egg whites**
> **Kosher (coarse) salt and pepper to taste**

1. Preheat the oven to 425° F. Grease a nonstick baking sheet with the vegetable oil.

---

8. There are a great many other sources of fat in the diet, most of which add up very quickly and most of which do not fit into the Best-Odds mold. For example, you can get 1 Fat serving and very little nutrition from: 1 typical croissant, doughnut, brownie, or Danish pastry; 1 slice of apple or ½ slice of pecan pie; ½ of a fast-food burger or a small fried chicken drumstick; ¼ cup premium ice cream (16% butterfat); 4 small biscuits. Be wary.

9. Since the fat content of salad dressings varies, read the labels; each 14 grams of fat is 1 Fat serving. In homemade dressings, each tablespoon of oil is equal to 1 Fat serving.

2. Scrub the potatoes thoroughly under running water; pat dry. Slice them lengthwise into ¼-inch-thick slices, then cut into fries of the desired size. Pat the fries dry.

3. In a medium-size bowl, beat the egg whites with a whisk until foamy. Add the potatoes and toss until coated with the egg whites.

4. Arrange the fries in a single layer on the prepared baking sheet. Leave some space between them so they don't stick together. Bake until crisp and lightly brown and tender, 30 to 35 minutes. Sprinkle with salt and pepper, and serve immediately.

1 serving = 1 Other Vegetable serving

POWER-PACKED OATMEAL

Makes 1 serving

> 1 ¼ cups water
> ½ cup rolled oats
> 2 tablespoons wheat germ (if constipation is a problem, substitute unprocessed bran for all or part of wheat germ)
> Salt to taste (optional)
> ⅓ cup instant nonfat dry milk

1. Bring the water to a boil in a small saucepan. Add the oats, wheat germ, and salt, if desired, stirring to mix thoroughly. Lower the heat and cook 5 minutes or longer, according to desired texture, adding more water if necessary.

2. Remove the pan from the heat and stir in the dry milk. Serve immediately.

SWEET VARIATION: Add 2 tablespoons raisins and 1 tablespoon apple juice concentrate (or to taste) when you add the oats, or during the last minute of cooking if you like firmer raisins; add ground cinnamon and/or salt to taste

(both optional) when you add the milk.

SAVORY VARIATION: Add pepper, grated Parmesan or Cheddar cheese (½ ounce = ½ Calcium serving) when you add the milk.

1 serving = 1 Protein serving; 1 Whole Grains serving; 1 Calcium serving; high fiber.

BRAN MUFFINS

Makes 12 to 16 muffins

> Vegetable cooking spray
> ⅔ cup raisins
> 1 cup apple juice concentrate
> ¼ cup orange juice concentrate
> 1 ½ cups whole-wheat flour
> ½ cup wheat germ
> 1 ½ cups unprocessed bran
> 1 ¼ teaspoons baking soda
> ½ cup chopped nuts
> 1 teaspoon ground cinnamon (optional)
> 1 ½ cups low-fat buttermilk
> 2 egg whites, slightly beaten
> ⅓ cup instant nonfat dry milk
> 2 tablespoons margarine or butter, melted and cooled

1. Preheat the oven to 350°F. Lightly grease nonstick muffin tins with vegetable cooking spray.

2. In a small saucepan, combine the raisins, ¼ cup of the apple juice concentrate, and the orange juice concentrate. Simmer, stirring occasionally, for 5 minutes.

3. Blend in a mixing bowl the flour, wheat germ, bran, baking soda, chopped nuts, and cinnamon.

4. In a separate bowl, beat together the buttermilk, egg whites, dry milk, margarine, and remaining apple juice concentrate.

5. Combine the dry and liquid ingredients, blending thoroughly in a few strokes. Fold in the raisins with their cooking juice. Fill the prepared muffin tins, or paper muffin cups placed in regular tins, two-thirds full.

6. Bake until a toothpick inserted in the center of a muffin comes out clean, about 20 minutes.

VARIATION: Add 2 medium apples or pears, diced, along with the nuts. If constipation is no problem, substitute 1 cup oats, oat bran, or barley flakes for the unprocessed bran.

1 large muffin (12 in a recipe) = 1½ Whole Grains servings; ½ Protein serving; very high fiber. Fruit Variation adds 1 Other Fruit serving.

WHOLE-WHEAT BUTTERMILK PANCAKES

Makes approximately 12 pancakes (3 servings)

Note: Allow 1 hour preparation time for batter to settle.

> 1 cup low-fat buttermilk
> 1 teaspoon apple juice concentrate
> ¾ cup whole-wheat flour
> 5 tablespoons wheat germ
> ⅓ cup nonfat dry milk
> Dash of salt, or to taste (optional)
> Ground cinnamon to taste (optional)
> 2 teaspoons baking powder
> 2 large egg whites
> Margarine or butter

Optional Garnishes
> Unsweetened applesauce (1 Other Fruit serving)
> Unsweetened (fruit only) preserves or apple butter
> ½ cup low-fat yogurt (½ Calcium serving)

1. Purée in a blender all the ingredients except the egg whites, margarine, and the garnishes.

2. In a mixing bowl, beat the egg whites until stiff. Quickly beat the buttermilk-flour mixture into the egg whites. Let the batter stand for 1 hour.

3. Heat a nonstick skillet, and when it is hot, lightly brush it with margarine or butter. Stir the batter, and spoon it onto the skillet to make 3-inch pancakes. When the surface of the pancakes begins to bubble and the undersides are lightly browned, turn and brown the other side. Continue making pancakes, brushing on additional margarine between batches, until the batter is used up. Serve the pancakes with any or all of the garnishes.

VARIATIONS: Add to the batter any of the following: ¼ cup raisins (½ Other Fruit serving); 6 whole dried apricots, diced (some Iron; 1 Yellow Fruit serving); ½ banana, pear, or apple, sliced (½ Other Fruit serving); ¼ cup chopped nuts (¼ Fat serving; some Protein).

⅓ recipe = 1 Whole Grains serving; 1 Protein serving; ½ Calcium serving; high fiber.

DOUBLE-THE-MILK SHAKE

Makes 1 serving

Note: Freeze an overripe banana, peeled and wrapped, 12 to 24 hours before making this shake.

> 1 cup skim or low-fat milk
> ⅓ cup nonfat dry milk
> 1 frozen overripe banana, cut into chunks
> 1 teaspoon vanilla extract
> Dash of ground cinnamon, or to taste (optional)

Purée all the ingredients in a blender. Serve immediately.

BERRY VARIATION: Add ½ cup berries, fresh or unsweetened frozen, and 1 tablespoon frozen apple juice concentrate (thawed) before blending; omit the cinnamon, if desired.

"CREAMSICLE" VARIATION: Add 2 tablespoons frozen orange juice concentrate (thawed); omit the cinnamon.

1 shake = 2 Calcium servings; ⅔ Protein serving; 1 Other Fruit serving. Berry Variation adds 1 Other Fruit serving, 1 Vitamin C serving if strawberries are used. "Creamsicle" Variation adds ½ Vitamin C serving.

FIG BARS

Makes about 36 cookie bars

> **Vegetable oil or vegetable cooking spray**
> **1 tablespoon fructose**
> **4 tablespoons (½ stick) margarine or butter**
> **1 cup plus 2 tablespoons apple juice concentrate, heated until warm**
> **1½ cups whole-wheat flour**
> **1 cup wheat germ**
> **1½ teaspoons vanilla extract**
> **1 pound dried figs, chopped**
> **2 tablespoons ground almonds or other nuts**

1. Preheat the oven to 350°F. Lightly grease a nonstick baking sheet with oil or vegetable cooking spray.

2. Cream the fructose and margarine together in a bowl. Add ½ cup plus 2 tablespoons of the apple juice concentrate, and continue to cream.

3. Add the flour, wheat germ, and vanilla, and mix to form a dough. Divide the dough in half, forming each half into a rectangular bar. Wrap them, separately, in waxed paper and chill for 1 hour.

4. Combine the figs and remaining apple juice concentrate in a saucepan, and cook over low heat until soft. Remove from the heat, and stir in the ground nuts until smooth.

5. Roll out one rectangular bar of dough on the prepared baking sheet until it is very thin, evening out the edges as much as possible. Spread the fig mixture evenly over the dough. Roll out the second rectangle of dough between two sheets of waxed paper to the same size as the first rectangle. Remove one sheet of waxed paper, and flip the dough as evenly as possible over the fig mixture. Press down lightly, and trim the ends as needed with a sharp knife.

6. Bake until lightly browned, 15 to 30 minutes. Cut into squares or diamond shapes while still hot.

3 cookies = 1 Whole Grains serving; 1 Other Fruit serving; some Iron; high fiber.

FRUITY OATMEAL COOKIES

Makes 24 2-inch cookies

> **Vegetable oil or vegetable cooking spray**
> **10 dates, pitted**
> **6 tablespoons apple juice concentrate**
> **2 tablespoons vegetable oil**
> **1½ cups rolled oats (or a mixture of oats and raw wheat flakes)**
> **1 cup raisins**
> **¼ to ½ cup chopped nuts**
> **Ground cinnamon to taste**
> **1 egg white**

1. Preheat the oven to 350°F. Lightly grease a nonstick baking sheet with the oil or vegetable cooking spray.

2. Combine the dates and the apple juice concentrate in a saucepan, and simmer until the fruit has softened. Purée the mixture in a blender or food

VEGETARIAN COMPLETE PROTEIN COMBINATIONS

The following selections are nutritious foods for all pregnant women; however, non-vegetarians should count only one serving a day as part of their protein allowance. Additional servings can count toward the Whole Grains and Legumes requirement. Strict vegetarians should have five of these protein servings daily.

Choose one serving (10 to 13 grams protein) from the legumes list plus one serving (10 to 13 grams protein) from the grains list for a complete protein combination.

LEGUMES

1 cup broad beans or black-eyed peas
¾ cup mung, black, Great Northern, lima, navy, pinto, or kidney beans
¾ cup soybeans or soy grits
1 cup chick-peas
⅔ cup lentils or split peas

GRAINS

1½ cups brown rice, groats, barley, millet, bulgur*
1⅓ cups wild rice
2 ounces (before cooking) soy pasta

2 to 4 ounces (before cooking; weight depending on protein content) whole-wheat pasta
2 ounces (before cooking) Superoni or soy pasta
⅔ cup (before cooking) oats
¾ cup seeds: sesame, sunflower, pumpkin
½ cup Brazil nuts or peanuts
2 ounces cashews, walnuts, or pistachios
⅓ cup wheat germ
2½ to 3 tablespoons peanut butter

DAIRY COMPLETE PROTEIN COMBINATIONS

Choose one serving (about 10 grams protein) from the legumes and grains list and one serving (about 12 grams protein) from the dairy foods list for a complete protein.

LEGUMES AND GRAINS

1 portion beans, peas, lentils, grains, pasta, noodles (see above)
4 slices whole-grain bread
⅔ cup cooked oatmeal
1½ ounces whole-grain ready-to-eat cereal

DAIRY FOODS

1¼ cups skim milk
1½ ounces Cheddar, American, Swiss, low-fat cheese
½ cup cottage cheese
¼ cup Parmesan cheese
⅓ cup nonfat dry milk plus 2 tablespoons wheat germ
1¼ cups yogurt
1 egg plus 2 egg whites

---

*These grains are low in protein; enrich with 2 tablespoons of wheat germ per serving.

processor, then pour it into a bowl. Add the 2 tablespoons oil and the oats, raisins, nuts, and cinnamon.

3. In a separate bowl, beat the egg white lightly. Fold it gently into the cookie mixture. Drop the batter in tablespoonsful onto the prepared sheet.

4. Bake until lightly browned, 10 to 12 minutes.

3 cookies = 1 Other Fruit serving; ½ Whole Grains serving; some Iron; high fiber.

FRUITED YOGURT

Makes about 1 cup

> ¾ cup plain low-fat yogurt
> ½ teaspoon freshly grated orange zest
> ½ cup fresh or frozen (thawed) unsweetened strawberries
> 1 tablespoon orange juice concentrate
> 5 teaspoons apple juice concentrate
> ½ teaspoon ground cinnamon, or to taste (optional)

Purée all the ingredients in a blender or food processor. Serve plain, or as a sauce for fruit, cake, or pancakes.

1 cup = 1 Vitamin C serving; ¾ Calcium serving.

MOCK STRAWBERRY DAIQUIRI

Makes 4 servings

> 2 cups washed, hulled fresh or frozen (unsweetened) strawberries (or substitute 2 very ripe bananas, cut into small pieces)

> 1 cup ice cubes, cracked (½ cup if using frozen berries)
> ¼ cup apple juice concentrate, or to taste
> 1 tablespoon fresh lime juice
> 1 teaspoon pure rum extract

Purée all the ingredients in a blender. Serve cold in tall glasses.

1 serving = 1 Other Fruit serving; 1 Vitamin C serving. Or 2 Other Fruit servings if bananas used.

VIRGIN SANGRIA

Makes 5 to 6 servings

> 3 cups unsweetened grape juice
> ¾ cup apple juice concentrate
> 1 tablespoon fresh lime juice
> 1 tablespoon fresh lemon juice
> 1 small unpeeled lemon, sliced and seeded
> 1 small unpeeled orange, sliced and seeded
> 1 small unpeeled McIntosh apple, cored, cut into eighths
> ¾ cup seltzer (unsalted club soda)

Combine all the ingredients except the seltzer in a large pitcher. Stir well, and chill. Add seltzer just before serving. Serve over ice in wineglasses.

1 serving = 1 Other Fruit serving.

Part 2

NINE MONTHS AND COUNTING:

From Conception to Delivery

5
The First Month

The first is the most comprehensive of all the prenatal visits.[1] A complete medical history will be taken, and certain tests and procedures will be performed only at this exam. One practitioner's routine may vary slightly from another's. In general, the examination will include:

Confirmation of Your Pregnancy. Your practitioner will want to check the following: the pregnancy symptoms you are experiencing; the date of your last normal menstrual period, to determine your estimated date of delivery (EDD), or due date (see page 6); your cervix and uterus, for signs and approximate age of the pregnancy. If there's any question, a pregnancy test may be ordered if you haven't already had one.

A Complete History. To give you the

1. See the Appendix for an explanation of the procedures and tests performed.

best care possible, your practitioner will want to know a great deal about you. Come prepared by checking home records and refreshing your memory, as necessary, on the following: your personal medical history (chronic illness, previous major illness or surgery, medications you are presently taking or have taken since conception, known allergies, including drug allergies); your family medical history (genetic disorders and chronic diseases); your social history (age, occupation, and habits, such as smoking, drinking, exercise, diet); your gynecological and obstetrical history (age at first menstrual period, usual length of menstrual cycle, duration and regularity of menstrual periods; past abortions, miscarriages, and live births; course of past pregnancies, labors, and deliveries); and factors in your personal life that might affect your pregnancy.

A Complete Physical Examination. This may include: assessment of your

WHAT YOU MAY LOOK LIKE

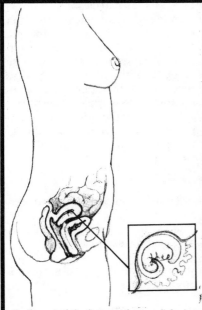

By the end of the first month, your baby is a tiny, tadpole-like embryo, smaller than a grain of rice. In the next two weeks, the neural tube (which becomes the brain and spinal cord), heart, digestive tract, sensory organs, and arm and leg buds will begin to form.

general health through examination of heart, lungs, breasts, abdomen; measurement of your blood pressure to serve as a baseline reading for comparison at subsequent visits; notation of your height and weight, usual and present; inspection of extremities for varicose veins and edema (swelling from excess fluid in tissues), to serve as a baseline for comparison at subsequent visits; inspection and palpation of external genitalia; internal examination of your vagina and cervix (with a speculum in place); examination of your pelvic organs bimanually (with one hand in the vagina and one on the abdomen) and also through the rectum and vagina; assessment of the size and shape of your bony pelvis.

A Battery of Tests. Some tests are routine for every pregnant woman; some are routine in some areas of the country or with some practitioners, and not others; some are performed only when circumstances warrant. The most common prenatal tests include:

❖ A blood test to determine blood type and check for anemia.

❖ Urinalysis to screen for sugar, protein, white blood cells, blood, and bacteria.

❖ Blood screens to determine immunity to such diseases as rubella.

❖ Tests to disclose the presence of such infections as syphilis, gonorrhea, hepatitis, chlamydia, and in some cases, AIDS.

❖ Genetic tests for sickle-cell anemia or Tay-Sachs disease.

❖ A Pap smear for the detection of cervical cancer.

❖ A gestational diabetic screening test to check for any tendency toward diabetes, particularly for women who have previously had an excessively large baby or gained excessive weight with an earlier pregnancy.

An Opportunity for Discussion. Come prepared with a list of questions, problems, and symptoms you would like to talk about. This is also a good time to bring up any special concerns that weren't addressed at an earlier consultation.

WHAT YOU MAY BE FEELING

You may experience all of these symptoms at one time or another, or only one or two.

PHYSICALLY:

❖ Absence of menstruation (though you may stain slightly when your period would have been expected or when the fertilized egg implants in the uterus)

❖ Fatigue and sleepiness

❖ Frequent urination

❖ Nausea, with or without vomiting, and/or excessive salivation (ptyalism)

❖ Heartburn, indigestion, flatulence, bloating

❖ Food aversions and cravings

❖ Breast changes (most pronounced in women who have breast changes prior to menstruation): fullness, heaviness, tenderness, tingling; darkening of the areola (the pigmented area surrounding the nipple). Sweat glands in the areola become prominent (Montgomery's tubercles), looking like large goose bumps; a network of bluish lines appear under the skin as blood supply to the breasts increases (though these lines may not appear until later)

EMOTIONALLY:

❖ Instability comparable to premenstrual syndrome, which may include irritability, mood swings, irrationality, weepiness

❖ Misgivings, fear, joy, elation—any or all of these

WHAT YOU MAY BE CONCERNED ABOUT

FATIGUE

"I'm tired all the time. I'm worried that I won't be able to continue working."

It would be surprising if you weren't tired. In some ways, your pregnant body is working harder even when you're resting than a nonpregnant body is when mountain-climbing; you just can't see its efforts. For one thing, it's manufacturing your baby's life-support system, the placenta, which won't be completed until the end of the first trimester. For another, it's adjusting to the many other physical and emotional demands of pregnancy, which are considerable. Once your body has adjusted and the placenta is complete (around the fourth month), you should have more energy. Until then, you may need to work fewer hours or take a few days off if you're really dragging. But if your pregnancy continues normally, there is absolutely no reason why you shouldn't stay at your job (assuming your doctor hasn't restricted your activity and/or the work isn't overly strenuous or hazardous; see page 72). Most pregnant women are happier and less anxious if they keep busy.

Since your fatigue is legitimate, don't fight it. Consider it a signal from your body that you need more rest. That, of course, is more easily suggested than done. But it is worth a try.

Baby Yourself. If you're a first-time expectant mother, enjoy what will probably be your last chance for a long while to focus on taking care of yourself without feeling guilty. If you already have one or more children at home, you will have to divide your focus. But either way, this is not a time to strive for Super-Mom-to-Be status. Getting adequate rest is more important than keeping your house white-glove-test clean or serving dinners worthy of four-star ratings. Keep evenings free of unessential activities. Spend them off your feet when you can, reading, watching TV, scouring baby-name books. If you have older children, read to them, play quiet games with them, or watch classic kiddie videos with them rather than traipsing off to the playground. (Fatigue may be more pronounced when there are older children at home, simply because there are so many more physical demands and so much less time to rest. On the other hand, it may be less noticed, since a mother of young children is usually accustomed to exhaustion and/or too busy to mind.)

And don't wait until nightfall to take it easy—if you can afford the luxury of an afternoon nap, by all means indulge. If you can't sleep, lie down with a good book. A nap at the office isn't a reasonable goal, of course, unless you have a flexible schedule and access to a comfortable sofa, but putting your feet up at your desk or in the ladies' lounge during breaks and lunch hours may be. (If you choose lunch hour to rest, don't forget to eat too.) Napping when you're mothering may also be difficult, but if you can time your rest with the children's nap-time, you may be able to get away with it—assuming you can tolerate the unwashed dishes and the dust balls under the bed.

Let Others Baby You. Accept your mother-in-law's offer to vacuum and dust the house when she's visiting. Let your dad take the older kids to the zoo on Sunday. Enlist your husband for chores like laundry and marketing.

Get an Hour or Two More Sleep Each Night. Skip the 11 o'clock news and turn in earlier; ask your husband to fix breakfast so you can turn out later.

Be Sure That Your Diet Isn't Deficient. First-trimester fatigue is often aggravated by a deficiency in iron, protein, or just plain calories. Double-check to make certain you're filling all of your requirements (see the Best-Odds Diet, page 80). And no matter how tired you're feeling, don't be tempted to rev up your body with caffeine, candy bars, and cake. It won't be fooled for long, and after the temporary lift, your blood sugar will plummet, leaving you more fatigued than ever.

Check Your Environment. Inadequate lighting, poor air quality (sick building syndrome), or excessive noise in your home or workplace can contribute to fatigue. Be alert to these problems and try to get them corrected.

Take a Hike. Or a slow jog. Or a stroll to the grocery store. Or the time to do a pregnancy exercise routine. Paradoxically, fatigue can be heightened by too much rest and not enough activity. But don't overdo the exercise. Stop before that exercise high dissolves into a low, and be sure to follow the precautionary guidelines on page 195.

Though fatigue will probably ease up by month four, you can expect it to return in the last trimester—probably as nature's way of preparing you for those long sleepless nights once the baby has arrived.

When fatigue is severe, especially if it is accompanied by fainting, pallor, breathlessness, and/or palpitations, it's wise to report it to your practitioner (see Anemia, page 154).

DEPRESSION

"I know I should feel happy about my pregnancy, but I seem to be suffering from postpartum depression prematurely."

First of all, you may be mistaking depression for the very normal mood swings of pregnancy. These swings may be more pronounced in the first trimester and, in general, in women who ordinarily suffer from emotional instability premenstrually. Feelings of ambivalence about the pregnancy once it's confirmed, which are common even when a pregnancy is planned, may exaggerate the swings still more. Though there's no cure for mood swings, avoiding sugar, chocolate, and caffeine (all of which can push a low even lower), following the Best-Odds Diet, getting a good balance of rest and exercise, and whenever possible talking your feelings out can all help to keep them from swinging too far.

If your lows are consistent or frequent, you may be one of the 10% of pregnant women who battle mild to moderate depression during pregnancy. Some of the factors that can put a woman at risk for such depression are:

❖ A personal or family history of mood disorder.

❖ Socioeconomic stress.

❖ Lack of emotional support from the baby's father.

❖ Hospitalization or bed rest because of pregnancy complications.

❖ Anxiety about her own health, especially if she experiences pregnancy complications or illness during pregnancy.

❖ Anxiety about her baby's health.

The most common symptoms of depression, in addition to feeling down, empty, and flat, include sleep disturbances; changed eating habits (not eating at all or eating endlessly); prolonged or unusual fatigue; extended loss of interest in work, play, and other activities or pleasures; and exaggerated mood swings. If that sounds like what you're experiencing, try those tips for dealing with postpartum depression that seem applicable to your life now (see page 398).

If the symptoms continue for longer than two weeks, speak to your practitioner about your depression or ask for a referral to a therapist. Except in extreme cases, antidepressant medication, the safety of which in pregnancy is not certain, will be bypassed in favor of supportive therapy, which can often be just as effective. Getting help is important, because your depression can lead to your not taking optimum care of yourself and your baby.

MORNING SICKNESS

"I haven't had any morning sickness. Can I still be pregnant?"

Morning sickness, like a craving for pickles and ice cream, is one of those truisms about pregnancy that ain't necessarily so. Only one-third to one-half of expectant women ever experience the nausea and/or vomiting of morning sickness. If you're among those who never suffer from it, you can consider yourself not only pregnant, but lucky too.

"My morning sickness lasts all day. I'm afraid I'm not able to keep down enough food to nourish my baby."

Fortunately, morning sickness (a misnamed malady, because it can strike morning, noon, or night—or even all day long) rarely interferes with proper nutrition enough to harm the developing fetus. And for most women, it doesn't last past the third month—though an occasional expectant mother won't experience it until well into the second trimester and a few, particularly those expecting twins, may enjoy its dubious pleasures for a full nine months.

What causes morning sickness? No one knows for sure, but there's no shortage of theories. It is known that the command post for nausea and vomiting is located in the brain stem. A myriad of physical reasons why this area may be overstimulated during pregnancy have been suggested, including the high level of the pregnancy hormone hCG in the blood in the first trimester, the rapid stretching of the uterine muscles, the relative relaxation of the muscle tissue in the digestive tract (which makes digestion less efficient), and the excess acid in the stomach caused by not eating or by eating the wrong foods.

But these physical triggers alone can't explain morning sickness, since most are common to all pregnancies and yet not all pregnant women experience nausea and vomiting. Several illuminating facts seem to support the theory that emotional factors augment the physical. For one thing, morning sickness is unknown in some more primitive societies where lifestyles are simpler, more relaxed, and less demanding (although it did exist in ancient Western civilization). For another, many women suffering from hyperemesis, or excessive vomiting, recover without treatment as soon as they are placed in the relatively tranquil environment of a hospital, away from their families and the problems of day-to-day living. And studies also show that many women with morning sickness are highly hypnotizable, indicating that they are very susceptible to the power of suggestion—and our society surely suggests that morning sickness is an expected part of pregnancy. Also quite revealing is the fact that some women suffer debilitating nausea and vomiting with unwanted, unplanned pregnancies, yet experience no morning sickness at all in pregnancies they are happy about. Physical or mental fatigue also seems to increase the possibility of nausea striking. As does carrying multiple fetuses—probably because of a multiplication of both physical and emotional stresses.

The fact that morning sickness is more common and tends to be more severe in first pregnancies supports the concept that both physical and psychological factors are involved. Physically, the novice pregnant body is less prepared for the onslaught of hormones and other changes than one that has been through it all before. Emotionally, those pregnant for the first time are more likely to be subject to the anxieties and fears that can turn a stomach, whereas women in subsequent pregnancies may be distracted from their worries and from their nausea by the demands of caring for older children.

Unfortunately, medical experts are even less certain of the cure for morning sickness than they are of its cause. They do, however, agree that there are many ways of alleviating its symptoms and minimizing its effects. See which work best for you:

❖ Eat a diet high in protein and complex carbohydrates (see the Best-Odds Diet, page 80)—both of which fight nausea. So does good nutrition, so eat as well as you can under the circumstances.

❖ Take plenty of fluids—especially if you're losing them through vomiting. If they are easier to get down than solids when your stomach is upset, use them to get your nutrients. Concentrate on any of the following you can handle: Double-the-Milk Shakes (see page 95); fruit or vegetable juices; soups, broths, and bouillons. If you find fluids make you queasier, eat solids with a high water content, such as fresh fruits and vegetables—particularly lettuce, melons, and citrus fruits. Some women find that drinking and eating at the same sitting puts too much strain on their digestive tract; if this is true for you, try taking your fluids only between meals.

❖ Take a prenatal vitamin supplement (see page 88) to compensate for nutrients you may not be getting. But take it at a time of day when you are least likely to chuck it back up—possibly before you go to bed. Your doctor may recommend an additional 50-milligram ration of B$_6$, which seems to help relieve nausea in some women. *Do not take any medication for morning sickness unless it is prescribed by your physician.* Such a prescription will almost certainly be written only when morning sickness is severe enough to be debilitating (see hyperemesis, page 343) and threatens to compromise your nutritional status and your baby's.

❖ Avoid the sight, smell, and taste of foods that make you feel queasy. Don't be a martyr and prepare a sausage and onion hero for your husband if it sends you rushing to the bathroom. And don't force-feed yourself foods that don't appeal, or worse still, that make you downright sick. Instead, with a little nutritional direction from your conscience, let your stomach be your guide in selecting your menus. Choose only sweet foods if they're all you can abide (get your vitamin A and protein from peaches and pancakes at dinner instead of from broccoli and chicken). Or only savories if they're your ticket to a less tumultuous tummy (have a grilled cheese and tomato sandwich for breakfast instead of cereal and orange juice.)

❖ Eat often—and before you feel hungry. When your stomach is empty, its acids have nothing to digest but its own lining. This can trigger nausea. So can the low blood sugar caused by long stretches between meals. Six small meals are better than three large. Carry nutritious snacks (dried fruit, whole-grain crackers) with you for snacking.

❖ Eat before nausea strikes. Food will be easier to get down and may prevent an attack.

❖ Eat in bed—for the same reasons you should eat often: to avoid an empty stomach and keep your blood sugar at an even keel. Before you go to sleep at night, have a snack that is high in protein and complex carbohydrates: a glass of milk and a bran muffin, for example. Twenty minutes before you plan to get out of bed in the morning, have a high-carbohydrate snack: a few whole-wheat crackers or rice cakes, or a handful of raisins. Keep them next to the bed so you don't have to get up for them, and in case you wake up hungry in the middle of the night.[2]

❖ Get some extra sleep and relaxation. Both emotional and physical fatigue can exacerbate morning sickness.

❖ Greet the morning in slow motion—rushing tends to aggra-

---

2. If you start to associate a particular carbohydrate snack (crackers, for instance) with your nausea, switch to a different snack.

vate nausea. Don't jump out of bed and dash out the door. Stay in bed digesting your crackers for 20 minutes, then rise slowly to a leisurely breakfast. This may seem impossible if you have other children, but try to wake up before they do to give yourself a little quiet time, or let your husband handle their early morning needs.

❖ Brush your teeth (with a toothpaste that doesn't increase your queasiness) or rinse your mouth (ask your dentist to recommend a good rinse, check with your practitioner to make sure it's okay to use) after each bout of vomiting, as well as after each meal. Not only will this help keep your mouth fresh and reduce nausea, it will decrease the risk of damage to teeth or gums that can occur when bacteria start working on that regurgitated material in your mouth.

❖ Minimize stress. Morning sickness is more common among women who are under a great deal of stress, either at work or at home. See page 113 for tips on dealing with stress during pregnancy.

❖ Try Sea-Bands. The 1-inch bands, worn on both wrists, put pressure on the inner wrist and often relieve nausea. They cause no side effects and are available at marine shops and pharmacies.

In an estimated 7 of every 2,000 pregnancies, nausea and vomiting become so severe that medical treatment is needed. If this seems to be the case with you, see page 343.

EXCESSIVE SALIVA

"My mouth seems to fill up with saliva all the time—and swallowing it makes me queasy. Does this have to do with pregnancy, or is it something else?"

An excess of saliva, also called ptyalism, is another common symptom of pregnancy. It's unpleasant but harmless. Happily, it usually disappears after the first few months. It's more common in women who are also experiencing morning sickness, and it seems to compound the queasiness. There's no sure cure, but brushing your teeth frequently with a minty toothpaste, rinsing with a minty mouthwash, or chewing gum can help dry things up a bit.

FREQUENT URINATION

"I'm in the bathroom every half hour. Is it normal to be urinating this often?"

Most—though by no means all—pregnant women do make frequent detours to the toilet in both the first and last trimesters. One of the reasons for an initial increase in urinary frequency is the increased volume of body fluids and the improved efficiency of the kidneys, which helps rid the body more quickly of waste products. Another is the pressure of the growing uterus, which is still in the pelvis next to the bladder. This pressure on the bladder is often relieved once the uterus rises into the abdominal cavity, around the fourth month. It probably won't return until the baby "drops" back down into the pelvis in the ninth month. But because the arrangement of internal organs varies slightly from woman to woman, the degree of urinary frequency in pregnancy may also vary.

Leaning forward when you urinate will help ensure that you empty your bladder completely and may reduce trips to the bathroom. If you find you go frequently during the night, try limiting fluids after 4 P.M. Don't, however, limit fluids otherwise.

"How come I'm not urinating fre-quently?"

No noticeable increase in the fre-quency of urination may be per-fectly normal for you, especially if you ordinarily urinate often. You should, however, be certain you're getting enough fluids (at least eight glasses a day). Not only can insuffi-cient fluid intake be the cause of infre-quent urination, it could also lead to urinary tract infection.

BREAST CHANGES

"I hardly recognize my breasts anymore—they're so huge. And they're tender too. Will they stay that way, and will they sag after I give birth?"

Get used to the chesty look for now. Although it may not always be in fashion, it's one of the hallmarks of pregnancy. Your breasts are swollen and tender because of the increased amounts of estrogen and progesterone your body is producing. (The same mechanism operates premenstrually, when many women experience breast changes—but the changes are more pronounced in pregnancy.) These changes are not random; they are aimed at preparing you to feed your baby when it arrives. If, however, they are less marked in a second or subse-quent pregnancy (as they often are), it doesn't mean that you will be less capable of breastfeeding.

In addition to their enlarging, you will probably notice other changes in your breasts. The areola (the pig-mented area around the nipple) will darken, spread, and may be spotted with even darker areas. This darken-ing may fade but not disappear en-tirely after birth. The little bumps you may notice on the areola are seba-ceous (sweat) glands, which become more prominent during pregnancy

and return to normal afterward. The complex road map of blue veins that traverses the breasts—often quite vivid on a fair-skinned woman—represents a mother-to-baby delivery system for nutrients and fluids. After delivery or sometime after nursing is discontinued, the appearance of the skin will return to normal.

What you won't have to get used to, fortunately, is the sometimes agoniz-ing sensitivity of your breasts. Though they will continue to grow through-out your pregnancy—possibly in-creasing as much as three cup sizes—they are not likely to remain tender to the touch past the third or fourth month. As for whether or not they will sag after the baby is born, that is at least partly up to you. Stretching and sagging of the breast tissue result from a lack of support during pregnancy—not from pregnancy itself—though the tendency to sag may be genetic. No matter how firm your breasts are now, protect them for the future by wearing a good support bra. If your breasts are particularly large or have a tendency to sag, it's a good idea to wear a bra even at night.

If your breasts enlarge early in preg-nancy and then suddenly diminish in size (and especially if other pregnancy symptoms also disappear without ex-planation), contact your practitioner.

"My breasts became very large in my first pregnancy, but they haven't seemed to change at all now that I'm in my second. Could something be wrong?"

Small-chested women who look forward to having their cups run-ning over in pregnancy are sometimes in for a disappointment, at least tem-porarily, the second or third time around. Though some experience as much enlargement early on as they did in the first pregnancy, others do not—perhaps because the breasts, thanks to their previous experience, don't need as much preparation and respond to the pregnancy hormones less dramatically. In these women, the breasts may gradually enlarge during pregnancy, or may hold off their expansion until after delivery, when milk production begins.

VITAMIN SUPPLEMENTS

"Should I be taking vitamins?"

Virtually no one gets a nutritionally perfect diet every day, especially early in pregnancy, when morning sickness is a common appetite suppressant and when what little nutrition some women manage to get down often comes right back up. A daily vitamin supplement, while it does not take the place of a good prenatal diet, can serve as your dietary insurance, guaranteeing that should your body not cooperate or should you slip up occasionally, your baby won't be cheated. In addition, some studies have shown that women who take vitamin supplements prior to pregnancy and during the first month significantly reduce the risk of neural tube defects (such as spina bifida) in their babies. Good formulations designed especially for expectant mothers are available by prescription or over the counter. (See page 88 for what the supplement should contain.) Do not take any kind of dietary supplements other than such a prenatal formula without your doctor's recommendation.

Many women find that taking a vitamin supplement increases nausea in early pregnancy, and sometimes beyond. Switching formulas may help, as may taking your pill after meals (unless that's when you usually throw up). If swallowing a standard-size pill is difficult for you, consider switching to a child-size formula, a chewable supplement, or a capsule that can be opened and sprinkled on food or drink. But be sure the formula you select approximates the requirements for supplements designed for pregnancy (see page 88). If your supplement was prescribed by your practitioner, check with him or her before switching.

In some women, the iron in a prenatal vitamin can cause constipation or diarrhea. Again, switching formulas may bring relief. Taking a pregnancy supplement without iron and a separate iron preparation (your doctor can prescribe one that dissolves in the intestines rather than in the more sensitive stomach) may also reduce irritation and relieve symptoms. Ask your practitioner for advice.

ECTOPIC PREGNANCY

"I've been having occasional cramping. Could I have an ectopic pregnancy without knowing it?"

The fear of ectopic, or tubal, pregnancy lurks somewhere in the mind of nearly every newly pregnant woman who has heard of this abnormal type of implantation. Fortunately, for the vast majority it's an unfounded fear—a fear that can be dismissed completely by the eighth week of pregnancy, by which time most tubal pregnancies have been diagnosed and terminated.

Only about 1 in 100 pregnancies are ectopic, that is, implanted outside the uterus, usually in the fallopian tubes.[3] A good many of these are diagnosed before a woman even realizes she is

---

3. This usually occurs because some irregularity in the tube blocks the passage of the egg down to the uterus. Rarely, the fertilized egg implants in the ovary, the abdominal cavity, or the cervix.

pregnant. So chances are that if your doctor has confirmed your pregnancy through a blood test and a physical exam and you've had no signs of ectopic pregnancy, then you can cross this worry off your list.

There are several factors that can make women more susceptible to ectopic pregnancy. They include:

❖ A previous ectopic pregnancy.

❖ Previous pelvic inflammatory disease.

❖ Previous abdominal or tubal surgery with postoperative scarring.

❖ Unsuccessful tubal ligation (sterilization surgery), or tubal ligation reversal.

❖ An IUD in place when conception occurs (an IUD is more likely to prevent conception in the uterus than outside it—increasing the risk of ectopics in IUD users).[4]

❖ Possibly, multiple induced abortions (the evidence isn't clear).

❖ Possibly, exposure to diethylstilbestrol (DES) in the womb, especially if it resulted in significant structural abnormalities of the reproductive tract.

Rare as ectopic pregnancies are, every pregnant woman—particularly those at high risk—should be familiar with the symptoms. Occasional cramping, probably the result of ligaments stretching as the uterus grows, is not one of them. But any or all of the following might be, and do require immediate evaluation by a physician. If you can't reach your physician, go at once to the hospital emergency room.

❖ Colicky, crampy pain with tenderness, usually in the lower

abdomen—on one side initially, though the pain can radiate throughout the abdomen. Pain may worsen on straining of bowels, coughing, or moving. If tubal rupture occurs, pain becomes very sharp and steady for a short time before diffusing throughout the pelvic region.

❖ Brown vaginal spotting or light bleeding (intermittent or continuous), which may precede pain by several days or weeks, though sometimes there is no bleeding unless the tube ruptures.

❖ Heavy bleeding if the tube ruptures.

❖ Nausea and vomiting—in about 25% to 50% of women—though this may be difficult to distinguish from morning sickness.

❖ Dizziness or weakness, in some women. If the tube ruptures, weak pulse, clammy skin, and fainting are common.

❖ Shoulder pain, in some women.

❖ Feeling of rectal pressure, in some women.

If an ectopic pregnancy is present, quick medical attention can often save the fallopian tube and the woman's fertility (see page 343 for the treatment of ectopic pregnancies).

THE CONDITION OF YOUR BABY

"I'm very nervous because I can't really feel my baby. Could it die without my knowing it?"

At this stage, with no noticeable enlargement of the abdomen or obvious fetal activity, it's hard to imagine that there's really a living, growing baby inside you. But the

---

4. But having worn an IUD in the past does not appear to increase risk.

death of a fetus or embryo that isn't expelled from the uterus in a miscarriage is very rare. When it does happen, a woman loses all signs of pregnancy, including breast tenderness and enlargement, and may develop a brownish discharge, though no actual bleeding. Upon examination, the physician will find that the uterus has diminished in size.

If at any time all of your pregnancy symptoms seem to have disappeared, call your doctor. That's a more positive approach than sitting around worrying.

MISCARRIAGE

"Between what I read and what my mother tells me, I'm afraid everything I've done, am doing, and will do might cause a miscarriage."

For many expectant women, the fear of miscarriage keeps their joy guarded in the first trimester. Some even refrain from spreading their happy news until the fourth month, when they begin to feel secure that the pregnancy will indeed continue. And for most of them—probably 90%—it will.[5]

There is still much to be learned about the reasons behind early miscarriage, but several factors are believed *not* to cause the problem. They include:

❖ Previous trouble with an IUD. Scarring of the endometrium (the lining of the uterus) caused by IUD-triggered infection could prevent a pregnancy from implanting in the uterus, but should not cause miscarriage once implantation is well established. Nor should previous difficulty holding an IUD in place affect a pregnancy.

❖ History of multiple abortions.[6] Scarring of the endometrium from multiple abortions, as from IUD-caused infections, could prevent implantation but should not otherwise be responsible for early miscarriage.

❖ Emotional upset—resulting from an argument, stress at work, or family problems.

❖ A fall or other minor accidental injury to the mother. But serious injury could result in miscarriage, so safety precautions—such as wearing a seat belt and not climbing on rickety chairs or ladders—should always be observed.

❖ Usual and accustomed physical activity, such as housework; lifting children, groceries, or other moderately heavy objects (see page 204); hanging curtains; moving light furniture; and moderate and safe exercise (see page 189).[7]

❖ Sexual intercourse—unless a woman has a history of miscarriage or is otherwise at high risk for pregnancy loss.

There are several factors, however, that *are* believed to increase the risk of spontaneous abortion. Some are not likely to recur and should not

---

5. Roughly 10% of diagnosed pregnancies end in clinically apparent miscarriage. Another 20% to 40% of pregnancies end before a pregnancy diagnosis is made; these are the miscarriages that usually go unnoticed.

6. Though not a direct cause of early miscarriage, repeated abortions or other procedures requiring dilation of the cervix may result in a weakened or incompetent cervix—often a cause of late miscarriage. (See page 177.)

7. In a high-risk pregnancy, the physician may limit these activities or even prescribe strict bed rest. But you need limit activity only on direction of your doctor.

Possible Signs of Miscarriage

When to Call Your Doctor Immediately, Just in Case

❖ When you experience bleeding with cramps or pain in the center of your lower abdomen. (Pain on one side in early pregnancy could be triggered by an ectopic pregnancy, and also warrants a call to the doctor.)

❖ When pain is severe or continues unabated for more than one day, even if it isn't accompanied by staining or bleeding.

❖ When bleeding is as heavy as a menstrual period, or light staining continues for more than three days.

When to Get Emergency Medical Attention

❖ When you have a history of miscarriage, and experience either bleed-ing or cramping or both.

❖ When bleeding is heavy enough to soak several pads in an hour, or when pain is so severe you can't bear it.

❖ When you pass clots or grayish or pink material—which may mean a miscarriage has already begun. If you can't reach your doctor, go to the nearest emergency room or to the one recommended by his or her office. The doctor may want you to save the material you pass (in a jar, plastic bag, or other clean container) so he or she can try to determine whether or not the miscarriage is simply threatening, is complete, or is incomplete and requires a D and C (dilation and curettage) to complete it.

---

affect future pregnancies. For example, exposure to rubella or other teratogenic disease, to radiation, or to drugs harmful to the fetus; a high fever; or an IUD in place at conception. Other risk factors, once identified, can be controlled or eliminated in future pregnancies (poor nutrition; smoking; hormonal insufficiency; and certain maternal medical problems). A few miscarriage risk factors are not easily overcome, such as a malformed uterus (though it can sometimes be surgically corrected) and certain chronic maternal illnesses.

Rarely, repeated miscarriages are traced to the mother's immune system rejecting the father's cells in the developing embryo. Immunotherapy may be able to correct this problem and allow for a normal pregnancy.

When Not to Worry. It's important to recognize that each cramp, ache, or bit of spotting isn't necessarily a warning of an impending miscarriage. Just about every normal pregnancy will include at least one of these usually innocuous symptoms at one time or another:[8]

❖ Mild cramps, achiness, or a pulling sensation on one or both sides of the abdomen. This is probably caused by the stretching of ligaments that support the uterus. Unless cramping is severe, constant, or accompanied by bleeding, there's no need to worry.

❖ Staining a bit around the time you

---

8. You should routinely tell your practitioner about *any* pains, cramping, or bleeding. In most cases his or her response will put your worries to rest.

would have expected your period, about seven to ten days after conception, when the little ball of cells that is going to develop into your baby attaches itself to the uterine wall. Slight bleeding at this time is common and doesn't necessarily indicate a problem with your pregnancy—as long as it isn't accompanied by lower abdominal pain.

If You Suspect Miscarriage. If you experience any of the symptoms listed in the box on page 112, put a call in to your practitioner. If your symptoms are listed under "When to Get Emergency Medical Attention" and your practitioner is not available, leave a message for him or her, and either call 911 or your local EMS (emergency medical service) or go straight to the nearest emergency room.

While waiting for help, lie down if you can, or rest in a chair with your feet up. This may not prevent a miscarriage if it's about to happen, but it should help you to relax. It should also help you to relax to know that most women who have episodes of bleeding in early pregnancy carry to term and deliver healthy babies.

If miscarriage is suspected or diagnosed, see page 346.

"I don't really feel pregnant. Could I have miscarried without knowing it?"

Fear of miscarrying without realizing it, though common, is unwarranted. Once a pregnancy is established, the signs that it is aborting are not easily overlooked. Simply "not feeling pregnant" is not usually a reason for concern—many women with normal pregnancies don't feel pregnant, at least until they begin to notice fetal movement. Share your concerns with your practitioner at your next visit; he or she will doubtless be able to reassure you.

If, however, you've been experiencing pregnancy symptoms and they all suddenly vanish without explanation, do give your practitioner a call.[9] Occasionally, an embryo dies and is not spontaneously expelled.

STRESS IN YOUR LIFE

"My job is a high-stress one. I wasn't planning to have a baby now, but I got pregnant. Should I quit work?"

Stress has, over the past couple of decades, become an important area for study because of the effect it can have on our lives. Depending on how we handle and respond to it, stress can be good for us (by sparking us to perform better, to function more effectively) or it can be bad for us (when it gets out of control, overwhelming and debilitating us). If the stress at work has you working at top efficiency, has you excited and challenged, then it shouldn't be harmful to your pregnancy. But if the stress makes you anxious, sleepless, or depressed, or if it is causing you to experience physical symptoms (such as headache, backache, or loss of appetite), then it could be. It could also be detrimental if it is exhausting you (see page 102 for tips on handling fatigue).

Negative reactions to stress can be compounded by the normal mood swings in pregnancy. And since such reactions as appetite loss, bingeing on the wrong foods, and sleeplessness can take a toll on you—and, if allowed

---

9. Don't forget, however, that by the end of the first trimester, morning sickness is usually gone, urinary frequency has lessened, and breast tenderness is less pronounced—all of which is normal.

Relaxation Made Easy

There are many routes to relaxation, including yoga. Here are a couple of relaxation techniques that are easy to learn and to do anywhere, anytime. If you find them helpful, you can do them when anxiety strikes, or regularly several times a day to try to ward it off.

1. Sit with your eyes closed. Relax your muscles, starting with those in your feet and working up slowly through the legs, torso, neck, and face. Breathe only through the nose (unless it's too stuffy, of course). As you breathe out, repeat the word "one" (or "peace," or any other simple word) to yourself. Continue the repetitions for 10 to 20 minutes.

2. Inhale slowly and deeply through your nose, pushing your abdomen out as you do. Count to four. Then, letting your shoulders and neck muscles relax, exhale slowly and comfortably to the count of six. Repeat this sequence four or five times to banish tension.

to continue into the second and third trimesters, on your baby—learning to handle the stress constructively should become a priority now. The following should help:

Talk About It. Allowing your anxieties to surface is the best way of making sure they don't get you down. Maintain open lines of communication with your spouse, spending some time at the end of each day airing concerns and frustrations. (Of course he, too, is probably in need of a friendly ear, so be prepared to do your fair share of listening.) Together you may be able to find some relief, even some humor, in your respective situations. If you find instead that you get on each other's nerves, talk to another family member, your practitioner, a friend, or a member of the clergy. If nothing seems to help, consider professional counseling.

Do Something About It. Identify sources of stress in your job and in other areas of your life, and determine how they can be modified to reduce the stress. If you're clearly trying to do too much, cut back in some areas.

If you've taken on too many responsibilities at home or at work, set priorities and then decide which can be postponed or passed to someone else. Learn to say no to new projects or activities before you're overloaded.

Sometimes sitting down with a notepad and making lists of the hundreds of things you need to get done (at home or at work), and the order you're planning to do them in, can help you feel more in control of the chaos in your life. Cross them off your list as they're taken care of for a rewarding sense of accomplishment.

Sleep It Off. Sleep is the ticket to regeneration—for mind and body. Often feelings of tension and anxiety are prompted by our not getting enough shut-eye. If you're having trouble sleeping, see the tips on page 140.

Nourish It. Hectic lifestyles can lead to hectic eating styles. Inadequate nutrition during pregnancy can be a double whammy: it can hamper your ability to handle stress as well as affect your baby's growth and development. So be sure to get three squares a day plus adequate snacks, within the Best-

Odds framework (see page 80).

Wash It Away. A warm bath (but not a hot tub) is an excellent way to relieve tension. Try one after a hectic day; it will also help you to sleep better.

Get Away from It Temporarily. Combat stress with any activity you find relaxing—sports (check first with your practitioner, and observe the guidelines on page 195); reading; moviegoing; listening to music (consider taking a cassette player with headphones to work, so you can listen to relaxing music during coffee breaks and lunch, or even while you work if that's feasible); long walks (or short ones during breaks or lunch—but be sure to leave time for eating); meditation (just close your eyes and picture a bucolic scene, or keep them open and gaze at a soothing picture or photo placed strategically in your office). Practice relaxation techniques (see page 114), not just because they'll come in handy during childbirth, but because they can help drain the strain anytime.

Get Away from It Permanently. Maybe the problem isn't worth the stress and anxiety it's generating. If it's your job, consider taking early maternity leave, cutting back to part-time, or switching positions for the time being to reduce stress to a manageable level.

Remember, your stress quotient is only going to increase once the baby is born; it makes sense to try to learn how to handle it now.

OVERWHELMING FEAR ABOUT BABY'S HEALTH

"I know it's probably irrational, but I can't sleep or eat or concentrate at work because I'm afraid my baby won't be normal."

Every expectant mother worries about whether her baby will be normal. But while even a moderate dose of worry that doesn't respond to reassurance (such as is found in this book) is an unavoidable side effect of pregnancy, worry that is so all-consuming that it interferes with functioning needs professional attention. Talk to your practitioner. Perhaps an ultrasound evaluation of the fetus can be arranged to help calm your fears. Many physicians are willing to order such an exam when a patient is extremely anxious, particularly if she feels she has a specific reason to fear for her baby's health (perhaps she spent a lot of time in a hot tub or had a few too many a few too many times before she found out she was pregnant), and even if her concerns seem unfounded or exaggerated. This is because the possible risks of the procedure to mother and fetus (research has yet to reveal any) are outweighed by the risks of such overwhelming anxiety (especially if it is keeping the mother-to-be from eating and sleeping).

Though ultrasound can't detect every potential problem, it can, once significant fetal development has taken place, show a great deal. Even the outline, as blurry as it is, of a normal baby—with all its limbs and organs in place—can offer enormous comfort. That, teamed with verbal reassurance from her own practitioner, and perhaps from the specialist who has evaluated the ultrasound, can help an expectant mother get on with the vital business at hand: caring for herself and nourishing her baby. If it doesn't, professional counseling may be necessary.

Other kinds of prenatal diagnosis, such as amniocentesis and chorionic villus sampling, which can also offer some reassurance, are usually recommended only when there is a valid medical reason (see pages 44 and 48), since the procedures themselves carry some risk.

PICKING UP OTHER CHILDREN

"I'm afraid to pick up my two-year-old daughter, who is pretty heavy, because I've heard physical strain can cause miscarriage."

You'll have to come up with a better excuse to get her to walk on her own two feet. Unless your physician has instructed you otherwise, carrying moderately heavy loads (even a strapping preschooler) is okay, though you should avoid exerting yourself to the point of exhaustion (see page 174 for tips on avoiding back strain when lifting). And in fact, blaming your child's as yet unborn sibling for your reluctance to carry her can needlessly set up feelings of rivalry and resentment toward the baby even before the pint-size competition arrives on the scene.

As your pregnancy progresses, however, your back may not be amenable to the strain of toting both a fetus and a toddler, and in that case, you should keep lifting of the latter to a minimum. But be sure you blame your back, and not the baby, for this slowdown in pickups, and that you compensate for it with plenty of holding and hugging in the sitting position.

WHAT IT'S IMPORTANT TO KNOW: GETTING REGULAR MEDICAL CARE

In the past decade, the self-care health movement has instructed Americans in everything from taking their own blood pressure and pulse to home-treating muscle strains and self-evaluating a scratchy throat or an aching ear. The impact this has had on the effectiveness of our health care has been unquestionably positive—cutting down on the number of trips we have to make to our doctors and making us better patients when we do go. Best of all, it's made us aware of the responsibility we each have for our own health, and it has the potential of making us a lot healthier in the years to come.

Even in pregnancy, as you can see throughout this book, there are countless steps you can take to make your own nine months safer and more comfortable, your labor and delivery easier, and your expected end product healthier. But to try to go it alone, even for a few months, is to abuse the concept of self-care—which is built on the foundation of a cooperative partnership between patient and health professional. Regular professional input in pregnancy is crucial. One major study found that women who had many prenatal visits (an average of 12.7) had bigger babies with better survival rates than those who had only a few prenatal visits (an average of 1.4).

A SCHEDULE OF PRENATAL VISITS

Ideally, your first visit to a physician or nurse-midwife should take place while that baby is still in the planning stages. That's an ideal many of us, especially those whose pregnancies are unplanned, can't always manage.

When to Call the Practitioner

It's best to set up an emergency protocol with your practitioner before an emergency strikes. If you haven't, and you are experiencing a symptom that requires immediate medical attention, try the following: First call the practitioner's office. If he or she isn't available and doesn't call back within a few minutes, call again and leave a message saying what your problem is and where you are headed. Then go directly to the nearest emergency room or call the emergency medical squad.

When you report any of the following, be sure to mention any other symptoms you may be experiencing, no matter how remote they may seem from the immediate problem. Also be specific, mentioning how long the symptom has existed, how frequently it recurs, what seems to relieve or exacerbate it, and how severe it is.

❖ Severe lower abdominal pain, on one or both sides, that doesn't subside: notify your practitioner the same day. If it is accompanied by bleeding, or nausea and vomiting: call immediately.

❖ Severe upper mid-abdominal pain, with or without nausea and swelling of hands and face: call immediately.

❖ Slight vaginal spotting: notify your practitioner the same day.

❖ Heavy vaginal bleeding (especially when combined with abdominal or back pain): call immediately.

❖ Bleeding from nipples, rectum, bladder: call the same day.

❖ Coughing up of blood: call immediately.

❖ A gush or steady leaking of fluid from the vagina: call immediately.

❖ A sudden increase in thirst, accompanied by a paucity of urination, or no urination at all for an entire day: call immediately.

❖ Swelling or puffiness of hands, face, eyes: call the same day. If very sudden and severe, or accompanied by headache or vision difficulties: call immediately.

❖ Severe headache that persists for more than two or three hours: call the same day. If accompanied by vision disturbances or puffiness of eyes, face, hands: call immediately.

❖ Painful or burning urination: call the same day. If accompanied by chills and fever over 102 degrees and/or backache: call immediately.

❖ Vision disturbances (blurring, dimming, double vision) that persist for two hours: call immediately.

❖ Fainting or dizziness: notify the doctor the same day.

❖ Chills and fever over 100 degrees (in the absence of cold or flu symptoms): call the same day. Fever over 102 degrees: call immediately.

❖ Severe nausea and vomiting, vomiting more often than two or three times a day in the first trimester, vomiting later in pregnancy when you haven't earlier: notify the doctor the same day. If vomiting is accompanied by pain and/or fever: call immediately.

❖ Sudden weight gain of more than two pounds not related to overeating: call the same day. If accompanied by swelling of the hands and face and/or headache or visual disturbances: call immediately.

❖ Absence of noticeable fetal movement for more than 24 hours after the 20th week: call the same day. Fewer than ten movements per hour (see page 201) after 28 weeks: call immediately.

When in Doubt

Sometimes the body's signals that something is wrong aren't clear. You feel unusually exhausted, achy, not quite right. But there are none of the clear-cut symptoms listed on page 117. If a good night's sleep and some extra rest don't team up to make you feel better in a day or two, don't be embarrassed to check with your physician. It's likely that you only need more rest than you're getting. But it is also possible that you are anemic or harboring an infection of some kind. Certain infections—cystitis, for one— can do their dirty work without showing any obvious symptoms.

Second best, and still very good, is a visit as soon as you suspect you have conceived. An internal exam will help to confirm your pregnancy, and a physical will uncover potential problems that may need monitoring. After that, the schedule of visits will vary depending on the practitioner you are seeing and whether or not yours is a high-risk pregnancy. In an uneventful low-risk pregnancy you can probably expect to see your practitioner monthly, or occasionally even less often, until the end of the 32nd week. After that you may begin going every two weeks until the last month, when weekly visits are customary.

For what you can expect at each prenatal visit, see the monthly chapters.

TAKING CARE OF THE REST OF YOU

You're understandably preoccupied with prenatal matters during pregnancy. But though your health care should begin with your belly, it shouldn't end there. And don't just wait for problems to drop into your lap. Pay a visit to your dentist; most dental work, particularly the preventive kind, can be done safely during pregnancy (see page 179). See your allergist, if necessary. You probably won't begin a course of allergy shots now, but if your allergies are severe, he or she may want to monitor your condition. Your family doctor or a specialist should also be monitoring any chronic illnesses or other medical problems that don't fall under the purview of the obstetrician; if you're seeing a nurse-midwife for pregnancy, you should see an obstetrician or your family physician for *all* medical problems.

If new medical problems come up while you're pregnant, don't ignore them. Even if you've noticed symptoms that seem relatively innocuous, it's more important now than ever to consult with your physician promptly. Your baby needs a *wholly* healthy mother.

6
The Second Month

WHAT YOU CAN EXPECT AT THIS MONTH'S CHECKUP

If this is your first prenatal visit, see What You Can Expect at Your First Prenatal Visit (page 100). If this is your second exam, you can expect your practitioner to check the following, though there may be variations depending upon your particular needs and your practitioner's style of practice:[1]

❖ Weight and blood pressure

❖ Urine, for sugar and protein

❖ Hands and feet for edema (swelling), and legs for varicose veins

❖ Symptoms you have been experiencing, especially unusual ones

❖ Questions or problems you want to discuss—have a list ready

WHAT YOU MAY BE FEELING

You may experience all of these symptoms at one time or another, or only one or two. Some may have continued from last month, others may be new. Don't be surprised, no matter what your symptoms, if you don't feel pregnant yet.

PHYSICALLY:

❖ Fatigue and sleepiness

❖ A need to urinate frequently

❖ Nausea, with or without vomiting, and/or excessive salivation (ptyalism)

❖ Constipation

❖ Heartburn, indigestion, flatulence, bloating

❖ Food aversions and cravings

❖ Breast changes: fullness, heaviness, tenderness, tingling; darkening of areola (the pigmented area around the nipple); sweat glands in the areola become prominent (Montgomery's tubercles), like large goose

1. See Appendix for an explanation of the procedures and tests performed.

bumps; a network of bluish lines appear under the skin as blood supply to the breasts increases

❖ Occasional headaches (similar to headaches in women taking birth control pills)

❖ Occasional faintness or dizziness

❖ Tightness of clothing around waist and bust; abdomen may appear en-

larged, probably due to bowel distention rather than uterine growth

EMOTIONALLY:

❖ Instability comparable to premenstrual syndrome, which may include irritability, mood swings, irrationality, weepiness

❖ Misgivings, fear, joy, elation—any or all of these

WHAT YOU MAY BE CONCERNED ABOUT

VENOUS CHANGES

"I have unsightly blue lines under the skin, on my breasts and abdomen. Is that normal?"

Very normal. What you see is part of the network of veins that has expanded to carry the increased blood supply of pregnancy. Not only are the veins nothing to worry about, they are a sign that your body is doing what it should. They may show up earliest in very slim or light-complexioned women. In some women this venous network may be less visible or not noticeable at all, or may not become obvious until later in pregnancy.

"Since I became pregnant I've got awful-looking spidery purplish-red lines on my thighs. Are they varicose veins?"

They aren't pretty, but they aren't varicose veins. They are probably spider nevi, or telangiectases, which can result from the hormone changes of pregnancy. They may fade and disappear after delivery; if they don't, they can be removed.

"My mother and grandmother both had varicose veins during pregnancy and had trouble with them ever after. Is there anything I can do to prevent the problem in my own pregnancy?"

Because varicosities often run in families, you're wise to think about prevention now—especially since varicose veins tend to worsen with subsequent pregnancies.

Normal, healthy veins carry blood from the extremities back to the heart. Because they must work against gravity, they are designed with a series of valves that prevent back flow. When these valves are missing or faulty, as they are in some people, blood tends to pool in the veins where the pressure of gravity is greatest (usually the legs, but sometimes the rectum or the vulva), resulting in the bulging of varicosities. Veins that are easily distended, or distensible, can further contribute to the condition. The problem is more common in people who are obese, and occurs four times more often in women than in men. In women who are susceptible, the condition often surfaces for the first time during pregnancy. There are several reasons for this: increased pressure from the uterus on the pelvic veins;

WHAT YOU MAY LOOK LIKE

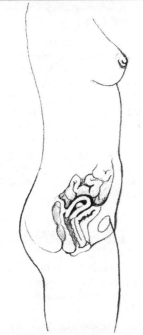

By the end of the second month, the embryo is more human-looking, about 1¼ inches long from head to buttocks (one-third of it is the head), and weighs about ⅓ ounce. It has a beating heart, and arms and legs with the beginnings of fingers and toes. Bone starts to replace cartilage.

increasing pressure on leg veins; expanded blood volume; and pregnancy-hormone-induced relaxation of the muscle tissue in the veins.

The symptoms of varicose veins aren't difficult to recognize, but they vary a great deal in severity. There may be severe pain, mild achiness, a sensation of heaviness, or none of these symptoms in the legs. A faint outline of bluish veins may be visible, or serpentine veins may bulge from ankle to upper thigh or vulva. In severe cases the skin overlying the veins becomes swollen, dry, and irritated. Occasionally, thrombophlebitis (the inflammation of a vein due to a blood clot) may develop at the site of a varicosity (see page 360).

Fortunately, varicose veins during pregnancy can often be prevented, or the symptoms minimized, by taking measures to eliminate unnecessary pressure on the leg veins.

❖ Avoid excessive weight gain.

❖ Avoid long periods of standing or sitting. When sitting, elevate your legs above the level of the hips when possible. When lying down, raise your legs by placing a pillow under your feet or lie on your side.

❖ Avoid heavy lifting.

❖ Avoid straining during bowel movements.

❖ Wear support pantyhose (light support hose seem to work well without being uncomfortable) or elastic stockings, putting them on before getting out of bed in the morning (before blood pools in your legs) and removing them at night before getting into bed.

❖ Don't wear restrictive clothing. Avoid tight belts or girdles, especially panty-leg girdles (even those designed for pregnancy); stockings and socks with elastic tops; garters; and snug shoes.

❖ Don't smoke. A possible correlation has been found between smoking and varicose veins (and of course a host of other health problems, including pregnancy complications; see page 54).

❖ Get some exercise—such as a brisk 20- to 30-minute walk—every day.

❖ Be sure to get enough vitamin C, which some physicians believe helps to keep veins healthy and elastic.

Surgical removal of varicose veins isn't recommended during pregnancy, although it can certainly be considered a few months after delivery. In most cases, however, the problem will clear up or improve spontaneously after delivery, usually by the time pre-pregnancy weight is reached.

COMPLEXION PROBLEMS

"My skin is breaking out the way it did when I was a teenager."

The glow of pregnancy that some women are lucky enough to radiate is caused not simply by joy over impending motherhood, but by an increased secretion of oils brought about by hormonal changes. And so, alas, are the less-than-glowing break-outs of pregnancy that some not-so-lucky women experience (particularly those whose skin ordinarily breaks out before their periods). Though such eruptions are hard to eliminate entirely, the following suggestions may help keep them to a minimum:

❖ Be faithful to the Best-Odds Diet—it's good for your skin as well as for your baby.

❖ Don't pass a tap without filling your glass. Water is one of the most effective pore-purifiers around.

❖ Wash your face two or three times a day with a gentle cleanser. Avoid skin-clogging creams and makeup.

❖ If your practitioner approves, take a vitamin B_6 supplement (no more than 25 to 50 milligrams). This vitamin is used in treating hormonally induced skin problems, though the evidence that it helps is not clear.

❖ If your skin problems are severe enough to warrant your seeing your internist and/or consulting a dermatologist, be sure to let him or her know you are expecting. Some drugs used for acne, particularly Accutane and possibly Retin-A, should not be used by pregnant women because they can be harmful to the fetus.

For some pregnant women, dry, often itchy, skin is a problem. Moisturizers may be helpful. (For optimum absorption, they should be applied while the skin is still damp after bath or shower.) So may drinking plenty of fluids and keeping rooms well humidified in the heating season. Too-frequent bathing, particularly with soap, tends to increase dryness. So cut down on bathing, and try using a mild soapless cleanser.

WAISTLINE EXPANSION

"Why does my waist seem to be expanding already? I thought I wouldn't 'show' until the third month at least."

Your expanding waistline may very well be a legitimate by-product of pregnancy, especially if you started out slender, with little excess flesh for your growing uterus to hide behind. Or it may be the result of bowel distention, very common in early pregnancy. On the other hand, it's also quite possible that your "show" may be an indication that you're gaining weight too quickly. If you've gained more than 3 pounds so far, analyze your diet—you are very likely taking in too many calories, possibly empty ones. Review the Best-Odds Diet, and read about weight gain on page 147.

LOSING YOUR FIGURE

"I'm worried that my figure will never be the same after I have a baby."

The 2 to 4 permanent pounds the average woman puts on with each pregnancy, and the flab that usually accompanies them, are not the inevitable result of being pregnant. They're the result of gaining too much weight, eating the wrong foods, and/or not getting enough exercise during those nine months.

The weight gain of pregnancy has just two legitimate purposes: to nourish the developing fetus now, and to store up reserves for breastfeeding to nourish the baby after delivery. If only enough weight to serve those purposes is gained and a woman keeps physically fit, her figure will generally return to prepregnancy form within a few months after her baby is born, especially if she is using up fat stores by breastfeeding.[2] So stop worrying and start taking action. Follow the Best-Odds Diet, and observe the recommendations about weight gain on page 147 and exercise on page 189.

With attention to diet and exercise now, you can look better than ever after pregnancy, because you will have learned how to take optimum care of your body. If your husband joins you in your healthier lifestyle, he can look better after your pregnancy too.

HEARTBURN AND INDIGESTION

"I have indigestion and heartburn all the time. Will this affect my baby?"

While you are painfully aware of your gastrointestinal discomfort, your baby is blissfully oblivious to and unaffected by it—as long as it isn't interfering with your eating the right foods.

Though indigestion can have the same cause (usually overindulgence) during pregnancy as when you're not pregnant, there are additional reasons

why it may be plaguing you now. Early in pregnancy, your body produces large amounts of progesterone and estrogen, which tend to relax smooth muscle tissue everywhere, including the gastrointestinal (GI) tract. As a result, food sometimes moves more slowly through your system, resulting in bloating and indigestion. This may be uncomfortable for you, but it is beneficial for your baby because this alimentary slowdown allows better absorption of nutrients into your bloodstream and subsequently through the placenta, into your baby's system.

Heartburn results when the ring of muscle that separates the esophagus from the stomach relaxes, allowing food and harsh digestive juices to back up from the stomach to the esophagus. These stomach acids irritate the sensitive esophageal lining, causing a burning sensation right about where the heart is; thus the term heartburn—which has nothing to do with your heart. During the last two trimesters the problem can be compounded by your blossoming uterus as it presses up on your stomach.

It's nearly impossible to have an indigestion-free nine months; it's just one of the less pleasant facts of pregnancy. There are, however, some pretty effective ways of avoiding heartburn and indigestion most of the time, and of minimizing the discomfort when it strikes:

❖ Avoid gaining too much weight; ex-

---

2. A few nursing mothers find they can shed very little weight while breastfeeding; they are usually able to return to prepregnancy weight soon after weaning their babies. If they don't, it is because they are consuming too many calories and burning too few. Bottle-feeding mothers will have to lose weight postpartum through diet and exercise.

cess weight puts excess pressure on the stomach.

❖ Don't wear clothing that is tight around your abdomen and waist.

❖ Eat many small meals rather than three big ones.

❖ Eat slowly, taking small mouthfuls and chewing thoroughly.

❖ Eliminate from your diet any food that causes GI discomfort. The most common offenders are hot and highly seasoned foods; fried or fatty foods; processed meats (hot dogs, bologna, sausage, bacon); chocolate, coffee, alcohol, carbonated beverages; spearmint and peppermint (even in gum).

❖ Don't smoke.

❖ Avoid bending over at the waist; bend instead with your knees.

❖ Sleep with your head elevated about 6 inches.

❖ Relax.

❖ If all else fails to relieve your symptoms, ask your doctor to recommend a low-sodium antacid or other over-the-counter medication that is safe for use in pregnancy. Avoid preparations containing sodium or sodium bicarbonate.

FOOD AVERSIONS AND CRAVINGS

"Certain foods—particularly green vegetables—that I've always liked taste funny now. Instead, I have cravings for foods that are less nutritious."

T he pregnancy cliché of a harried husband running out in the middle of the night, raincoat over his pajamas, for a pint of ice cream and a jar of pickles to satisfy his wife's cravings is probably played out more often in the heads of cartoonists than in real life. Not many pregnant women's cravings carry them—or their husbands—that far.

But most of us do find that our tastes in food change somewhat in pregnancy. Studies show that between 76% and 90% of expectant mothers experience a craving for at least one food during pregnancy, and between 50% and 85% have at least one food aversion. To a certain extent, these sudden gastronomic eccentricities can be blamed on hormonal havoc— which probably explains why food aversions and cravings are most common in the first trimester of first pregnancies, when that havoc is at its height.

Hormones, however, don't offer the only explanation for pregnancy food aversions and cravings. The long-favored theory that these are sensible signals from our bodies—that when we develop a distaste for something, it's usually bad for us, and that when we crave something, it's usually something we need—has some merit. Such a signal comes when the black coffee that used to be the mainstay of your workday becomes totally unappealing. Or the cocktail before dinner seems too strong even when it's weak. Or you suddenly can't get enough citrus fruit. On the other hand, when you can't stand the sight of fish, or broccoli suddenly tastes bitter, or you crave ice-cream sundaes, you can't credit your body with sending accurate signals.

The fact is that body signals relating to food are notoriously unreliable, probably because we've departed so significantly from the food chain in nature that we can no longer interpret these signals correctly. Before ice-cream sundaes were invented, when food came from nature, a craving for carbohydrates and calcium would have steered us toward fruits or berries and milk or cheese. With the wide variety of tempting (but often unwholesome) foods available today, it's no wonder our bodies are confused.

You can't totally ignore cravings and aversions. But you can respond to them without putting your baby's nutritional needs in jeopardy. If you crave something that's good for you and baby, by all means go ahead and enjoy it. If you crave something that you really shouldn't have, then seek a substitute that satisfies the craving without sabotaging your baby's nutritional interests: raisins, dried apricots, or a fruit-juice-sweetened muffin, cookie, or chocolate bar instead of sugary candies; lightly salted whole-wheat pretzels instead of the usually oversalted, nutritionally vacant variety. When substitutes don't satisfy, sublimation may be helpful—try exercise, knitting, reading, a leisurely bath, or other distractions when unwholesome urges strike. And, of course, occasionally give in to your cravings and cheat (see page 129).

If you experience a sudden aversion to coffee or alcohol or chocolate ice cream, great. It will make giving them up for the duration all the easier. If it's fish or broccoli or milk you can't tolerate, you don't have to force-feed yourself, but you do have to find compensating sources of the nutrients they supply. (See the Best-Odds Diet for appropriate substitutions.)

Most cravings and aversions disappear or weaken by the fourth month. Cravings that hang in there longer may be triggered by emotional needs—the need for a little extra attention, for example. If both you and your spouse are aware of this need, it should be easy to satisfy. You might, instead of requesting a middle-of-the-night pint of Rocky Road, settle for some quiet cuddling or a romantic bath-for-two.

Some women find themselves craving, even eating, such peculiar substances as clay, ashes, and laundry starch. Since this habit, known as pica, can be a sign of nutritional deficiency, particularly of iron, it should be reported to your practitioner.

MILK AVERSION OR INTOLERANCE

"I can't tolerate milk, and drinking four cups a day would make me ill. Will my baby suffer if I don't drink milk?"

First of all, it's not milk your baby needs, it's calcium. Since milk is the most convenient source of calcium in the American diet, it's the one most often recommended for filling the greatly increased requirement during pregnancy. But there are many substitutes that fill the nutritional bill just as well. Many people who are lactose-intolerant (can't digest the milk sugar, lactose) can tolerate some kinds of dairy products, such as hard cheeses, fully processed yogurts, and the new lactose-reduced milk, in which 70% of the lactose has been converted to a more easily digested form. If you can't tolerate any dairy products, you can still get all the calcium your baby requires by eating the nondairy foods listed under Calcium-Rich Foods on page 90.

You may find, however, that even though you have been lactose-intolerant for years, you are able to handle some dairy products during the second and third trimesters, when fetal needs for calcium are the greatest. Even if that's so, don't overdo it; try to stick primarily to those products that are less likely to provoke a reaction.

If your problem with milk isn't physiological but just a matter of distaste, there are many sources of calcium that should not offend your taste buds. You'll find them all in the

Calcium-Rich Foods list. Or you can try to fool your taste buds with non-fat dry milk that comes to your table incognito (in oatmeal, soups, muffins, sauces, shakes, frozen desserts, puddings, and so on).

If, in spite of all your best efforts, you can't seem to get enough calcium into your diet, ask your practitioner about prescribing a calcium supplement.

CHOLESTEROL

"My husband and I are very careful about our diets, and we limit our cholesterol and fat intake. Should I continue to do this while I'm pregnant?"

Pregnant women, and to a lesser extent nonpregnant women of childbearing age, are in an enviable position: they do not have to limit their cholesterol intake as drastically as do men and older women. In fact, cholesterol is necessary for fetal development, so much so that the mother's body automatically increases its production, raising blood cholesterol levels by anywhere from 25% to 40%.[3] Though you don't have to eat a high-cholesterol diet to help your body step up production, you can feel free to indulge a bit. Have an egg every day[4] if you like, use cheese to meet your calcium requirement, and enjoy an occasional steak—all without guilt. But don't overdo, because many high-cholesterol foods are high in fat and

calories, and an excess of them could send the numbers on your scale soaring. Too much fat could also put you over your fat quota (see page 87). And remember that many foods high in cholesterol are also high in animal fats that may be contaminated by undesirable chemicals (see page 131).

But while you don't necessarily have to hold the mayo (and the butter, and the egg yolks, and the lamb chops), everyone else in your household (except for under-two-year-olds)[5] should, most of the time. That goes most emphatically for adult men, both those with borderline-to-high cholesterol counts and those who just want to avoid developing a problem. Because serving two sets of breakfasts, lunches, and dinners—one cholesterol-lenient and one cholesterol-trimmed—is not only a strain on the cook but also unfair to those being denied, it's wise to continue, or to institute, a healthy heart regimen for family meals. Lean toward lean meats, poultry without the skin, low-fat dairy products, cholesterol-combating oils (such as olive and canola), and the white of the egg rather than the yolk. Enjoy your cholesterol on the sly, when no one else is around to drool.

A MEATLESS DIET

"I eat chicken and fish but no red meat. Can I supply my baby with all the nutrients he needs without meat?"

Your baby can be just as happy and healthy as any beef-eating mother's offspring. Fish and poultry, in fact, give you more protein and less fat

---

3. Women who have hypercholesteremia, a familial type of high blood cholesterol, are exceptions to the loosening of the cholesterol reins in pregnancy. These women should continue to follow their doctors' advice about diet.

4. Not raw, however, or even undercooked, because of the risk of salmonella poisoning.

---

5. Babies under two need fat and cholesterol for proper growth and brain development, and should never be placed on a fat- and cholesterol-restricted diet except under medical supervision.

for your calories than beef, pork, lamb, and organ meats. A red-meatless diet also contains less cholesterol, which may not make a big difference to you while you're pregnant, but represents a plus for your spouse and perhaps other family members.

A VEGETARIAN DIET

"I'm a vegetarian and in perfect health. But everyone—including my doctor—says that I have to eat meat and fish, eggs, and milk products to have a healthy baby. Is this true?"

Vegetarians of every variety can have healthy babies without compromising their dietary principles. But they have to be even more careful in planning their diets than meat-eating mothers-to-be, being particularly sure to get all of the following:

Adequate Protein. For the ovo-lacto vegetarian, who eats eggs and milk products, adequate protein intake can be ensured by taking ample quantities of both. A vegan (a strict vegetarian who eats neither milk nor eggs) has to depend on combinations of vegetable proteins to meet her five-serving protein allowance (see Vegetarian Complete Protein Combinations, page 97). Some meat substitutes are good protein sources; others are low in protein and high in fat and calories. Read the labels.

Adequate Calcium. This is no problem for the vegetarian who eats dairy products, but adroit maneuvering is needed for those who don't. Many soy products are fairly high in calcium, but beware of soy milks loaded with sucrose (sugar, corn syrup, honey); look for a pure soybean product instead. For tofu to be counted as a calcium food, it must have been coagulated with calcium; otherwise it will contain little or none of that mineral. Some brands of stone-ground corn tortillas are good nondairy sources of calcium, providing as much as half a calcium serving per piece (check the labels). Another easy-to-take nondairy source of calcium is calcium-added orange juice. For yet others, see the Calcium-Rich Foods list on page 91. For added insurance, it is recommended that vegans also take a prescribed calcium supplement (vegetarian formulas are available).

Vitamin B$_{12}$. Vegetarians, particularly vegans, often don't get enough of this vitamin because it is found primarily in animal foods. So they should be certain to take a vitamin supplement that includes B$_{12}$ as well as folic acid and iron.

Vitamin D. This important vitamin occurs naturally only in fish liver oils. It is also produced by our skin when we are exposed to sunlight, though because of the vagaries of weather, cover-up clothing, and the dangers of spending too much time in the sun, this is an unreliable source of the vitamin for most women. To ensure adequate intake of vitamin D, particularly for children and pregnant women, U.S. law requires that milk be fortified with 400 mg of vitamin D per quart. If you don't drink milk, be sure that there is vitamin D in the supplement you are taking (see page 88). Be careful, however, not to take vitamin D in doses beyond pregnancy requirements, since it can be toxic in excessive amounts.

JUNK-FOOD JUNKIE

"I'm addicted to junk foods—doughnuts for breakfast; fast-food burgers, fries, and Cokes for lunch. I'm afraid that if I can't break these bad habits, my baby will be undernourished."

You're right to worry. Before you became pregnant, your dietary indiscretions could hurt only you; now they can hurt your baby as well. Make a daily diet of doughnuts, fast-food burgers, and Cokes, and you'll be denying your baby adequate nourishment during the most important nine months of his or her life. Eat the junk food on top of a balanced diet, and your baby won't be the only one growing.

Happily, addictions can be broken. Heroin. Tobacco. Even junk food. Here are several ways to make your withdrawal almost as painless as it is worthwhile:

Change the Locale of Your Meals. If breakfast usually consists of a danish at your desk, have a better breakfast before you leave for work. If you can't resist a burger at lunch, go to a restaurant that doesn't serve burgers, or order in a nutritious sandwich from the local deli or bring one from home.

Stop Thinking of Eating as a Catch-as-Catch-Can Proposition. Rather than settling for what's easiest, select what's best for your baby. Plan meals and snacks ahead of time to be sure you get all of your Daily Dozen.

Don't Give Temptation a Tumble. Keep candy, chips, sugary cookies made with refined flours, and sugar-sweetened soft drinks out of the house (other family members will survive without them, and in fact will benefit from their absence). When the coffee wagon bell chimes at work, don't answer it. Stock home and workplace with such wholesome snacks as fresh and dried fruit, nuts, fruit-juice-sweetened baked goods, whole-wheat breadsticks and crackers, juices, hard-cooked eggs, and string cheese (the last two will need refrigeration at work, or the company of an ice pack in your lunch box).

Don't Use Lack of Time as an Excuse for Sloppy Eating. It takes no more time to make a tuna sandwich to take to work than to stand on line at Burger King. Or to slice a fresh peach into a container of yogurt than to cut a slab of peach pie. If the prospect of preparing a real dinner every night seems overwhelming, cook enough for two or three dinners at one time and give yourself alternate nights off. And keep it simple: fancy sauces aren't nutritious, only high in fat and calories. Utilize frozen vegetables or the fresh, prewashed, cut-up vegetables at salad bars or in supermarket produce sections when you don't have the time to do it yourself (raw vegetables can be quickly steamed or stir-fried at home).

Don't Use a Tight Budget as an Excuse for Eating Junk Foods. A glass of orange juice or milk is cheaper than a can of Coke. A homemade broiled chicken breast and baked potato cost a lot less than a Big Mac and fries.

Quit Cold Turkey. Don't tell yourself you can have just one cola today or just one doughnut. That approach almost never works when you're trying to break an addiction. Just tell yourself that junk food is out—at least until you deliver. You may be surprised to find, once the baby's born, that your new good eating habits are as hard to break as your old bad ones—which will make setting a good example for your child all the easier.

Study the Best-Odds Diet. Make it part of your life.

EATING FAST FOOD

"I go out with friends for fast food after a movie about once a month. Do I have to skip this for the rest of my pregnancy?"

Best-Odds Cheating

Unless you have a food allergy or sensitivity, no food need be completely off limits, even during pregnancy. The Best-Odds Diet recognizes that all of us slip up—really *need* to slip up—every once in a while. To eliminate guilt, the diet allows for cheating. So once a week give in to something that is not quite perfect but not totally terrible: a bagel, some bread, or pancakes made with refined flour; frozen yogurt or ice milk made with sugar; french fries or fried chicken; a fast-food burger; a bran or whole-grain muffin made with sugar or honey. Once a month, treat yourself to something terribly wicked: a slice of cake or pie; an ice-cream sundae; a candy bar. Always try to cheat selectively—choose carrot cake or cheesecake over butter-cream-frosted yellow cake; ice cream over milkless frozen desserts (unless you can't tolerate milk); cookies made with oats, raisins, or nuts rather than chocolate chips. Cheat only on something you really want and love. And don't cheat at all if you find that you can't stop once you get started.

Though fast food still can't be called health food, the major chains have gone a long way recently to improve the nutritive quality of the fare they offer. Still, you have to pick and choose to be sure you get the best of the offerings. At some fast-food establishments you can get help from the nutrition information posted or available on request. Look for grilled chicken, broiled or baked fish, baked potatoes (without the fat-rich toppings), a taco, a slice of pizza, occasionally a plain burger, salads that aren't swimming in oily dressings (select fresh vegetables instead, and lightly dress them and sprinkle with cheese), or other main-course items that are not excessively high in fat and sodium. Avoid the fries (though they may no longer be made with beef fat, they're still high in fat and calories), double burgers, processed cheese toppings for potatoes (use some fresh cheese from the salad bar instead), sugary canned fruits and puddings, sodas, and fruit pies. If the shakes or frozen desserts are made with real milk, treat yourself occasionally—but avoid those that are primarily sugar, saturated fat, and chemicals. Drink juice, milk, soda water, or plain water, and bring along your own dessert (a couple of fruit-juice-sweetened cookies or a piece of fruit) if you fear your sweet tooth may get the better of you if it isn't appeased. If you come away without having had a single green leafy or yellow vegetable, munch a carrot or enjoy a slice of cantaloupe when you get home.

CHEMICALS IN FOODS

"With additives in packaged foods, insecticides on vegetables, PCBs in fish, DES in meat, and nitrates in hot dogs, is there anything I can safely eat during pregnancy?"

Reports of hazardous chemicals in just about every item in the American diet are enough to scare the appetite out of anyone—and especially a pregnant woman afraid not only for her own health but for that of her unborn child. Thanks to the media, "chemical" has become synonymous with "dangerous," and "natural" with "safe." But neither generalization is true. Everything we eat is made up of chemicals. Some chemicals are harmful, some are not; some are even beneficial. And although "natural" is often better than artificial or unnatural, it can also be deadly. A "natural" mushroom can be poisonous; "natural" eggs, butter, and animal fats are associated with heart disease; and "natural" sugar and honey cause cavities.

That's not to say that you have to give up eating altogether in order to protect your baby from danger at the table. In spite of anything you might have heard, no food or additive presently in use has been shown to cause birth defects. And in fact, most American women fill their shopping carts without giving safety a second thought and have perfectly normal babies. Clearly, the danger that exists from the chemical additives in food is remote.

If you want to do your best to eliminate even this remote risk, use the following as a guide to help you decide what to drop into your shopping cart and what to pass up.

❖ Use the Best-Odds Diet as the foundation for food selection; it steers you clear of most potential perils. It also supplies Green Leafies and Yellows that are rich in protective beta-carotene, which may counteract the negative effects of toxins in our food.

❖ Use sweeteners wisely. Entirely avoid foods sweetened with saccharin; it crosses the placenta and its long-term effects on the fetus are unknown. If you do not have difficulty handling the amino acid phenylalanine, you can, however, use aspartame (Equal, NutraSweet). The components of this sweetener do not appear to cross the placenta in any significant amounts, and studies show no harm to the fetus with moderate maternal use in nor-

mal women. (But there are reasons why foods made with aspartame may not be the best ones for you; see page 62.) Sweeteners made of slowly absorbed carbohydrates, such as sorbitol and mannitol, are also believed safe, but be aware that they are not low in calories and that even moderate doses can cause diarrhea.

❖ Whenever possible, cook from scratch with fresh ingredients. You'll avoid many questionable additives found in processed foods, and your meals will be more nutritious too.

❖ Contact your local Environmental Protection Agency (EPA) or health department for a list of fish in your area that have not been contaminated with PCBs or other chemicals. If the fish you are planning to enjoy is the bounty of a family fishing expedition or a prize that was reeled in by a neighbor, be especially careful to check on its safety. Because it may have inhabited polluted waters, it is more suspect than most commercially caught fish.

There is some disagreement about how safe or unsafe fish and seafood are these days, with consumer advocates issuing dire warnings and the industry insisting they are unfounded. As a general rule, ocean fish are less likely to be contaminated than river and lake dwellers (though levels of contamination vary from lake to lake). Bluefish and striped bass, it is generally agreed, pose the greatest risk and should be avoided by pregnant women. Whether mercury in fish is really a danger or not isn't clear, but some experts recommend avoiding swordfish (which tends to contain the highest concentrations of mercury) altogether during pregnancy, and eating no more than half a pound of tuna or halibut (which also have relatively high levels) in any one week. Beware, too, of eating fish from waters that are grossly contaminated with microorganisms—from sewage dumping, for example.[6]

❖ Generally avoid foods preserved with nitrates and nitrites: frankfurters, salami, luncheon meats, smoked fish and meats.

❖ Whenever you have a choice between a product with artificial colorings, flavorings, preservatives, and other additives and one without, opt for the one that's additive-free.

❖ In cooking, don't use MSG or flavor enhancers that contain it. In Chinese restaurants, request no MSG when ordering.

❖ Choose lean cuts of meat and poultry and remove visible fat and skin before cooking, since chemicals that are fed to livestock tend to concentrate in these parts of the animal. Don't eat organ meats (liver, kidneys, etc.) very often, for the same reason. When possible, buy poultry and meat that has been raised organically, without hormones or antibiotics. Free-range chickens, for example, are not only less likely to be contaminated with these chemicals, they are also less likely to carry such infections as salmonella because the birds are not kept in cramped disease-breeding quarters.

❖ As a precaution, give all your non-organic fruits and vegetables a de-tergent bath (in the same detergent you use to hand-wash dishes) just before using them. Scrub skins when possible, and be sure to rinse thoroughly. Peel when practical, to remove surface chemical residues, especially when a vegetable has a waxy coating (as cucumbers, and sometimes tomatoes, apples, and eggplants, often do).

❖ Beware of picture-perfect produce. Fruits and vegetables that appear to have been embalmed, so unblemished are they, may very well have been heavily protected by pesticides in the fields. The less pretty produce may be the healthier bet.

❖ Buy organic produce when possible and practical. Produce that is certified organic usually is as close as possible to being free of all chemical residues. Transitional produce may still contain some residues from soil contamination, but should be safer than conventionally grown produce. If organic produce is available locally and you can afford the premium price, make it your choice. If it isn't available, ask the produce manager at your favorite market to order it.

❖ Favor domestic produce. Imported produce (and foods made from such produce) may contain higher levels of pesticides than that grown in the U.S., since pesticide regulation in other countries is often lax or nonexistent. Bananas, all of which are imported, are apparently safe, however; government monitoring sources have found them virtually free of pesticides.

❖ Vary your diet. Variety ensures not only a more interesting gastronomic experience and better nutrition, but also better odds of avoiding excessive exposure to any one potentially toxic substance. Switch between broccoli, kale, and car-

---

6. For the latest information on fish safety from the industry, call the American Seafood Institute: 1-800-EAT-FISH (in Rhode Island, dial 401-783-4200), between 9 A.M. and 5 P.M. Monday through Friday.

rots, for instance; melon, peaches, and strawberries; salmon, tuna, and sole; wheat, oats, and rice.

❖ Don't be fanatic. Though trying to avoid theoretical hazards in food is a commendable goal, making your life stressful in order to do so is not.

READING LABELS

"I'm eager to eat well, but it's difficult to figure out what's in the products I buy."

Labels aren't designed to help you as much as to sell you. Keep this in mind when food shopping, and learn to read the small print, especially the ingredients list and the nutrition label.

The ingredients listing will tell you, in order of predominance (with the first ingredient the most plentiful and the last the least), exactly what is in the product. A quick perusal will tell you whether the major ingredient in a cereal is sugar or a wholegrain. It will also tell you when a product is high in salt, fat, or additives.

Nutritional labels appear on more than half the products on your grocer's shelves, and these are particu-larly valuable for a pregnant woman counting her protein and watching her calories, as they provide the grams of the former and the number of the latter in each serving. The listing of percentages of the government's recommended daily allowance, however, is less useful, because the RDA for pregnant women is different from the RDA used on package labels. Still, a food high in a wide variety of nutrients is a good product to purchase.

While it's important to pay attention to the small print, it's sometimes just as important to ignore the large print. When a box of English muffins trumpets boldly, "Made with whole wheat, bran, and honey," reading the small print may reveal that that the major ingredient (first on the list) is *white,* not whole-wheat, flour, that the muffins contain precious little bran (it's near the bottom of the ingredients list), and that there's a lot more sugar (it's high on the list) than honey (it's low).

"Enriched" and "fortified" are also banners to be wary of. Adding a few vitamins to a poor food doesn't make it a good food. You'd be much better off with a bowl of oatmeal, which comes by its vitamins honestly, than with a refined cereal that is 50% sugar

Eating Safe

A more immediate threat than the chemicals in your food are the little microorganisms—bacteria and parasites—that can contaminate it. These villains can cause anything from mild stomach upset to severe illness, and in very rare instances even death. So beware of dishes (particularly those containing poultry, meat, fish, or eggs) that have been prepared under less than sanitary conditions; cooked food that has been left standing unrefrigera-ted for more than a couple of hours; food from cans that are leaky or swollen; undercooked or raw eggs and any kind of raw, or even undercooked, meat, fish, or poultry. To be sure that you don't contaminate food yourself, carefully wash your hands with soap and water before cooking or eating.*

---

*For more on safe food preparation, see *What to Eat When You're Expecting.*

(the nutrition label usually lists the percentage of sugar) but has a few pennies' worth of vitamins and minerals added.

WHAT IT'S IMPORTANT TO KNOW: PLAYING IT SAFE

The home. The highway. The backyard. The most significant risks faced by pregnant women are from pregnancy complications, not from accidents.

Accidents often seem "accidental," that is, to happen by chance. Yet most are the direct result of carelessness—often on the part of the victim herself—and many can be avoided with a little extra caution and common sense. There are a wide variety of steps you can take to prevent injuries and accidents:

❖ Recognize that you're not as graceful as you were prepregnancy. As your abdomen grows, your center of gravity will shift, making it easier for you to lose your balance. You will also find it increasingly difficult to see your feet. These changes can contribute to your becoming accident-prone.

❖ Always fasten your seat belt—and keep it fastened—in autos and on airplanes.

❖ Never climb on a shaky chair or ladder, or better still, don't climb at all.

❖ Don't wear high spiky heels, sloppy slippers, or thongs that can snap, all of which encourage falls and twisted ankles. Don't walk on slippery floors in your stocking feet or in smooth-soled shoes.

❖ Be careful getting in and out of the tub; be sure your tub and shower are equipped with nonskid surfaces and sturdy grab bars.

❖ Check your house and backyard for hazards: rugs without skidproof bottoms, especially at the top of stairs; toys or junk on stairways; poorly lit stairs and hallways; wires strung across the floor; overwaxed floors; icy sidewalks and steps.

❖ Observe the safety rules of whatever sport you play; follow all the tips for safe exercise and activity on page 195.

❖ Don't overdo. Fatigue is a major contributor to accidents.

7
The Third Month

WHAT YOU CAN EXPECT AT THIS MONTH'S CHECKUP

This month you can expect your practitioner to check the following, though there may be variations depending upon your particular needs and your practitioner's style of practice:[1]

❖ Weight and blood pressure

❖ Urine, for sugar and protein

❖ Fetal heartbeat

❖ Size of uterus, by external palpa-tion, to see how it correlates to estimated date of delivery (EDD), or due date

❖ Height of fundus (the top of the uterus)

❖ Hands and feet for edema (swelling), and legs for varicose veins

❖ Questions or problems you want to discuss—have a list ready

WHAT YOU MAY BE FEELING

You may experience all of these symptoms at one time or another, or only a few of them. Some may have continued from last month, others may be new. You may also have additional, less common, symptoms.

PHYSICALLY:

❖ Fatigue and sleepiness

---

1. See Appendix for an explanation of the procedures and tests performed.

❖ A need to urinate frequently

❖ Nausea, with or without vomiting, and/or excessive salivation

❖ Constipation

❖ Heartburn, indigestion, flatulence, bloating

❖ Food aversions and cravings

❖ Breast changes: fullness, heaviness, tenderness, tingling; darkening of the areola (the pigmented area surrounding the nipple); sweat glands

WHAT YOU MAY LOOK LIKE

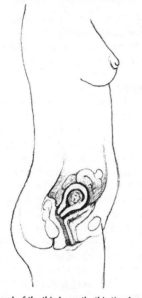

By the end of the third month, this tiny human, now a fetus, is 2½ to 3 inches long and weighs about ½ ounce. More organs are developing; circulatory and urinary systems are operating; the liver produces bile. Reproductive organs are developed, but the gender of the fetus is difficult to distinguish externally.

in the areola become prominent (Montgomery's tubercles), like large goose bumps; network of bluish lines under the skin expands

❖ Additional veins visible elsewhere, as blood supply to abdomen and legs also increases

❖ Occasional headaches

❖ Occasional faintness or dizziness

❖ Tightness of clothing around waist and bust, if it wasn't tight already; abdomen may appear enlarged by end of month

❖ Increasing appetite

EMOTIONALLY:

❖ Instability comparable to premenstrual syndrome, which may include irritability, mood swings, irrationality, weepiness

❖ Misgivings, fear, joy, elation—any or all

❖ A new sense of calmness

WHAT YOU MAY BE CONCERNED ABOUT

CONSTIPATION

"I've been terribly constipated for the past few weeks. Is this common?"

Very common. And there are sound reasons why. For one, increased relaxation of the musculature of the bowel, due to the high levels of certain hormones circulating during pregnancy, makes elimination sluggish. For another, the pressure from

the growing uterus on the bowels inhibits their normal activity.

But there's no sound reason for accepting constipation as inevitable with every pregnancy. Irregularity can be overcome by taking the following measures, which can also head off a common result of irregularity, hemorrhoids (see page 203):

Fight Back with Fiber. Avoid constipating refined foods and focus on such fiber-rich items as fresh fruit and vegetables (raw or lightly cooked, with skin left on when possible); whole-grain cereals, breads, and other baked goods; legumes (dried beans and peas); and dried fruit (raisins, prunes, apricots, figs). If you normally eat little fiber, add these high-fiber foods to your diet gradually or you may find your stomach unsettled. (You may find it unsettled for a while anyway, since flatulence is a frequent but usually temporary side effect of a fiber-infused diet, as well as a common complaint of pregnancy.) Spreading your daily fare out over six small meals rather than trying to squeeze everything into three overly filling ones may make you less uncomfortable.

If your case is a desperate one that doesn't seem to respond to such dietary manipulation or to the tactics below, add some wheat bran to your diet, starting with a sprinkle and working up to a couple of tablespoons. But avoid larger quantities of wheat bran; as it moves speedily through your system, it can carry away important nutrients before they've had a chance to be absorbed.

Drown Your Opponent. Constipation doesn't stand a chance against an ample fluid intake. Most fluids—particularly water and fruit and vegetable juices—are effective in softening stool and keeping food moving along the digestive tract. Some people find cups of hot water flavored with lemon (but no sugar) especially helpful. If constipation is severe, prune juice may do the trick.

Start an Exercise Campaign. Fit a brisk walk of at least half an hour into your daily routine; supplement it with any exercise you enjoy that is safe during pregnancy (see Exercise During Pregnancy, page 189).

If your efforts don't seem to be productive, consult with your practitioner. He or she may prescribe a bulk-forming stool softener for occasional use.

"All my pregnant friends seem to have problems with constipation. I don't; in fact, I've been more regular than ever. Is my system working right?"

Pregnant women are so programmed by mothers, friends, books, even doctors, to expect constipation that those who do become constipated accept it as normal and inevitable, and those who don't worry that there's something wrong.

But from the sound of things, your system couldn't be working better. Chances are your new digestive efficiency is attributable to a change in your diet—almost undoubtedly a change for the better.[2] Stepping up your consumption of fruits, vegetables, whole grains and other complex carbohydrates, and fluids, as recommended by the Best-Odds Diet, is bound to counteract the natural digestive slowdown of pregnancy and keep things moving smoothly. As your system gets used to the rough stuff, its productivity may decrease a little (and flatulence, which often temporarily accompanies such dietary changes, may ease up), but you will probably continue to be "regular."

If your stools are either very frequent (more than twice a day), or loose, watery, bloody, or mucousy, however, consult with your practitioner. Diarrhea during pregnancy requires prompt intervention.

---

2. Iron supplements may contribute to diarrhea *or* to constipation. If your supplement seems to unsettle your system, ask your practitioner to suggest a different formula.

FLATULENCE (GAS)

"I'm very bloated from gas and worry that the pressure, which is so uncomfortable for me, might also be hurting the baby."

S nug and safe in a uterine cocoon, protected on all sides by impact-absorbing amniotic fluid, your baby is impervious to your intestinal distress. If anything, he or she probably is soothed by the bubbling and gurgling of your gastric Muzak.

The only possible threat to your baby's well-being is if bloating—which often worsens late in the day—is preventing you from eating regularly and properly. To avoid this risk (and to minimize your own discomfort), take the following measures:

Stay Regular. Constipation is a common cause of gas and bloating.

Don't Gorge. Large meals just add to the bloated feeling. They also overload your digestive system, which isn't at its most efficient to begin with during pregnancy. Instead of three large meals a day, eat six small ones.

Don't Gulp. When you rush through meals or eat on the run, you're bound to swallow as much air as food. This captured air forms painful pockets of gas in your gut.

Keep Calm. Particularly during meals: Tension and anxiety can cause you to swallow air.

Steer Clear of Gas-Producers. Your stomach knows what they are—possibly onions, cabbage and cabbage-family members such as Brussels sprouts and broccoli, fried foods and sugary sweets (which you shouldn't be having now anyway), and of course the notorious beans.

WEIGHT GAIN

"I'm concerned that I didn't gain any weight in my first trimester."

M any women have trouble putting on an ounce in the early weeks; some even lose a few, usually courtesy of morning sickness. Fortunately, nature offers some protection for the babies of mothers who are too queasy to eat well during the first trimester: the fetus's need for calories and certain nutrients during this time is not as great as it will be later, so not gaining early on isn't likely to have an effect. But not gaining weight from here on in *can* have an effect—a significant one—because calories and nutrients will be more and more in demand as your baby-making factory picks up steam.

So don't worry, but do eat. And start watching your weight carefully to make sure it begins to move upward at a satisfactory rate (about 1 pound a week through the eighth month). If you continue to have trouble gaining weight, try packing more of a nutritional wallop with the calories you take in, through efficient eating (see page 81). Try, too, to eat a little more food each day, by adding more frequent snacks. But don't try to add pounds by adding junk food to your diet—that kind of weight gain will round out your hips and thighs, not your baby.

"I was shocked to find out that I'd already gained 13 pounds in the first trimester. What should I do now?"

Y ou can't turn back the scales— that weight is there to stay for now, at least until some time after delivery. And you can't apply the extra pounds toward next trimester's gain, either. Your fetus needs a steady supply of calories and nutrients, particularly during the months to come. You can't cut back on calories now, expecting it to get sufficient nourishment from the excess weight you've already accumulated. Dieting to lose or maintain weight is never appropriate during pregnancy, and it is an especially dangerous game during the second and third trimesters, when fetal growth is dramatically swift and significant.

But while you can't do anything about the weight you've gained so far, there's plenty you can do to ensure that you don't continue putting on pounds at an excessive rate. Some women experience an early weight gain blitz because they overindulge in the kinds of starchy sweets they find comforting to their morning-sick tummies. If that was your problem, it should be less and less of one as queasiness tapers off and an appetite for a more varied diet returns. Other women gain too much in the first trimester because they've bought into the misconception that no-holds-barred eating is a pregnant woman's right and responsibility. Review the Best-Odds Diet (see page 80 and *What to Eat When You're Expecting*) to find out why it isn't, and to learn how you can eat for your baby's health without munching your way to a 60-pound weight gain. Gaining efficiently, on the highest-quality foods possible, will not only accomplish that goal but will make the weight you do gain easier to shed in the postpartum period.

HEADACHES

"I find that I'm getting a lot more headaches than ever before. Do I have to suffer with them because I can't take pain relievers?"

That women are more susceptible to headaches during the time they're supposed to stay away from pain relievers is one of the ironies of pregnancy. Although it may be one you'll have to live with, it's not necessarily one you'll have to suffer excessively with. While it's true that you can't turn to your medicine cabinet for a quick cure (see Appendix), prevention, teamed with home remedies, can offer some relief from the recurrent headaches of pregnancy. The best way of preventing and treating the headache depends on the cause or causes. Pregnancy headaches are most commonly the result of hormonal changes (which are responsible for the increased frequency and severity of many types of headaches, including sinus headaches), fatigue, tension, hunger, physical or emotional stress, or any combination of these.

With many of the following ways of overcoming and preventing headaches, you can fit the cure to the cause:

Relax. Pregnancy can be a time of high anxiety, with tension headaches a common result. Some women find relief through meditation and yoga. You can take a course or read a book on these or other relaxation techniques, or try those on page 114.

Of course, relaxation exercises don't work for everyone—some women find that they increase tension instead of alleviating it. For them, lying down in a dark, quiet room, or stretching out on the sofa or with their feet up at their desk for 10 or 15 minutes is a better foil for tension and tension headaches.

See the other tips for stress reduction on page 113.

Get Enough Rest. Pregnancy can also be a time of high fatigue, particularly in the first and last trimesters, and often for the full nine months for women who work long hours at a job or caring for their other children.

Sleep can be elusive once the belly starts burgeoning (how will I ever get comfortable?) and the mind starts racing (how will I ever get everything done before the baby comes?), compounding fatigue. Making a conscious effort to get more rest, day *and* night, can help keep headaches at bay. But be careful not to sleep *too much,* as excess sleep can also give you a headache.

Eat Regularly. To avoid hunger headaches triggered by low blood sugar, be sure not to miss meals. Carry high-energy snacks (complex carbohydrates and protein will work most effectively) with you in your purse, stash them in the glove compartment of your car and in your office desk drawer, and always keep a supply on hand at home.

Seek Some Peace and Quiet. If you're "allergic" to noise, stay away from it whenever possible. Avoid loud music, noisy restaurants, roaring parties, and crowded department stores. At home, lower the volume on the telephone's ring, the TV, and the radio.

Don't Get Stuffy. If an overheated, smoke-filled, unventilated room touches off headaches, leave it for a stroll outdoors now and then—or better still, avoid such locations entirely. Dress in layers when you know you're going somewhere stuffy, and keep comfortable by removing layers as needed. If your workplace is poorly ventilated, move to a better-ventilated office or area if that's possible; take frequent breaks if it isn't.

Go Hot and Cold. For relief of sinus headaches, apply hot and cold compresses to the aching area, alternating 30 seconds of each for a total of 10 minutes, four times a day. For tension headaches, try ice applied to the back of the neck for 20 minutes while you close your eyes and relax. (Use an ordinary ice pack or a special neck pillow that holds a gel-based cold pack.)

Straighten Up. Slouching or looking down to read, sew, or do other close work for long stretches of time can also cause headaches, so watch your posture.

If an unexplained headache persists for more than a few hours, returns very often, is the result of fever, or is accompanied by visual disturbances or puffiness of the hands and face, notify your practitioner at once.

"I suffer from migraine headaches. I heard they are more common in pregnancy. Is this true?"

Some women find their migraines strike more frequently during pregnancy. Others find they are less frequent. It isn't known why this should be so, or even why some people have recurrent migraines and others never have a single one.

Migraines are headaches that are in a class by themselves. Their development is related to constriction, or narrowing, of the blood vessels in the head, followed by their sudden dilation, or opening. This interferes with blood flow and causes pain and other symptoms. Though symptoms vary from person to person, a migraine is usually preceded by fatigue. The fatigue may then be followed by nausea with or without vomiting and diarrhea, sensitivity to light, and possibly a misting or zigzagging over one or, occasionally, both eyes. When the headache finally arrives, anywhere from minutes to hours after the first warning symptom, the pain, which is intense and throbbing, is usually localized on one side, but it can spread to the other side. Some people also experience tingling or numbness in one arm or side of the body, dizziness, ringing in the ears, runny nose, runny and/or bloodshot eyes, and temporary mental confusion.

If you've had migraines in the past, be prepared for dealing with them during pregnancy, preferably through prevention. If you know what brings on an attack, you can try to avoid the culprit. Stress is a common one (see page 113 for tips on handling it), as are chocolate, cheese, coffee, and red wine (not an approved pregnancy beverage, anyway). Try to determine what, if anything, can stave off a full-blown attack once the warning signs appear. For some people, splashing the face with cold water helps, or lying down in a darkened room for two or three hours, eyes covered (napping, meditating, or listening to music, but not reading or watching TV). Discuss with your physician which migraine medications are safe to take during pregnancy, and which might be most effective.

If you experience for the first time what seems like a migraine, call your doctor immediately. The same symptoms could also be indicative of a pregnancy complication. If an unexplained headache persists for more than a few hours, returns very often, is the result of fever, or is accompanied by visual disturbances or puffiness of the hands and face, also notify your practitioner at once.

TROUBLE SLEEPING

"I've never had a sleep problem in my life—until now. I can't seem to settle in at night."

Your mind is racing, your belly burgeoning—it's no wonder you can't settle in for a good night's sleep. You could write this insomnia off as good preparation for the sleepless nights that likely lie ahead in the first

months of your baby's life, or you could try the following tips:

❖ Get enough exercise. A body that gets a workout by day (see page 189 for guidelines) will be a sleepier body at night. But don't exercise too close to bedtime, since the exercise-induced high could keep you from crashing when your head hits the pillow.

❖ Set a leisurely pace at dinner. Don't gobble your meals on a television tray; partake at the table, with your spouse and a healthy helping of relaxing conversation.

❖ Develop a bedtime routine and stick with it. After dinner, maintain the easy pace, focusing on activities that relax you. Indulge in light reading (but nothing you can't put down) or television (no violent or emotionally wrenching dramas), soothing music, relaxation exercises (see page 114), a warm bath, a backrub, some lovemaking.

❖ Have a light snack to keep your blood sugar level up. Too much food or none at all before bedtime can interfere with sleep. Good soporific snacks include whole-grain fruit-sweetened cookies and milk; fruit and cheese; cottage cheese and unsweetened applesauce.

❖ Get comfortable. Be sure your bedroom is neither too hot nor too cold, that your mattress is firm and your pillow supportive. See page 173 for comfortable sleep positions; the sooner in pregnancy you learn to sleep comfortably on your side, the easier it will be for you to do it later on.

❖ Get some air. A stuffy environment is not a good sleeping environment. So open a window in all but the coldest or hottest weather (when a fan or air conditioning can help circulate the air). And don't sleep with the covers over your head. This will decrease the oxygen and increase the carbon dioxide you breathe in, which can cause headaches and even abnormal heart rhythms.

❖ Stay out of your bedroom except to sleep.

❖ If frequent trips to the bathroom are interfering with your sleep, limit fluids after 4 P.M. and stand as little as possible during the day, since standing increases nighttime urination.

❖ Clear your mind. If you've been losing sleep over problems at work or at home, try to solve them during the day, or at least talk about them with your spouse early in the evening. But put any worries out of your mind in the hours just before bedtime. (See other tension relief tips on page 113.)

❖ Don't use such crutches as medications or alcohol to assist you in falling asleep. These could be harmful in pregnancy, and they don't help in the long run anyway. Avoid caffeine (in tea, coffee, colas) and/or large quantities of chocolate (not very Best-Odds anyway) after noontime. These can interfere with sleep in the short run.

❖ Stay up later. You may need less sleep than you think you do. Putting off your bedtime may, paradoxically, help you sleep better. Avoiding daytime napping may help, too.

❖ Judge the adequacy of your sleep by how you feel, not by how many hours you stay in bed. Remember that most people with sleep problems actually get more sleep than they think. You're getting enough rest if you're not chronically tired (beyond the normal fatigue of pregnancy).

❖ Don't worry about your insomnia —it won't hurt you or your baby. When you can't sleep, get up and read, knit, or watch TV until you get drowsy. Worrying about not sleeping will certainly be more stressful than lack of sleep itself.

STRETCH MARKS

"I'm afraid I'm going to get stretch marks. Can they be prevented?"

For many women—especially those who favor bikinis—stretch marks are more to be dreaded than flabby thighs. Nevertheless, 90% of all women will develop these pink or reddish, slightly indented, sometimes itchy streaks on their breasts, hips, and/or abdomen sometime during pregnancy.

As their name implies, stretch marks are caused by the skin stretching, generally due to a large and/or rapid increase in weight. Expectant mothers who have good, elastic skin tone (because they either inherited it or earned it through years of excellent nutrition and exercise) may slip through several pregnancies without a single telltale striation. Others may be able to minimize, if not prevent, stretch marks by keeping weight gain steady, gradual, and moderate. Promoting elasticity in your skin by nourishing it with the Best-Odds Diet (page 80) may help, but no cream, lotion, or oil, no matter how expensive, will prevent or alleviate stretch marks—although they may be fun for your husband to rub on your tummy, and will prevent your skin from drying.

If you do develop stretch marks during pregnancy, you can console yourself with the knowledge that they will gradually fade to a silvery sheen some months after delivery. It may also help to think of them less as a disfigurement than as a medal of motherhood.

BABY'S HEARTBEAT

"My friend heard her baby's heartbeat at 2½ months. I'm a week ahead of her and my doctor hasn't picked up my baby's yet."

It's possible to pick up the fetal heartbeat as early as the 10th or 12th week with a highly sensitive instrument called a Doppler (a hand-held ultrasound device that amplifies the sound). But an ordinary stethoscope isn't powerful enough to detect the heartbeat until the 17th or 18th week at the earliest. Even with sophisticated instruments, the heartbeat may not be audible this early because of the baby's position or other interfering factors, such as excess layers of maternal fat. It's also possible that a slightly miscalculated due date may be causing the delay. Wait until next month. By your 18th week, the miraculous sound of your baby's heartbeat is certain to be available for your listening pleasure. If it isn't, or if you are very anxious, your doctor may order an ultrasound, which will pick up a heartbeat that, for some reason, is difficult to hear with a stethoscope.

SEXUAL DESIRE

"All of my pregnant friends say that they had an increased desire for sex early in pregnancy—some had orgasms and multiple orgasms for the first time. How come I feel so unsexy?"

Pregnancy is a time of change in many aspects of your life, not the least of them sexual. Some women who have never had either orgasm or much of a taste for sex suddenly experience both for the first time when

pregnant. Other women, accustomed to having a voracious appetite for sex and to being easily orgasmic, suddenly find that they are completely lacking in desire and are difficult to arouse. These changes in sexuality can be disconcerting, guilt-provoking, wonderful, or a confusing combination of all three. And they are perfectly normal.

As you will see by reading Making Love During Pregnancy (page 164), there are many logical explanations for such changes and for the feelings that they may provoke. Some of these factors may be strongest early in pregnancy, when nausea and fatigue make you feel understandably unsexy, when being able to make love without worrying about trying to get (or trying not to get) pregnant frees you of inhibitions and makes you sexier than ever, when guilt results because you're feeling sexy and you think you should be feeling motherly instead. Other factors, such as physical alterations that may make orgasm easier to achieve, more powerful, or more elusive, continue throughout gestation.

Most important is recognizing that your sexual feelings—and your husband's as well—during pregnancy may be more erratic than erotic; you may feel sexy one day and not the next. Mutual understanding and open communication will see you through.

ORAL SEX

"I've heard that oral sex is dangerous during pregnancy. Is this true?"

Cunnilingus is safe throughout pregnancy as long as your mate is careful not to blow any air into your vagina. Doing this could force air into your bloodstream and cause an air embolism (obstructing a blood vessel), which might prove deadly to both mother and baby.

Fellatio, because it doesn't involve the female genitalia, is always safe during pregnancy and for some couples is a very satisfactory substitute when intercourse isn't permitted.

CRAMP AFTER ORGASM

"I get an abdominal cramp after orgasm. Is this a sign that sex is hurting my baby? Will it cause a miscarriage?"

Cramping—both during and after orgasm, and sometimes accompanied by backache—is very common and harmless during a normal, low-risk pregnancy. Its cause can be physical: a combination of the normal venous congestion in the pelvic area during pregnancy and the equally normal congestion of the sexual organs during arousal and orgasm. Or it can be psychological: a result of the common fear of hurting the baby during intercourse.

The cramping is not a sign that sex is hurting the fetus. Most experts agree that sexual relations and orgasm during a normal, low-risk pregnancy are perfectly safe and are not a cause of miscarriage. If the cramps bother you, ask your husband for a gentle low back rub. It may relieve not only the cramps but any tension that might be triggering them, too.[3] (see Making Love During Pregnancy, page 164.)

TWINS AND MORE

"I'm already very big. Could I be carrying twins?"

It's more likely that you're just carrying a little extra weight because you gained more than your share in the first trimester. Or that you're small-boned to begin with and on you, uterine expansion is noticeable earlier than it would be on a larger frame. A relatively large abdomen in and of itself is not generally considered a sign that an expectant mother is carrying multiple fetuses; in making the diagnosis, a practitioner will look at other factors, including:

❖ A large-for-date uterus. The size of the uterus, not of the abdomen, is what counts in the diagnosis of multiple fetuses. If your uterus seems to be growing more rapidly than expected for your due date, a multiple pregnancy would be suspected. Other possible explanations for a large-for-date uterus include a miscalculated due date or an excessive amount of amniotic fluid (polyhydramnios).

❖ Exaggerated pregnancy symptoms. When twins are being carried, the troubles of pregnancy (morning sickness, indigestion, edema, and so on) can be doubled, or seem that way. But all of these can also be exaggerated in a singleton pregnancy.

❖ More than one heartbeat. Depending on the position the babies are in, a practitioner may be able to hear two (or more) distinctly separate heartbeats. But because the heartbeat of a single fetus may be heard at several locations, the locating of two (or more) confirms twins (or more) only if the heartbeats are different in rate. So twins aren't often diagnosed this way.

❖ Predisposition. Though there are no factors that increase the chances of having identical twins, there are several that make a woman more likely to have nonidentical twins. These include nonidentical twins in the mother's family, advanced

---

3. Some women also experience crampiness in the legs after intercourse. See page 202 for tips on relieving such discomfort.

age (women over 35 more frequently release more than one egg), the use of drugs to stimulate ovulation (fertility drugs), and in-vitro fertilization. Twins are also more common among black women than white, and less common among Asians.

If one or more of these factors lead the practitioner to the conclusion that there's a possibility of more than one fetus, an ultrasound exam will be ordered. In virtually every case (except in the rare instance where one camera-shy fetus remains stubbornly hidden behind the other), this technique will accurately diagnose a multiple pregnancy.

"We'd barely adjusted to the fact that I was pregnant when we found out I'm carrying twins. I'm worried about the risks involved for them—and for me."

Multiple births are multiplying at a fantastic rate; 2 in 100 sets of parents can expect to see double (or triple, or more) in the delivery room, up from 1 in 100 a generation ago. And although some multiple births are still conceived the old-fashioned way—as a result of random throws of nature's dice or because of an inherited predisposition—scientists point to several new factors in explaining the current baby-baby boom. One is the increase in older mothers: women over 35, because their ovulation tends to be erratic (with greater chances of more than one egg being released at a time), are more likely to conceive a multiple birth. Another is the use of such fertility drugs as Pergonal and Clomiphene (again, more often by older women, since fertility decreases with age), which increase the likelihood of multiple birth. Still another is the use of in-vitro fertilization, a procedure wherein eggs fertilized in a test tube are implanted into the uterus,

which, since several ova are involved, also yields an increased risk of multiple birth.

But if today's mother is more likely to conceive twins, she is also more likely to deliver those twins in good condition. Better than 90% of twin pregnancies, studies show, have happy endings. Much of this success is attributable to the advance-warning capabilities of ultrasound; rare is the couple nowadays who is taken by surprise by twins in the delivery room. Advance warning makes not only for fewer practical and logistical complications after birth (having to go back to the store at the last minute for an extra crib and layette), but also for fewer medical complications during pregnancy and at delivery. Armed with the knowledge that she is carrying more than one baby, an expectant mother and her practitioner can take many precautions that can reduce her risk of certain pregnancy complications (hypertension, anemia, and abruptio placenta are more common in multiple pregnancies) and improve her chances of carrying the babies to term and delivering them in top-notch condition:

Extra Medical Care. Much of the higher risk a multiple pregnancy carries can be reduced with expert medical monitoring by an obstetrician (high-risk pregnancies should not be overseen by a midwife). You will be scheduled for more frequent appointments than will the woman carrying a single fetus—often seeing the doctor every other week after the 20th week and weekly after the 30th. And you will be watched more closely for signs of complications so that if one develops, it can be treated quickly.

Extra Nutrition. Eating for three (or more) is at least double the responsibility of eating for two. On top of all the other good things it can do for all babies (see page 80), excellent nutrition can have a dramatic impact on one of the most common problems of multiple pregnancies: low birthweight. Instead of being born at 5 pounds and less (once the standard in multiple births), twins who are nourished on a superior diet can weigh in at a much healthier 6 to 7 pounds or more.

Many of the Best-Odds dietary requirements are multiplied with each fetus you're carrying. Specifically, that translates to approximately 300 additional calories, one additional Protein serving, one additional Calcium serving, and one additional Whole Grain serving. Because that's a lot of food to fit into a stomach cramped by a rapidly growing uterus, and because prenatal gastrointestinal discomforts, such as morning sickness and indigestion, are often multiplied in multiple pregnancies, the quality of the food you eat will be particularly important. Avoiding nutritionless frills will help ensure that you'll have room for the good stuff. Eating efficiently (see page 81) and spreading your requirements out over at least six small meals and many snacks, rather than trying to get your Daily Dozen and then some in at three sittings, should help too.

Extra Weight Gain. An additional baby means additional weight gain—not just because of the baby itself, but because of the extra baby by-products (often including an extra placenta and additional amniotic fluid). Your physician will probably advise a carefully monitored weight gain of at least 35 to 45 pounds above your prepregnancy weight (unless you're very overweight), or about 50% more than is recommended in a singleton pregnancy. That means about 1½ pounds a week after the 12th week. Particularly if this weight is gained on an excellent diet, it will go a long way toward producing healthier babies.

Extra Vitamins and Minerals. An additional fetus also means an increased need for such nutrients as iron and folic acid (needed to prevent anemia; see page 154), zinc, copper, calcium, B$_6$, vitamin C, and vitamin D. Because of this increased need, it's been stated by the Food and Nutrition Board of the American Academy of Sciences that women carrying more than one fetus are in the high-risk group that should take a prenatal vitamin-mineral supplement daily. So be sure you do. *Do not,* however, take any supplements beyond that, unless recommended by your physician.

Extra Rest. Your body will be working twice as hard at baby building, so it's going to need twice as much rest for its efforts. It's your job to make sure it gets it whenever it needs it. Make time for a nap or a rest with your feet up by depending more on others for help around the house and with errands, and by relying more on modern conveniences (use frozen vegetables, which are just as nutritious as fresh, or precut ones from a salad bar or supermarket produce section). And, if at all possible, work fewer hours at your job, or even stop work early if fatigue is severe.

Extra Caution. Depending on how your pregnancy is going, the doctor may prescribe taking an early leave from work (as early as the 24th week in some cases), getting help with the housework, and, sometimes, complete bed rest at home. Hospital bed rest during the last months of pregnancy is usually reserved for complicated multiple pregnancies; most studies show that for normal twin pregnancies, routine hospital admission at this time does not prevent preterm labor. Following doctor's orders to the letter, no matter how difficult that might be, is one of the best ways you can help your babies go to term.

Extra Help for the Extra Symptoms of Multiple Pregnancies. Since the common discomforts of pregnancy (including morning sickness, indigestion, backache, constipation, hemorrhoids, edema, varicose veins, shortness of breath, and fatigue) are likely to be exaggerated in a mom carrying more than one fetus, she needs to be aware of the various routes to relief. Though relief may be more elusive in a twin pregnancy, the suggestions in this book for dealing with these complaints apply to all mothers, whether they are expecting one baby or more than one (refer to the complaints individually; see the index). Consult with your doctor for additional advice, or if symptoms seem particularly severe.

An extremely uncommon complaint that occasionally complicates a multiple pregnancy is separation of the symphysis pubis, or the lower joint of the pelvic bone. This separation can cause limited mobility and severe localized pain in the pelvic area; contact your obstetrician if you experience either of these symptoms.

"Everybody thinks it's so exciting that we're going to have twins—except us. We're disappointed and scared. What's wrong with us?"

Nothing. Our prenatal daydreams rarely involve two cribs, two diaper pails, two high chairs, two strollers, or two babies. We prepare ourselves psychologically, as well as physically, for the arrival of one baby; when we hear that we're going to have two, feelings of disappointment are not unusual. Nor is fear. The impending responsibilities of caring for one new infant are daunting enough without having them doubled.

So accept the fact that you are ambivalent about the dual arrivals, and don't burden yourself with guilt. Instead, use this time before delivery to get used to the idea of twins. Talk to each other and to anyone you know who has twins. Your practitioner may also be able to provide the name of a local parents-of-twins support group or the name of a mother of twins in your area. Sharing your feelings, and recognizing that you're not the first expectant parents to experience them, will help you feel more accepting of, and in time even excited about, this pregnancy.

A CORPUS LUTEUM CYST

"My doctor said that I have a corpus luteum cyst on my ovary. She said that it won't be a problem, but I'm concerned."

Every month of a woman's reproductive life, a small yellowish body of cells forms after ovulation. Called a corpus luteum (literally "yellow body"), it occupies the space in the Graafian follicle formerly occupied by the ovum, or egg. The corpus luteum produces progesterone and estrogen, and is programmed by nature to disintegrate in about 14 days. When it does, diminishing hormone levels trigger menstruation. In pregnancy the corpus luteum, sustained by the hormone hCG (human Chorionic Gonadotropin) that is generated by the trophoblast (the cells that develop into the placenta), continues to grow and produce progesterone and estrogen to nourish and support the new pregnancy until the placenta takes over. In most cases, the corpus luteum starts to shrink about six or seven weeks after the last menstrual period and ceases to function at about 10 weeks, when its work of providing bed and board for the baby is done.

In an estimated 1 in 10 pregnancies, however, the corpus luteum fails to regress at the expected time and develops into a corpus luteum cyst. Usually, as your doctor has already assured you, the cyst won't present a problem. But just as a precaution, the physician will monitor its size and condition regularly via ultrasound, and if it becomes unusually large or if it threatens to twist or rupture, will consider removing it surgically. Such intervention is necessary with only about 1% of all corpus luteum cysts, and after the 12th week the surgery rarely threatens the pregnancy.

WHAT IT'S IMPORTANT TO KNOW:
WEIGHT GAIN DURING PREGNANCY

Put two pregnant women together anywhere—in a doctor's waiting room, on a bus, at a business meeting—and the questions are certain to start flying. "When are you due?" "Have you felt the baby kicking yet?" "Have you been feeling sick?" And perhaps the favorite query of all: "How much weight have you gained?"

The comparisons are inevitable, and sometimes a little disturbing. Women who started off with a bang, enthusiastically eating their way to 10-pound first-trimester gains, wonder "how much is too much?" Others who, appetites daunted by bouts with morning sickness, ended up with net gains that barely registered on the practitioner's scale (perhaps even with a slight weight loss), wonder "what's too little?" All wonder "how much is just right?"

Total Increase. Though it was once in medical vogue to limit a woman's pregnancy weight gain to 15 pounds, it is now recognized that this kind of weight gain was insufficient. Babies whose mothers gain under 20 pounds are more likely to be premature, small for their gestational age, and to suffer growth retardation in the uterus.

Almost as hazardous, however, was the next vogue, which urged women to eat to their hearts' and souls' content and gain any amount of weight. There are serious risks in gaining too much weight: assessment and measurement of the fetus become more difficult; excess weight overworks muscles and results in backache, leg pain, increased fatigue, and varicose veins; the baby may become so large that a vaginal delivery becomes difficult or impossible; if surgery, such as cesarean section, is needed, it becomes more difficult, and postoperative complications more common; and after pregnancy the excess weight may be hard to shed.

Though there's a good chance that a woman with an enormous weight gain may have an oversized baby, the mother's weight gain and the weight of her infant don't always correlate. It's possible to gain 40 pounds and deliver a 6-pound baby, and to gain 20 and have an 8-pounder. The quality of the food that contributes to the weight gain is more important than the quantity.

The sensible and safe pregnancy weight gain for the average woman is between 25 and 35 pounds, with a petite, small-boned woman's gain likely to fall at the lower end of the range and a larger, big-boned woman's gain likely to fall on the high end. That gain allows about 6 to 8 pounds for baby and 14 to 24 pounds for placenta, breasts, fluids, and other byproducts (see page 148). It also ensures a speedier return to prepregnancy weight for mom.

The formula changes for women with special needs. Women who begin pregnancy extremely underweight should try to gain enough weight during the first trimester so that they start the second trimester at or close to their ideal weight; then they should aim to gain the requisite 25 to 35 pounds on top of that. Women who start pregnancy 10% to 20% or more overweight can probably safely gain somewhat less weight on average, though only on the best-quality food and only under the careful supervision of their physicians. Pregnancy is never a time for weight loss or maintenance because a fetus can't survive on a mother's fat stores alone since they provide calories but no nutrients.

Women who are carrying more than one fetus also need to have their weight gain goal adjusted by their physicians. Though it doesn't double for twins or triple for triplets, it does increase significantly—to 35 to 45 pounds for twins, and more when there are more than two fetuses.

Rate of Increase. The average-weight woman should gain approximately 3 to 4 pounds during the first trimester, and about a pound a week, 12 to 14 pounds in all, during the second trimester. Weight gain should continue at a rate of about 1 pound a week during the seventh and eighth months, and in the ninth month drop off to a pound or 2—or even none at all—for a total of 8 to 10 pounds during the third trimester.

Rare is the woman who can tailor her weight gain precisely to the ideal formula. And it's fine to fluctuate a little—a ½ pound gain one week, 1½ pounds the next. But the goal of every pregnant woman should be to keep weight gain as steady as possible, without any sudden jumps or drops. If you don't gain any weight for two weeks or more during the fourth to eighth months, if you gain more than 3 pounds in any one week in the second trimester, or if you gain more than 2 pounds in any week in the third trimester, especially if it doesn't seem to be related to overeating or excessive intake of sodium, check with

Breakdown of Your Weight Gain

(All weights are approximate)

Baby	7½ pounds
Placenta	1½ pounds
Amniotic fluid	1¾ pounds
Uterine enlargement	2 pounds
Maternal breast tissue	1 pound
Maternal blood volume	2¾ pounds
Fluids in maternal tissue	3 pounds
Maternal fat	7 pounds
Total average	26½-pound overall weight gain

your doctor. Check, too, if you gain no weight for more than two weeks in a row.

If you find that your weight gain has strayed significantly from what you planned (for instance, that you gained 14 pounds in the first trimester instead of 3 or 4, or that you gained 20 pounds in the second trimester instead of 12), take action to see that it gets back on a sensible track, but don't try to stop it in its tracks. With your practitioner, readjust your goal to include the excess you've already gained (which your baby can't thrive on) and the weight you still have to gain (which your baby needs). Keep in mind that your baby requires a steady daily shipment of nutrients throughout the pregnancy. Watch your diet carefully, but never diet. Monitor your weight from the beginning, and you'll never have to put your baby on a diet to keep yourself from getting fat.

8
The Fourth Month

WHAT YOU CAN EXPECT AT THIS MONTH'S CHECKUP

This month you can expect your practitioner to check the following, though there may be variations depending upon your particular needs and upon your practitioner's style of practice:[1]

❖ Weight and blood pressure

❖ Urine, for sugar and protein

❖ Fetal heartbeat

❖ Size of uterus, by external palpation

❖ Height of fundus (top of the uterus)

❖ Hands and feet for edema (swelling), and legs for varicose veins

❖ Symptoms you've been experiencing, especially unusual ones

❖ Questions or problems you want to discuss—have a list ready

WHAT YOU MAY BE FEELING

You may experience all of these symptoms at one time or another, or only a few of them. Some may have continued from last month, others may be new. You may

---

1. See Appendix for an explanation of the procedures and tests performed.

also have other, less common, symptoms.

PHYSICALLY:

❖ Fatigue

❖ Decreased urinary frequency

❖ An end to, or a decrease in, nausea

and vomiting (in a few women, "morning sickness" will continue; in a very few it is just beginning)

❖ Constipation

❖ Heartburn, indigestion, flatulence, bloating

❖ Continued breast enlargement, but usually decreased tenderness and swelling

❖ Occasional headaches

❖ Occasional faintness or dizziness, particularly with sudden change of position

❖ Nasal congestion and occasional nosebleeds; ear stuffiness

❖ "Pink toothbrush" from bleeding gums

❖ Increase in appetite

❖ Mild swelling of ankles and feet, and occasionally of hands and face

❖ Varicose veins of legs and/or hemorrhoids

❖ Slight whitish vaginal discharge (leukorrhea)

❖ Fetal movement near the end of the month (but usually this early only if you are very slender or if this is not your first pregnancy)

EMOTIONALLY:

❖ Instability comparable to premenstrual syndrome, which may include irritability, mood swings, irrationality, weepiness

❖ Joy and/or apprehension—if you have started to feel pregnant at last

❖ Frustration—if you don't really feel pregnant yet but are too big for

WHAT YOU MAY LOOK LIKE

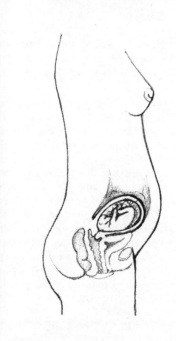

By the end of the fourth month, the 4-inch fetus, now nourished by the placenta, is developing reflexes, such as sucking and swallowing. Body growth begins to outstrip that of the head; tooth buds appear; fingers and toes are well defined. Though human-looking, it cannot survive outside the uterus.

your regular wardrobe and too small for maternity clothes

❖ A feeling you're not quite together. You're a scatterbrain, you forget things, drop things, have trouble concentrating

WHAT YOU MAY BE CONCERNED ABOUT

ELEVATED BLOOD PRESSURE

"At my last visit with the doctor, she said that my blood pressure was up a little bit. I've been worried ever since."

Worrying about your blood pressure will only send the readings higher, and a slight increase at one visit probably doesn't mean much of anything. Perhaps you were just nervous, or were late for your appointment and ran all the way, or were worrying about a report you had to finish at work. If your pressure had been taken the next day, or even later that same day, it might very well have been normal. But because it is often difficult to determine the cause of an isolated elevated reading, your practitioner may advise you to take it easy until the next visit.

If your blood pressure remains slightly elevated, however, you may be among the 1% to 2% of pregnant women who develop transient high blood pressure during pregnancy. This type of hypertension is perfectly harmless, as far as is known, and disappears after delivery.

What is considered normal blood pressure in pregnancy varies somewhat over the course of nine months. A baseline reading (what is normal for you) is obtained at the first prenatal visit. Generally blood pressure drops a little over the next several months. But as delivery nears, somewhere about the seventh month, it usually begins to rise a bit.

During the first or second trimester, if systolic pressure (the upper number) rises 30 mmHg or the diastolic pressure (the lower number) rises 15 mmHg over the baseline reading, and

stays up for at least two readings taken at least six hours apart, close observation, and possibly treatment, is warranted. In the third trimester, treatment is usually begun only if the rise is greater than that.

If such an increase in blood pressure is accompanied by sudden weight gain (more than 3 pounds in one week in the second trimester, or more than 2 pounds in one week in the third), severe edema (swelling due to water retention), particularly of hands and face, as well as ankles, and/or protein in the urine,[2] the problem may turn out to be preeclampsia (also called pregnancy-induced hypertension—PIH; see page 351). In women who receive regular medical care, this condition is generally diagnosed before it progresses to more serious symptoms, which include blurred vision, headaches, irritability, and gastric pain. If you should experience any of the symptoms of preeclampsia, call your doctor immediately (see page 204).

SUGAR IN THE URINE

"At my last office visit the doctor said that there was sugar in my urine. She said not to worry, but I'm convinced I have diabetes."

Take your doctor's advice—don't worry. A small amount of sugar in the urine on one occasion during pregnancy does not a diabetic make. Your body is probably doing just what it's supposed to do: making sure that your fetus, which depends on you for its fuel supply, is getting enough glucose (sugar).

---

2. See Appendix for an explanation of protein in the urine.

Since it is insulin that regulates the level of glucose in your blood and ensures that enough is taken in by your body cells for nourishment, pregnancy triggers *anti*-insulin mechanisms to make sure enough sugar remains circulating in your bloodstream to nourish your fetus. It's a perfect idea that doesn't always work perfectly. Sometimes the anti-insulin effect is so strong that it leaves more than enough sugar in the blood to meet the needs of both mother and child—more than can be handled by the kidneys. The excess is "spilled" into the urine. Thus your "sugar in the urine"—a not uncommon occurrence in pregnancy, especially in the second trimester, when the anti-insulin effect increases. In fact, roughly half of all pregnant women show some sugar in the urine at some point in their pregnancies.

In most women, the body responds to an increase in blood sugar with an increased production of insulin, which will usually eliminate the excess sugar by the next office visit. This may well be the case with you. But some women, especially those who are diabetic or have tendencies toward diabetes, may be unable to produce enough insulin at one time to handle the increase in blood sugar, or they may be unable to use the insulin they do produce efficiently. Either way, these women continue to show high levels of sugar in both blood and urine. In those who were not previously diabetic, this is known as gestational diabetes.

If sugar appears in your urine at your next visit, your doctor may test your blood for sugar and may order a glucose-tolerance test, a procedure that accurately reflects the body's response to sugar in the bloodstream and identifies individuals with diabetes. Symptoms that may suggest gestational diabetes include excessive hunger and thirst; frequent urination,

even in the second trimester; recurrent vaginal monilial infections; and an increase in blood pressure.

About 1% to 2% (some estimates are as high as 10%) of pregnant women develop this condition—which probably could more appropriately be called "carbohydrate intolerance of pregnancy" rather than the alarming "gestational diabetes"—making it the most common pregnancy complication. Because it is so common, most doctors now screen for it routinely with a blood sugar test between the 24th and 28th weeks of pregnancy. Higher-risk mothers-to-be are screened earlier and more often. Those at higher risk include older mothers (since the tendency toward diabetes increases as we get older) and women with a family history of diabetes mellitus; women with a history of sugar in the urine during pregnancy or of glucose intolerance outside of pregnancy; women who are obese, were large babies themselves (over 9 pounds), or have had one or more large babies previously; and women who have a poor obstetrical history (including previous gestational diabetes, toxemia, repeated urinary tract infection, excessive amniotic fluid, recurrent miscarriage, unexplained stillbirth, or a baby with a congenital anomaly).

Though diabetic mothers-to-be and their fetuses were once at great risk, thanks to modern medicine this is no longer the case. When blood sugar is closely controlled through diet and, if needed, medication, women with diabetes can have normal pregnancies and healthy babies. If you should de-

---

3. Women with abnormal blood glucose but normal glucose-tolerance tests may still be at risk for having large babies and may need to control their diets carefully. If you have an abnormal blood sugar screening, consult your physician.

velop gestational diabetes, see pages 325 and page 350.

Blood sugar abnormalities disappear after delivery in about 97% to 98% of women with gestational diabetes, but some of these women, particularly those who are obese, may develop diabetes later in life. To reduce this risk, those with gestational diabetes should take the following preventive measures: have regular medical checkups, maintain ideal weight, cultivate good diet and exercise habits, and learn the symptoms of the disease so they can be reported promptly to the physician.

ANEMIA

"A friend of mine became anemic during pregnancy. How can I tell if I am, and can I prevent it?"

As blood volume builds during pregnancy, the amount of iron needed for producing red blood cells gradually increases. Because not all pregnant women get the iron they need, nearly 20% become iron-deficient. Fortunately iron-deficiency anemia is easily corrected—in most cases simply by following a varied and nutritious diet and by taking an iron supplement.

A blood test for anemia is administered at the first prenatal visit, but few women turn out to be iron-deficient at this time. Some may have come into pregnancy with the condition (common during the childbearing years because of monthly menstrual blood loss). But with conception and the cessation of menstruation, iron stores—if dietary intake is adequate—are replenished. It isn't until the 20th week (when expanding maternal blood volume and a growing fetus increases the need for iron significantly) that most cases of iron-deficiency anemia develop.

When the iron deficiency is mild, there may be no symptoms; but as oxygen-carrying red blood cells are further depleted, the mother begins to exhibit such symptoms as pallor, extreme fatigue, weakness, palpitations, breathlessness, and even fainting spells. This may be one of the few instances where the fetus's nutritional needs are met before the mother's, since the baby of an anemic mother is rarely iron-deficient at birth. However, there is some evidence, not yet conclusive, that babies of anemic mothers who don't take iron supplements may be at a slightly increased risk of being small or premature.

While all pregnant women are susceptible to iron-deficiency anemia, certain groups are at particularly high risk: those who have had several babies in quick succession, those who are carrying more than one fetus, those who have been vomiting a lot or eating little because of morning sickness, and those who came to pregnancy undernourished and/or have been eating poorly since they conceived. Not surprisingly, low-income women often fall into this last category, making them much more likely than middle- and upper-income women to become anemic.

To prevent iron-deficiency anemia, it is generally recommended that expectant mothers eat a diet rich in iron (see the Iron-Rich Food Selection list, page 92). But because it is difficult to impossible to get adequate iron from dietary sources alone, daily iron supplementation of 30 mg is also usually prescribed (see page 86). Additional supplementation, usually another 30 mg, is recommended when iron-deficiency anemia is diagnosed.

Sometimes, when iron deficiency is ruled out as a cause of anemia in pregnancy, testing may be needed to check for the presence of one of the other types of anemia, such as folic acid deficiency, sickle-cell, or thalassemia.

BREATHLESSNESS

"Sometimes I feel like I am having trouble breathing. Is this because of my pregnancy?"

P robably. Many pregnant women experience a mild breathlessness beginning in the second trimester. Once again, pregnancy hormones are at work. The hormones swell the capillaries of the respiratory tract as they do other capillaries in the body and relax the muscles of the lungs and bronchial tubes as they do other muscles. As pregnancy progresses, another factor comes into play and it becomes more of an effort to take a deep breath because the growing uterus pushes up against the diaphragm, crowding the lungs and making it difficult for them to expand fully. Such breathlessness is normal.

Severe breathlessness, on the other hand, especially when breathing is rapid, lips or fingertips seem to be turning bluish, and/or there is chest pain and rapid pulse, could be a sign of trouble and requires an immediate call to the doctor or trip to the emergency room.

FORGETFULNESS

"Last week I left the house without my wallet; this morning I completely forgot an important business meeting. I can't focus on anything, and I'm beginning to think I'm losing my mind."

Y ou're not alone. Many pregnant women begin to feel that as they're gaining pounds, they're losing brain cells. Even women who pride themselves on their organizational skills, their capacity to deal with complicated issues, and their ability to maintain their composure suddenly find themselves forgetting appoint-

ments, having trouble concentrating, and losing their cool. Fortunately the scatterbrain syndrome (similar to one that many women experience premenstrually) is only temporary. Like numerous other symptoms, it's caused by the hormonal changes wrought by pregnancy.

Feeling tense about this intellectual fogginess will only compound it. Recognizing that it is normal, even accepting it with a sense of humor, may help to ease it. Reducing the stresses in your life as much as possible will also help (see page 113). It just may not be feasible to do as much as efficiently as you did before you took on the added job of baby-making. Taking informal inventory or keeping written checklists at home and at work (and referring to them before leaving home or work) can help contain the mental chaos as well as keep you from making potentially dangerous mistakes (such as forgetting to lock the door or turn off the burner under the tea kettle before leaving the house).

And you might as well get used to working at a little below peak efficiency. The fog may well continue through the early weeks after your baby's arrival (due to fatigue, not hormones) and perhaps may not lift completely until baby is sleeping through the night.

HAIR DYES AND PERMANENTS

"As if the weight I've been putting on hasn't been depressing enough, my hair has started to lose all its body. Is it safe to get a permanent?"

T hough the pregnant belly is the most obvious physical effect a gestating fetus has on its mother, it's by no means the only one. The changes are evident everywhere—

from the palms of the hands (which may temporarily turn a ruddy red) to the inside of the mouth (gums may swell and bleed). The hair is no exception. It can take a turn for the better (as when lackluster hair suddenly takes on a brilliant shine) or for the worse (as when once bouncy hair goes limp).

Ordinarily, a permanent or a body wave would be the obvious answer to hair that has taken a wrong turn, but it isn't during pregnancy. For one thing, hair responds unpredictably under the influence of pregnancy hormones; a permanent might not take at all, or might result in an unflattering frizz instead of bouncy waves. For another thing, the chemical solutions used in permanents are absorbed through the scalp into the bloodstream, raising questions about the safety of their use during pregnancy. So far, studies of the effects of such chemicals on the fetus have been extremely reassuring: no link has been found between the use of permanents and the development of birth defects. But since more study will be necessary before these substances are completely exonerated, the very cautious may wish to stay "straight" until after delivery. Don't be concerned, however, about a permanent you've already had—the risk is only theoretical, and certainly not worth worrying about. (The same can be said for hair relaxers and prescription dandruff shampoos. Avoid using them from now on, but don't worry about any previous use.)

Excellent nutrition may help revive some of your hair's luster; "extra body" shampoos and curling irons may help restore the bounce. But by and large, your hair will probably continue to limp its way through your pregnancy. So, it might make sense to switch to a style that doesn't depend on fullness, such as a very short cut, or one that builds fullness in, such as a blunt cut.

"After I went for my three-month coloring appointment last week, I was horrified to hear from a friend that hair dyes can cause birth defects. What should I do?"

Relax. As with permanents, there has been no solid evidence that hair dyes cause birth defects. Since the risk is only theoretical, there's no point in worrying about applications you've already had. But since it's wise to be extra prudent during pregnancy, at least when that's possible and practical, you might not want to schedule any more appointments until after delivery.

If you're determined to "hide that gray" or those pesty roots and want to be totally cautious at the same time, ask your hairdresser about using pure vegetable colorings.

NOSEBLEEDS AND NASAL STUFFINESS

"My nose has been congested a lot, and sometimes it bleeds for no apparent reason. I'm worried because I know bleeding can be a sign of illness."

Nasal congestion, often with associated nosebleeds, is a common complaint in pregnancy, probably because the high levels of estrogen and progesterone circulating in the body bring increased blood flow to the mucous membranes of the nose, causing them to soften and swell—much as the cervix does in preparation for childbirth.

You can expect the stuffiness to get worse before it gets better—which won't be until after delivery. You may also develop a postnasal drip, which can occasionally lead to nocturnal coughing or gagging. Don't use medication or nasal sprays (unless prescribed by your doctor) to deal with the problem.

The congestion and bleeding are more common in winter, when heating systems force hot, dry air into the house, drying delicate nasal passages. Using a humidifier may help overcome this dryness. You might also try lubricating each nostril with a dab of petroleum jelly.

Taking an extra 250 mg of vitamin C (with your practitioner's approval), in addition to your required vitamin C foods, may help to strengthen your capillaries and reduce the chance of bleeding. (But don't take megadoses of the vitamin.)

Sometimes a nosebleed will follow overly energetic nose-blowing. Correct nose-blowing is an art, which you would do well to master: First gently close one nostril with the thumb, and then carefully blow the mucus out the opposite side. Repeat with the other nostril, continuing to alternate until you can breathe through your nose.

To stem a nosebleed, sit or stand leaning slightly forward, rather than lying down or leaning backward. Press your nostrils together with your thumb and forefinger and hold for five minutes; repeat if the bleeding continues. If the bleeding isn't controlled after three tries, or if the bleeding is frequent and heavy, call your doctor.

ALLERGIES

"My allergies seem to have worsened since my pregnancy began. My nose is runny and my eyes tear all the time."

You may be mistaking the normal nasal stuffiness of pregnancy for allergies. Or, though some fortunate women find temporary relief during this time, pregnancy may have indeed aggravated your allergies. If this is the case, check with your physician to see what you can safely use to relieve any severe symptoms. Some antihista-mines and other medications appear to be relatively safe for use in pregnancy (your usual medication may not be one of these). But, because no tests for safety are absolutely conclusive, drugs should be used only when all else fails. If your nose is very runny, the secretions are thick, or you're sneezing a lot, increase your fluid intake to compensate for any loss and to thin the secretions.

In general, however, the best approach to dealing with allergies in pregnancy is preventive—avoiding the offending substance or substances, assuming you know what they are:

❖ If pollens or other outdoor allergens trouble you, stay indoors in an air-conditioned and air-filtered environment as much as you can during your susceptible season. Wash your hands and face if you've been outdoors, and wear large curved sunglasses to keep pollens from floating into your eyes.

❖ If dust is a culprit, try to have someone do the dusting and sweeping for you. A vacuum cleaner, damp mop, or a damp cloth-covered broom kicks up less dust than an ordinary broom, and an absorbent cloth will do better than a feather duster. Stay away from musty places like attics and libraries full of old books. Have someone pack away dust collectors in your home, such as draperies and rugs.

❖ If you're allergic to certain foods, stay away from them, even if they are good foods for pregnancy. Consult the Best-Odds Diet (page 80) for substitutes.

❖ If animals bring on allergy attacks, let friends know of the problem in advance so that they can rid a room of both pets and their dander before you visit. And of course, if your own pet is suddenly triggering an allergic response, try to keep one or more areas in your home (particularly your bedroom) pet-free.

❖ Tobacco-smoke allergy is easier to control these days, since fewer people smoke and more smokers oblige if they are asked to refrain. To ease your allergy, as well as for the benefit of your baby, you should avoid exposure to cigarette, pipe, and cigar smoke. Don't be embarrassed to say, "Yes, I mind very much if you smoke."

VAGINAL DISCHARGE

"I've noticed a slight vaginal discharge that is thin and whitish. I'm afraid I have an infection."

A thin, milky, mild-smelling discharge (leukorrhea) is normal throughout pregnancy. It's much like the discharge many women have prior to their menstrual periods. Since it increases until term and may become quite heavy, some women are more comfortable wearing sanitary pads during the last months of pregnancy. Do not use tampons, which could introduce unwanted germs into the vagina.

Aside from offending your esthetic sensibilities (and possibly your husband's—who may be turned off oral sex by the unusual taste and odor), the discharge should be of no concern. It is important to keep the genital area clean and dry; cotton, or cotton-crotched, underwear may help to do this. Avoid tight pants, jeans, leotards, and spandex exercise suits. Rinse the vaginal area thoroughly after soaping during a bath or shower, and avoid exposing it to such irritants as deodorant soaps, bubble baths, and perfumes.

Do *not* use a douche unless it is prescribed by your doctor. (Even then, *do not use a bulb syringe,* such as the disposable variety. Use a douche bag or can, and hold it *no higher than 2 feet above the nozzle* to keep the water pressure low. The tip should not be inserted more than 1 inch past the entrance of the vagina, and the labia should be held open, allowing the fluid to run freely out. These precautions should be followed to reduce the risk of introducing air and causing a life-threatening air embolism.)

If you develop a vaginal discharge that is yellowish, greenish, or thick and cheesy, has a foul odor, or is accompanied by burning, itching, redness, or soreness, infection is likely. Notify your doctor or nurse-midwife so that the infection can be treated (probably with vaginal suppositories or gels, ointments, or creams inserted with an applicator). Unfortunately, though medication may banish the infection temporarily, it often returns off and on until after delivery. Though it may require retreatment, simple vaginitis is not cause for worry and does not pose a risk to your baby.

If your vaginitis is caused by a yeast called monilia, your doctor will be careful to treat it with medication so you won't pass the infection on to your baby during delivery (in the form of thrush, a yeast infection of the mouth)—although the infection is not hazardous to the newborn and is easily treated.

You may be able to hasten your recovery and prevent reinfection by maintaining scrupulous cleanliness, especially after going to the bathroom (always wipe from front to back), and by following the Best-Odds Diet— being especially careful to avoid refined sugars, which may help to create a breeding ground for infectious organisms. Recent research indicates that eating 1 cup of yogurt containing live lactobacillus acidophilus cultures (check the label) daily can reduce the risk of vaginal infections dramatically.

If the infection is a sexually transmittable one, avoiding intercourse and any other sexual contact until both you and your spouse are infection-free is generally recommended. Condoms may be suggested for six months after the condition has cleared. To prevent reinfection, care should be exercised to avoid transferring germs from anus to vagina (with fingers, penis, or tongue).

FETAL MOVEMENT

"I haven't felt the baby moving yet; could something be wrong? Or could I just not be recognizing the kicking?"

Fetal movement may be the greatest source of joy in your pregnancy, and lack of it the greatest cause of anxiety. More than a positive pregnancy test, an expanding belly, or even the sound of the fetal heartbeat, the presence of fetal movement affirms that you've got a new life growing inside you. Its absence breeds terror that the new life is not thriving.

Though the embryo begins to make spontaneous movements by the seventh week, these movements do not become apparent to the mother until much later. That first momentous sensation of life, or "quickening," can occur anywhere between the 14th and 26th weeks, but generally closer to the average of the 18th to 22nd week. Variations on that average are common. A woman who's had a baby before is likely to recognize movement earlier (because she knows what to expect and because her uterine muscles are laxer, making it easier to feel a kick) than one who is expecting her first child. A very slender woman may notice very early, weak movements, whereas an overweight woman may not be aware of movements until they've become more vigorous.

Sometimes the first perception of movement is delayed slightly because of a miscalculated due date. Or sometimes it's delayed because a woman has failed to recognize fetal movement when she felt it.

Nobody can tell a first-time mother-to-be exactly what she can expect to feel; a hundred pregnant women may describe that first movement in a hundred different ways. Perhaps the most common descriptions are "a fluttering in the abdomen" and "butterflies in the stomach." But early fetal movements have also been described as "a bumping or nudging," "a twitch," "a growling stomach," "someone hitting my stomach," "a bubble bursting," "the squirmies," "like being turned upside down on an amusement park ride." Often the first noticeable movements are mistaken for gas or hunger pains. And one woman recalls, "I thought a bug was on my shirt, but when I went to brush it off, I realized it was the baby moving."

Although it isn't unusual to be unaware of fetal movements until the 20th week or later, your practitioner may order a sonogram to check on the baby's condition if you haven't felt anything—and he or she hasn't been able to elicit fetal response by prodding—by the 22nd week. If the fetal heartbeat is strong, however, and everything else seems to be progressing normally, the practitioner may hold off even longer on testing.

"I felt little movements every day last week, but I haven't felt anything at all today. What's wrong?"

Anxiety over when the first movement will be felt is often replaced by anxiety that fetal movements don't seem frequent enough, or that they haven't been noticed for a while. At this stage of pregnancy, however, these anxieties, while understandable, are usually unnecessary. The frequency of noticeable movements at this point may vary a great deal; patterns of movement are erratic at best. Though the fetus is stirring almost continuously, only some of these movements are strong enough for you to feel. Others may be missed because of the fetal position (facing and kicking inward, for instance, instead of outward). Or because of your own activity (when you're walking or moving about a lot, your fetus may be rocked to sleep; or it may be awake, but you may be too busy to notice its movements). It's also possible that you're sleeping right through your baby's most active period—which for many babies is in the middle of the night.

One way to elicit fetal movement if you haven't noticed any all day is to lie down for an hour or two in the evening, preferably after a glass of milk or other snack; the combination of your inactivity and the jolt of food energy may be able to get the fetus going. If that doesn't work, try again in a few hours, but don't worry. Many mothers find they don't notice movement for a day or two at a time, or even three or four, before the 20th week. After that time, though there's still no need to panic, it's probably a good idea to call your practitioner for reassurance if 24 hours go by without perceptible fetal activity (assuming, of course, that you've already started feeling movement).

After the 28th week fetal movements become more consistent, and studies show that it's a good idea for mothers to get into the habit of checking fetal activity daily (see page 202).

APPEARANCE

"I get depressed when I look in the mirror or step on a scale—I'm so fat."

In a society as obsessed with slenderness as ours, where those who can "pinch an inch" despair, the weight gain of pregnancy can easily become a source of depression. It shouldn't. There's an important difference between pounds added for no good reason (willpower gone astray) and pounds gained for the best and most beautiful of reasons: your child and its support system growing inside you.

Yet in the eyes of many beholders, a pregnant woman isn't just beautiful inside but outside as well. Many women and their husbands consider the rounded pregnant reflection to be the most lovely—and sensuous—of feminine shapes.

As long as you're eating right and not exceeding the recommended limits for pregnancy weight gain (see page 147), you needn't feel "fat"—just pregnant. The added inches you're seeing are all legitimate byproducts of pregnancy and will disappear soon after the baby is born. If you *are* exceeding the limits, self-defeating depression won't keep you from getting fatter (and may even fuel your appetite), but careful scrutiny of your eating habits might. Remember, however, that dieting to lose or keep from gaining weight during pregnancy is extremely unsafe. Never cut back on the Best-Odds Diet requirements because you're afraid of putting on too much weight.

Watching your weight gain isn't the only way to give your appearance an edge. Wearing clothes that flatter your changing figure will also help; choose from the growing selection of creative maternity styles available instead of trying to squeeze into outfits in your prepregnancy wardrobe (see below).

You'll like your mirror image better, too, if you get an easy-care hairstyle (one that doesn't require a permanent; see page 155), take care of your complexion, and take the time to apply makeup if you ordinarily wear it.

MATERNITY CLOTHES

"I can't squeeze into my baggy jeans anymore, but I dread buying maternity clothes."

There's never been a more fashionable time to be pregnant. Gone are the days when pregnancy wardrobes were limited to dowdy smocks and overblouses. Not only are today's maternity clothes a lot more interesting to look at and practical to wear, but pregnant women can supplement and mix-and-match these specialized purchases with a variety of other items that they can continue to wear even after they get their shape back.

Consider the following when preparing to make your pregnancy fashion statement:

❖ You've still got a way to grow. Don't go on a whirlwind spending spree at the local maternity boutique on the first day you can't button your jeans. Maternity clothes can be costly, especially when you consider the relatively short period of time they can be worn. So buy as you grow, and then buy only as much as you need (once you've checked what you can use that's already in your closet, you may end up needing a lot less than you'd figured). Though the pregnancy pillows available in try-on rooms in maternity stores can give a good indication of how things will fit later, they can't predict how you will carry (high, low, big, small) and which outfits will end up being the most comfortable when you need comfort most.

❖ You're not limited to maternity clothes. If it fits, wear it, even if it isn't from the maternity department. Buying nonmaternity clothing for maternity use (or using items you already own) is, of course, the best way of getting your money's worth. And depending on what the designers are showing in a particular season, anywhere from a few to many of the fashions on the regular racks may be suitable for pregnant shapes. But be wary of spending a lot on such purchases. Though you may love the clothes now, you may love them considerably less after you've worn them throughout your pregnancy; postpartum, the impulse may be great to pack them away like so many maternity clothes.

❖ Your personal sense of style counts when you're pregnant too. If you normally dress in tailored clothes, or casual clothes, don't try to talk yourself into a wardrobe of frilly smocked maternity dresses. Though the novelty of looking the part of the lady-in-waiting may carry you contentedly through a month or two, it's doomed to fizzle out long before you're able to relinquish the maternity clothes, leaving you to face the rest of your pregnancy in clothes you despise.

❖ Accessories deserve a starring role. When you're not pregnant, accessories are a nice touch. When you are pregnant, they're essential. The boost you get from an interesting scarf, an exotic pair of earrings, an electric shade of hosiery, even a bright-colored pair of sneakers, will compensate for a lot of the inevitable fashion compromises expectant mothers have to make.

❖ Among your most important accessories are the ones the public never sees. A well-fitting, supportive bra is vital during pregnancy, when breast expansion generally makes your old bras useless. Bypass the sale racks and put yourself in the hands of an experienced fitter at a well-stocked lingerie department or shop. With any luck, she will be able to tell you approximately how much extra room and support you need and which kind of bra will provide it. But don't stock up. Buy just a couple (one to wear and one to wash), and then go back for another fitting when you start growing out of them.

Special maternity underwear isn't usually necessary and, unless you're used to high-waisted briefs, won't be terribly comfortable. A nice alternative is bikini underwear, bought in a larger than usual size, that you can wear *under* your belly. Buy them in favorite colors and/or sexy fabrics to give your spirits a lift (but make sure crotches are cotton).

❖ A pregnant woman's best friend can be her husband's closet. It's all there for the taking (though it's probably a good idea to ask first): oversized T-shirts and regular shirts that look great over pants or under jumpers (try belting them under the belly for an interesting silhouette), sweatpants that will accommodate more inches than yours will, running shorts that will keep up with your waistline for at least a couple more months, belts with the few extra notches you need.

❖ Both a borrower and a lender be. Accept all offers of used maternity clothes, even if the offerings don't suit your usual style. In a pinch, any extra dress, jumper, or pair of slacks may do—you can make any borrowed item more "yours" with accessories. When your term is over, offer to lend those maternity

outfits you can't or don't want to wear postpartum to newly pregnant friends; between you and your friends, you'll be getting your money's worth from your maternity clothes.

❖ Cool is in. Hot stuff (fabrics that don't breathe, such as nylon and other synthetics) isn't so hot when you're pregnant. Since your metabolic rate is higher than usual, making you warmer, you'll feel more comfortable in cottons. Light colors, mesh weaves, and loose garments will also help to keep you cool. Knee-highs are more comfortable than pantyhose, but avoid those that have a narrow constrictive band at the top. When the weather turns cold, dressing in layers is ideal, since you can selectively peel off as you heat up or when you go indoors.

REALITY OF PREGNANCY

"Now that my abdomen is swelling, the fact that I'm really pregnant has finally sunk in. Even though we planned this pregnancy, I suddenly feel scared, trapped by the baby—even antagonistic toward it."

E ven the most eager of expectant parents may be surprised (and guilt-ridden) to find themselves with second thoughts as their pregnancy starts to become a reality. An unseen little intruder has suddenly come between them, turning their lives upside down, depriving them of freedoms they'd always taken for granted, making more demands on them—both physically and emotionally—than anyone ever has before. Every aspect of the lifestyle they had become accustomed to—from how they spent their evenings, to what they ate and drank, to how often they made love—is being altered by this child even before its birth. And the knowledge that these changes will become still more imposing after delivery compounds their mixed feelings, deepens their apprehension.

Studies show that not only is a little ambivalence, a little fear, even a little antagonism, normal, it's healthy—as long as these feelings are acknowledged and confronted. And now is the best time to do that. Work out any resentments now (over not being free to stay out late on Saturday nights, to pick up and go on a weekend trip when the spirit moves you, to work full time, or to spend your money any way you please), and you won't find yourself venting them at your baby after he or she's arrived. Sharing your feelings with your partner is the best way to do this—and encourage him to do likewise.

Although the lifestyle changes may be greater or lesser, depending on how you and your spouse decide to order your priorities, it's true that your life is never going to be the same again once your "two" becomes "three." But as some parts of your world become more constricted, others will open up. You may find yourself reborn with your baby's birth. And this new life may turn out to be the best yet.

UNWANTED ADVICE

"Now that it's obvious I'm expecting, everyone—from my mother-in-law to strangers on the elevator—has advice for me. It drives me crazy."

Short of taking up a reclusive existence on a desert island, there's no way for a pregnant woman to escape the unsolicited advice of those around her. There's just something about a bulging belly that brings out the "expert" in all of us. Take your morning jog around the park and someone is sure to chide: "You shouldn't be running in your condition!" Lug home

two bags of groceries from the supermarket and you're bound to hear: "Do you think you ought to be carrying such heavy bundles?" Or reach up for a subway strap and you may even be warned: "If you stretch that way the cord will wrap around your baby's neck and strangle it."

Between such gratuitous advice and the inevitable predictions about the sex of the baby, what's an expectant mother to do? First of all, keep in mind that most of what you hear is probably nonsense. Old wives' tales that *do* have foundation in fact have been scientifically substantiated and have become part of standard medical practice. Those that do not, though still tightly woven into the tapestry of pregnancy mythology, can be confidently dismissed. Those recommendations that leave you with a nagging doubt—"What if they are right?"— and are therefore impossible to dismiss are best checked with your doctor, nurse-midwife, or childbirth educator.

Whether it's possibly plausible or obviously ridiculous, however, don't let unwanted advice get your dander up. Neither you nor your baby will profit from the added tension. Instead, keeping your sense of humor handy, you can take one of two approaches: Politely inform the well-meaning stranger, friend, or relative that you have a trusted physician who counsels you on your pregnancy and that you can't accept advice from anyone else. Or, just as politely, smile, say thank you, and go on your way, letting their comments go in one ear and out the other—without making any stops in between.

But no matter how you choose to handle unwanted advice, you'd also do well to get used to it. If there's anyone who attracts a crowd of advice-givers faster than a pregnant woman, it's a woman with a new baby.

WHAT IT'S IMPORTANT TO KNOW:
MAKING LOVE DURING PREGNANCY

Religious and medical miracles aside, every pregnancy begins with the sexual act. So why is it that what got you into this situation in the first place may now have become one of your biggest problems?

Whether sex becomes virtually nonexistent, just a little uncomfortable, or better than ever, almost every expectant couple finds that their sexual relationship undergoes some kind of change during the nine months of pregnancy.

Variations in sexual appetite and response before conception are wide to begin with. What constitutes a satisfying sex life to one couple—"obligatory" relations once a week, for instance—would be completely unsatisfactory for another, for whom once a day might not always be enough. After conception, such variations may be even more exaggerated. And to further complicate matters sexual, physical and emotional upheaval sometimes leaves the once-a-day couple less in the mood for love than the once-a-week couple, and vice versa.

Though there are variations from couple to couple, a general down-up-down pattern of sexual interest during the three trimesters of pregnancy is common. It's not surprising that a diminution of sexual interest may occur early in pregnancy (in one survey, 54% of women reported reduced libido in the first trimester). After all, fatigue, nausea, vomiting, and painfully tender breasts do make less than ideal bedfellows. In women with comfortable first trimesters, however, sexual desire often remains more or less the same. And a sizable minority of expectant women find it increases significantly—often because the hormonal changes of early pregnancy leave the vulva engorged and ultrasensitive, and/or because the heightened breast sensitivity that is painful for other women is pleasurable for them. These women may experience orgasms or multiple orgasms for the first time.

Interest often—but not always—picks up during the midtrimester, when a couple is physically and psychologically better adjusted to the pregnancy. It usually wanes again as delivery nears, even more drastically than in the first trimester—for obvious reasons: first, the bulk of the abdomen is more and more difficult to get around; second, the aches and discomforts of advancing pregnancy are capable of cooling the hottest passion; and third, late in the trimester it's hard to concentrate on anything but that eagerly and anxiously awaited event.

Sexual pleasure, like sexual interest, seems to diminish in some—but certainly not all—couples. In one group of women, only 21% received little or no pleasure from sex before conception. The percentage of these women finding sex not pleasurable rose to 41% at 12 weeks of gestation, and to 59% going into the ninth month. The same study found that at 12 weeks, about 1 in 10 couples were not having sex at all; by the ninth month, more than a third were abstaining. But encouragingly, the study also found that more than 4 in 10 women were still enjoying sex at this point—more than half of these with *no* problems.

So you may find that sex during pregnancy is the best you've ever had. Or something you wish you could enjoy but can't. Or it may become an uncomfortable obligation. You may even abandon it altogether. Normalcy in pregnancy lovemaking, as in so many other aspects of pregnancy, is what is right for you.

UNDERSTANDING SEXUALITY DURING PREGNANCY

U nfortunately, some practitioners are as inhibited about sexuality as the rest of us. Often they don't tell expectant couples what to expect, or not to expect, in the intimate part of their relationship. And that leaves many couples uncertain how to proceed.

Understanding why making love during pregnancy is different than it is at other times can help ease fears and worries, and can make having intercourse (or not having it) more acceptable and more pleasurable.

First of all, there are many physical changes that affect desire and actual sexual pleasure both positively and negatively. Some negative factors can be dealt with to minimize their interference in your sex life; others you may just have to learn to live with—and love with.

Nausea and Vomiting. If your morning sickness stays with you day and night, you may just have to wait its symptoms out. (In most cases, queasiness will start letting up by the end of the first trimester.) If it strikes just at certain hours, keep your schedules flexible, and put the good times to good use. Don't pressure yourself to feel sexy when you're feeling lousy; morning sickness can be aggravated by emotional stress. (See page 104 for tips on minimizing morning sickness.)

Fatigue. This, too, should pass by the fourth month. Until then, make love while the sun shines (when the opportunity presents itself), instead of trying to force yourself to stay up late for romance. If your weekend afternoons are free, cap off a nap with a lovemaking session. (See page 102 for more on easing fatigue.)

The Changing Shape. Making love can be both awkward and uncomfortable when a bulging belly seems to loom as large and forbidding as a Himalayan mountain. As pregnancy progresses, the gymnastics required to scale that growing abdomen may not seem, to some couples, worth the effort. (But there are ways to get around the mountain; see page 169.) In addition, the woman's full-figured silhouette may actually turn off one or both partners. You may be able to psych yourself out of this socially conditioned reflex by thinking: big (in pregnancy) is beautiful.

The Engorgement of Genitals. Increased blood flow to the pelvic area, caused by the hormonal changes of pregnancy, can heighten sexual response in some women. But it can also make sex less satisfying (especially later in pregnancy) if a residual fullness persists after orgasm, leaving a woman feeling as though she didn't quite make it. For the male, too, the engorgement of the pregnant woman's genitalia may increase pleasure (if he feels pleasantly and snugly caressed) or decrease it (if the fit is so tight he loses his erection).

Leakage of Colostrum. Late in pregnancy, some women begin producing the premilk called colostrum. Colostrum can leak from the breasts during sexual stimulation, and it can be disconcerting in the middle of foreplay. It's nothing to worry about, of course, but if it bothers you or your partner, it can easily be avoided by refraining from breast play.

Breast Tenderness. Some fortunate couples revel throughout pregnancy in the fun of full-and-firm-for-the-first-time breasts. But many find that in early pregnancy, the breasts may have to be neglected during love play because they are painfully tender. (Be certain to communicate your discomfort to your partner, rather than suffering, and resenting, his touch in silence.) However, as the tenderness diminishes toward the end of the first trimester, the extreme sensitivity of the breasts enhances sex for some couples.

Alterations in Vaginal Secretions. These secretions increase in volume and change in consistency, odor, and taste. The increased lubrication may make intercourse more enjoyable for a couple if the woman's vagina has always been dry and/or uncomfortably narrow. Or it might make the vaginal canal so wet and slippery that a man may have trouble holding an erection. The heavier scent and taste of the secretions may also make oral sex unpleasant to some men. Massaging scented oils into the pubic area or the inner thighs may help to disguise the problem.

Bleeding Caused by the Sensitivity of the Cervix. The mouth of the uterus also becomes engorged during pregnancy—crisscrossed with many additional blood vessels to accommodate increased blood flow to the uterus—and much softer than before pregnancy. This means that deep penetration can occasionally cause bleeding, particularly late in pregnancy when the cervix begins to ripen for delivery. If this occurs (and threatened miscarriage or any other complications that require abstinence from intercourse are ruled out by your practitioner), simply avoid deep penetration.

There is a full complement of psychological hangups that can interfere with sexual enjoyment during pregnancy. These, too, can be minimized.

Fear of Hurting the Fetus or Causing a Miscarriage. In normal pregnancies sexual intercourse will do neither. The fetus is well cushioned and protected inside the amniotic sac and uterus, and the uterus is securely sealed off from the outside world with a mucous plug in the mouth of the cervix.

Fear That Having an Orgasm Will Stimulate Miscarriage or Early Labor. Although the uterus does contract following orgasm—and these contractions can be quite pronounced in some women, lasting as long as half an hour after intercourse—such contractions are not a sign of labor and pose no danger in a normal pregnancy. However, orgasm, particularly the more intense kind triggered by masturbation, may be prohibited in pregnancies at high risk for miscarriage or premature labor.

Fear That the Fetus Is "Watching" or "Aware." Though a fetus may enjoy the gentle rocking of uterine contractions during orgasm, neither can it see what you're doing nor has it any idea what is happening during intercourse, and your baby will certainly have no memory of it. Fetal reactions (slowed movement during intercourse, then furious kicking and squirming and speeded-up heartbeat after orgasm) are responses solely to hormonal and uterine activity.

Fear That the Introduction of the Penis into the Vagina Will Cause Infection. As long as the male does not have a sexually transmittable disease, there appears to be no danger of infection to either mother or fetus through intercourse during the first seven or eight months—in the amniotic sac, the baby is safe from both semen and infectious organisms. Most physicians believe this is true even during the ninth month—as long as the sac remains intact (the membranes haven't ruptured). But because they could rupture at any time, some suggest that a condom be worn during intercourse in the last four to eight weeks of pregnancy, as added insurance against infection.

Anxiety Over the Coming Attraction. Both the mother- and father-to-be are subject to mixed feelings over the upcoming blessed event; thoughts about the responsibilities and lifestyle changes and the financial and emotional cost of bringing up a baby can inhibit relaxed lovemaking. This ambivalence, which many expectant parents experience, should be confronted and talked through openly rather than being brought to bed.

The Changing Relationship Between Husband and Wife. A couple may have trouble adjusting to the idea that they will no longer be just lovers, or husband and wife, but mother and father as well. After all, many of us still avoid associating our own parents with sex, though we are living proof that such an association exists. On the other hand, some couples may discover that the new dimension in their relationship brings a new intimacy into bed with them—and with it, a new excitement.

Subconscious Hostility. Of the expectant father toward the expectant mother, because he is jealous that she has become the center of attention. Or of mom-to-be toward dad-to-be because she feels she is doing all the suffering (particularly if the pregnancy has been a rough one) for the baby they both want and will both enjoy. Such feelings are important to

talk out, but not in bed.

Belief That Intercourse During the Last Six Weeks of Pregnancy Will Cause Labor to Begin. It *is* true that the uterine contractions triggered by orgasm become stronger as pregnancy proceeds. But unless the cervix is "ripe," these contractions do not appear to bring on labor—as many hopeful and eager overdue couples can attest. However, since no one knows exactly what mechanism initiates labor, and because some studies do show an increase in premature births among couples having intercourse in the last weeks of pregnancy, abstinence is often prescribed for women with a tendency toward preterm delivery.

Fear of "Hitting" the Baby Once the Head Is Engaged in the Pelvis. Even couples who were relaxed about having intercourse earlier can tighten up now because the baby is too close for comfort. Many doctors suggest that though you can't hurt the baby, deep penetration won't be comfortable at this time and should be avoided.

Psychological factors can also affect sexual relations for the better:

Switching from Procreational to Recreational Sex. Some couples who worked hard at becoming pregnant may be delighted at being able to have sex for its own sake—free from thermometers, charts, calendars, and anxiety. For them, sex becomes really enjoyable for the first time in months, or even years.

Though sexual intercourse during pregnancy may be different from what you've experienced before, it is in most cases perfectly safe. In fact, it can be good for you, both physically and emotionally: it can keep you and your spouse close; it can help you get in shape, preparing your pelvic muscles for delivery; and it's relaxing—which is beneficial for everyone concerned, baby included.

WHEN SEXUAL RELATIONS MAY BE LIMITED

Since lovemaking has so much to offer the expectant couple, it would be ideal if every couple could take advantage of it throughout pregnancy. Alas, for some this isn't possible. In high-risk pregnancies, intercourse may be restricted at certain times, or even for nine months. Or, intercourse may be permitted without orgasm for the wife, or petting may be allowed as long as penetration is avoided. Knowing precisely *what* is safe and *when* is essential; if your doctor instructs you to abstain, ask why and whether he or she is referring to intercourse, orgasm, or both, and whether the restrictions are temporary or apply for the entire gestation.

Intercourse will probably be restricted under the following circumstances:

❖ Any time unexplained bleeding occurs.

❖ During the first trimester if a woman has a history of miscarriages or threatened miscarriage, or shows signs of a threatened miscarriage.

❖ During the last 8 to 12 weeks if a woman has a history of premature or threatened premature labor, or is experiencing signs of early labor.

❖ If amniotic membranes (the bag of waters) have ruptured.

❖ When placenta previa is known to exist (the placenta is located near or over the cervix, where it could be prematurely dislodged during intercourse, causing bleeding and threatening mother and baby).

❖ In the last trimester if multiple fetuses are being carried.

ENJOYING IT MORE, EVEN IF YOU'RE DOING IT LESS

Good, lasting sexual relationships —like good, lasting marriages— are rarely built in a day (or even a really terrific night). They grow with practice, patience, understanding, and love. This is true, too, of an already established sexual relationship that undergoes the emotional and physical assaults of pregnancy. Here are a few ways to "stay on top":

❖ Never allow how frequently or infrequently you have intercourse to interfere with other aspects of your relationship. The quality of lovemaking is always more important than the quantity—and never more so than during pregnancy.

❖ Keep the emphasis on love, rather than lovemaking. If one or both of you don't feel like having intercourse, or if intercourse is frustrating because it isn't fully satisfying, find alternative routes to intimacy. The possibilities are far more numerous than positions in a sex manual. For example: old-fashioned kissing and necking, hand holding, back rubs, foot massage, sharing a milkshake in bed (see page 95 for a recipe), reading love poems, watching television while cuddling under the blanket, taking a shower together, going out (or staying in) for a romantic dinner by candlelight, meeting for a quiet lunch—or whatever else makes the lovebird in you coo.

❖ Recognize the possible strains that expectant parenthood may have placed on your relationship, and acknowledge any changes in the intensity of sexual desire that either or both of you may be feeling. Discuss any problems openly; don't sweep them under the bedcovers. If any problems seem too big to handle by yourselves, seek professional help.

❖ Think positive: Making love is good physical preparation for labor and delivery. (Not many athletes have this much fun in training.)

❖ Think of having to try new positions during pregnancy as an adventure. But give yourselves time to adjust to each position you try. (You might even consider a "dry run"—trying out a new position fully clothed first, so that it'll be more familiar when you try it for real.) Usually comfortable positions include: male on top, but off to one side or supported by his arms (to keep his weight off the woman); woman on top (but avoid deep penetration); both partners on their side—front-to-front or front-to-back.

❖ Keep your expectations within reality's reach. Though some women

achieve orgasm for the first time during pregnancy, at least one study showed that most women are less likely to achieve orgasm *regularly* during pregnancy than before conception—particularly in the last trimester, when only 1 out of 4 women reach climax consistently. Your goal doesn't always have to be orgasm; sometimes just physical closeness can satisfy.

❖ If the doctor has ruled out sexual intercourse during any period of your pregnancy, ask if orgasm is okay—via mutual masturbation. If it's taboo for you, you might still get pleasure out of pleasuring your husband in this way.

❖ If the doctor has prohibited orgasm for you but not coitus, you might still be able to enjoy lovemaking without your reaching climax. Though this may not be completely satisfying, it can provide a sense of intimacy. Another possibility: intercourse between the thighs.

Even if the quality, or quantity, of your sexual relations isn't quite what it once was, understanding the dynamics of sexuality during pregnancy can keep the relationship strong—even strengthen it—without spectacular or frequent intercourse.

9
The Fifth Month

WHAT YOU CAN EXPECT AT THIS MONTH'S CHECKUP

This month, you can expect your practitioner to check the following, though there may be variations depending upon your particular needs and upon your practitioner's style of practice:[1]

❖ Weight and blood pressure

❖ Urine, for sugar and protein

❖ Fetal heartbeat

❖ Size and shape of uterus, by external palpation

❖ Height of fundus (top of uterus)

❖ Feet and hands, for edema (swelling), and legs for varicose veins

❖ Symptoms you have been experiencing, especially unusual ones

❖ Questions and problems you want to discuss—have a list ready

WHAT YOU MAY BE FEELING

You may experience all of these symptoms at one time or another, or only a few of them. Some may have continued from last month, others may be new. Still others may hardly be noticed because you've become so used to them. You may also have other, less common, symptoms.

PHYSICALLY:

❖ Fetal movement

❖ Increasing whitish vaginal discharge (leukorrhea)

❖ Lower abdominal achiness (from stretching of the ligaments supporting the uterus)

❖ Constipation

❖ Heartburn, indigestion, flatulence, bloating

---

1. See Appendix for an explanation of the procedures and tests performed.

WHAT YOU MAY LOOK LIKE

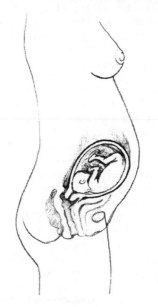

By the end of the fifth month, the activity of this 8- to 10-inch fetus is strong enough to be felt by its mother. Soft downy lanugo covers its body; hair begins to grow on its head; brows and white eyelashes appear. A protective vernix coating covers the fetus.

❖ Occasional headaches, faintness or dizziness

❖ Nasal congestion and occasional nosebleeds; ear stuffiness

❖ "Pink toothbrush" from bleeding gums

❖ Hearty appetite

❖ Leg cramps

❖ Mild swelling of ankles and feet, and occasionally of hands and face

❖ Varicose veins of legs and/or hemorrhoids

❖ Increased pulse (heart rate)

❖ Easier—or more difficult—orgasm

❖ Backache

❖ Skin pigmentation changes on abdomen and/or face

EMOTIONALLY:

❖ An acceptance of the reality of pregnancy

❖ Fewer mood swings, but irritability still occasionally occurs; continued absentmindedness

WHAT YOU MAY BE CONCERNED ABOUT

FATIGUE

"I get tired when I am exercising or doing heavy cleaning; should I stop?"

Not only should you stop when you get tired, you should, whenever possible, stop before then. Exerting yourself to the point of exhaustion is never a good idea. During pregnancy it's a particularly bad one, since overwork takes its toll not only on

you but on the baby as well. Pay careful attention to your body's signals. If you become breathless when you're jogging, or find the vacuum suddenly feels as if it weighs a ton, take a break.

Instead of marathon activity sessions, pace yourself. Work or exercise a bit, rest a bit. Most of the time the work, or the workout, will get done, and you won't feel drained afterward. If occasionally something doesn't get done, you're getting good training for the days when the demands of parenthood will often keep you from finishing what you start. See page 102 for tips on dealing with fatigue.

FAINTNESS AND DIZZINESS

"I feel dizzy when I get up from a sitting or lying-down position. And yesterday I nearly fainted while I was shopping. Am I okay? Can this hurt my baby?"

On late-show movies, a fainting spell is a more reliable indicator of pregnancy than a dead rabbit. Screenwriters in the '40s were, however, off the mark. Though dizziness is fairly common in pregnancy, fainting, also called syncope, is less so. There are a variety of reasons, known or suspected, for a pregnant woman feeling lightheaded or dizzy.

In the first trimester, dizziness may be related to a blood supply that is inadequate to fill the rapidly expanding circulatory system; in the second trimester, it may be caused by the pressure of the expanding uterus on maternal blood vessels. Dizziness can occur anytime you rise from a sitting or prone position. This is called postural hypotension. It's caused by a sudden shifting of blood away from the brain when blood pressure drops rapidly. The cure is simple: Always get up very gradually. Jumping up quickly to answer the phone is likely to land you right back on the sofa.

You might also feel dizzy because your blood sugar is low. Generally this is caused by going too long without food and can be avoided by getting some protein (which helps keep blood sugar level) at every meal and by taking more frequent, smaller meals or eating snacks between your usual mealtimes. Carry a box of raisins, a piece of fruit, or some whole-wheat crackers or breadsticks in your bag for quick blood-sugar lifts.

Dizziness can strike, too, in an overheated store, office, or bus, especially if you are overdressed. The best way to handle such dizziness is to get some fresh air by going outside or opening a window. Taking off your coat and loosening your clothes—especially around the neck and waist—should help, too.

If you feel lightheaded and/or think you are going to faint, try to increase circulation to your brain by lying down, if possible, with your feet (not your head) elevated, or by sitting down with your head between your knees, until the dizziness subsides. If there's no place to lie or sit, kneel on one knee and bend forward as though you were trying to tie your shoelace. Actual fainting is rare, but if you do faint, there is no need for worry or concern—although the flow of blood to your brain is temporarily being reduced, this will not affect your baby.[2]

Tell your practitioner about any dizziness or faintness you experience when you see him or her next. Report actual fainting promptly. Frequent fainting—occasionally a sign of severe anemia or other illness—needs to be evaluated by a physician.

HEPATITIS TESTING

"I'm in my fifth month and my obstetrician just tested me for hepatitis B. Why?"

As a routine precaution, it's now recommended that all women be tested for hepatitis B at least once during their pregnancy, usually late in the second trimester. That's because hepatitis B, unlike hepatitis A, can be passed on to the fetus, almost always during childbirth, though very occa-

---

2. First aid for mothers-to-be who've actually fainted is the same as the preventive measures.

sionally during pregnancy itself. Nearly 9 in 10 infected babies, if untreated, will become chronic carriers of hepatitis B, and are at risk of later developing liver inflammation or more serious liver disease. Routine testing allows doctors to diagnose the disease in infected mothers so that their babies can be treated at birth (see page 318), which almost always prevents the infection from taking hold.

SLEEPING POSITION

"I've always slept on my stomach. Now I'm afraid to. And I just can't seem to get comfortable any other way."

Giving up your favorite sleeping position during pregnancy can be as traumatic as giving up your teddy bear was when you were six. You're bound to lose some sleep over it—but only until you get used to the new position. And the time to get used to it is now, before your expanding belly makes getting comfortable even more difficult.

Two common favorite sleeping positions—on the belly and on the back—are not the best choices during pregnancy. The belly position, for obvious reasons: as your stomach grows, sleeping on it would be about as

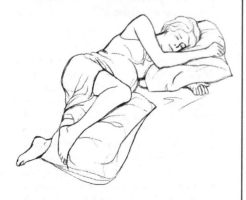

Sleep on your left side.

comfy as sleeping on a watermelon. The back position, though more comfortable, rests the entire weight of your pregnant uterus on your back, your intestines, and the inferior vena cava (the vein responsible for returning blood from the lower body to the heart). This can aggravate backaches and hemorrhoids, inhibit digestive function, interfere with breathing and circulation, and possibly cause hypotension, or low blood pressure.

This doesn't mean you have to sleep standing up. Curling up or stretching out on your side—preferably the left side—with one leg crossed over the other and with a pillow between them, is best for both you and your fetus. It not only allows maximum flow of blood and nutrients to the placenta but also enhances efficient kidney function, which means better elimination of waste products and fluids and less edema (swelling) of ankles, feet, and hands.

Very few people, however, manage to stay in one position through the night. Don't be alarmed if you wake up and find yourself on your back or abdomen. No harm done—just turn back to your side. You may feel uncomfortable for a few nights, but your body will soon adjust to the new position.

BACKACHE

"I'm having a lot of backaches. I'm afraid I won't be able to stand up at all by the ninth month."

The aches and discomforts of pregnancy are not designed to make you miserable. They are the side effects of the preparations your body is making for that momentous moment when your baby is born. Backache is no exception. During pregnancy, the usually stable joints of the pelvis begin to loosen up to allow easier passage for the baby at delivery. This, along with your oversized abdomen, throws your body off balance. To compensate, you tend to bring your shoulders back and arch your neck. Standing with your belly thrust forward—to be sure that no one who passes fails to notice you're pregnant—compounds the problem. The result: a deeply curved lower back, strained back muscles, and pain.

Even pain with a purpose hurts. But without defeating the purpose, you can conquer (or at least subdue) the pain. The best approach, as usual, is prevention: coming into pregnancy with strong abdominal muscles, good posture, and graceful body mechanics. But it's not too late to learn body mechanics that will minimize pregnancy backache. To align your body properly, practice the pelvic tilt, as shown on page 191. The following should also help:

❖ Try to keep weight gain within the recommended parameters (see

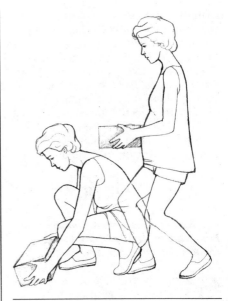

Bend at the knees.

page 147). Excess poundage will only add to the load your back is struggling under.

❖ Don't wear very high heels, or even very flat ones without proper support. Some doctors recommend wide 2-inch heels to help keep the body properly aligned. There are shoes and shoe inserts especially designed to help alleviate leg and back problems during pregnancy; ask your practitioner or a salesperson at a good shoe store.

❖ Learn the proper way to lift heavy loads (packages, children, laundry, books, etc.). Don't lift abruptly. Stabilize your body first by assuming a wide stance (feet shoulder-width apart) and tucking your buttocks in. Bend at the knees, not at the waist, and lift with your arms and legs rather than your back. (See illustration, above.) If backache is a problem, try to limit the carrying you do. If you're forced to carry a heavy load of groceries, divide them between two shopping bags

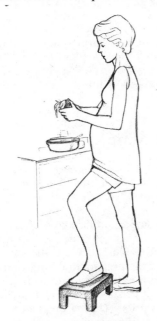

Take an anti-backache position.

and carry one in each arm, rather than carrying the lot in front of you.

❖ Try not to stand for long periods. If you must, keep one foot up on a stool with your knee bent to prevent strain on your lower back. (See illustration, facing page.) When standing on a hard-surfaced floor, as when cooking or washing dishes, put a small skid-proof rug underfoot.

❖ Sit smart. Sitting puts more stress on your spine than almost any other activity, so it pays to do it right. That means sitting, when possible, in a chair that offers adequate support, preferably one with a straight back, arms (use them for assistance when you rise from the chair), and a firm cushion that doesn't allow you to sink down into it. Avoid backless stools and benches. And wherever you're sitting, never cross your legs. Not only can leg crossing promote circulation problems, it can cause you to tilt your pelvis too far forward, aggravating backache. Whenever possible, sit with your legs slightly elevated (see illustration, right); when driving, keep your seat forward so you can keep one knee higher and bent.

Sitting too long can be as bad as sitting the wrong way. Try not to sit for more than an hour without taking a walking/stretching break; setting a half-hour limit would be even better.

❖ Sleep on a firm mattress, or put a board under an overly soft one. A comfortable sleeping position (see page 173) will help minimize aches and pains when you're awake. When getting out of bed in the morning, swing your legs over the side of the bed to the floor, rather than twisting to get up.

❖ Ask your practitioner if a pregnancy girdle or a crisscross support sling for your belly will be helpful in lessening the strain on your lower back.

❖ Don't stretch to put dishes back into the cupboard or to hang a painting. Instead, use a low, steady footstool. Reaching above your head puts a strain on the back muscles.

❖ Use a heating pad (wrapped in a towel) or warm (but not hot) baths to temporarily relieve sore muscles.

❖ Learn to relax. Many back problems are aggravated by stress. If you think yours might be, try some relaxation exercises when pain strikes. Also follow the suggestions beginning on page 113 for dealing with stress in your life.

❖ Do simple exercises that strengthen your abdominal muscles, such as the Dromedary Droop (page 192) and the Pelvic Tilt (page 191).

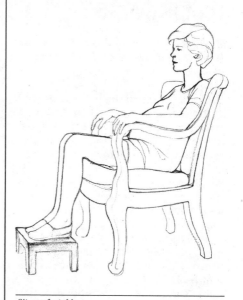

Sit comfortably.

CARRYING OLDER CHILDREN

"I have a 3½-year-old who always wants to be carried up the stairs. But my back is breaking from her weight."

It would be a good idea to break her habit rather than continue breaking your back; the strain of carrying a growing fetus is enough without adding some 30 or 40 pounds of preschooler. Be careful not to blame her sibling-to-be for the change in parental policy, however—blame your back instead. And make much ado about her efforts when she does agree to walk on her own.

Of course there will be times when your child won't take "walk" for an answer. So learn the proper way to lift (see page 174), and be assured that such lifting in no way compromises your unborn baby, unless your practitioner has restricted such strenuous activities.

FOOT PROBLEMS

"My shoes are all beginning to feel uncomfortably tight. Could my feet be growing along with my belly?"

Not growing in the usual sense, but they may indeed be getting larger. First of all there is the swelling, or edema, caused by the normal fluid retention of pregnancy. There may also be extra fat on the feet if your weight gain is excessive. Then there is the spreading of your foot joints (along with all your other joints) as the hormone relaxin sets about its job of loosening up your pelvis for delivery. The swelling in your feet will go down after delivery and the weight will probably be lost. But though the joints will tighten up, it's possible that your feet will be permanently larger—

by as much as a full shoe size.

In the meantime, try the tips for reducing excessive swelling (see page 217) if that seems to be your problem, and get a couple of pairs of shoes that fit you comfortably now—one for walking and working, and one for dress wear. Both should have heels no more than 2 inches high, nonskid soles, and plenty of space for your feet to spread out in (try them on at the end of the day, when your feet are the most swollen); and both should be made of leather or canvas so your feet can breathe. If you choose carefully, you can find not just walking shoes, but dress shoes too, that meet these requirements.

Shoes, or orthotic inserts, that are designed to correct the distorted center of gravity of pregnancy can not only make your feet more comfortable but reduce back and leg pain as well. They are available in two different designs, one to take you through the first six months of pregnancy and the other to take you through the final trimester. Ask your practitioner for a recommendation.

Elasticized slippers worn for several hours a day have also been useful in reducing fatigue and achiness in feet and lower legs, though they don't seem to reduce swelling. If your legs are aching and tired at the end of the day, wearing such slippers while you are at home—or even at work, if that's feasible—may help.

FAST-GROWING HAIR AND NAILS

"It seems to me that my hair and nails have never grown so fast before."

The bounteous circulation and increased metabolism caused by pregnancy hormones is nourishing your skin cells well. Happy effects of this increased nourishment are nails that grow faster than you can manicure them, and hair that grows faster (and if you're really lucky, is thicker and more lustrous) than you can secure appointments with your stylist.

The extra nourishment can, however, also have less happy effects. It can cause hair to grow in places women would rather it didn't. Facial areas (lips, chin, and cheeks) are most commonly plagued with this pregnancy-induced hirsutism, but arms, legs, back, and belly can be affected too. Much of the excess hair disappears within six months postpartum, though some may linger longer.

Though there's no known risk, it's probably not a good idea to use depilatories or bleach cream once you find out you're pregnant. Your skin may not react well to the chemicals, and it's even possible that they may be absorbed into your bloodstream. Plucking facial hair and shaving legs and underarms present no problem.

LATE MISCARRIAGE

"I know they say that once you pass the third month, you don't have to worry about miscarriage. But I know someone who lost her baby in the fifth month."

While it's essentially true that there's little reason to worry about miscarriage after the first trimester, it does occasionally happen that a fetus is lost between the 12th and 20th weeks. This is known as a *late* miscarriage, and accounts for fewer than 25% of all spontaneous abortions; it is rare in an uneventful, low-risk pregnancy. After the 20th week, when the fetus usually weighs over 500 grams (17½ ounces) and there is the possibility that it can survive with specialized care, its delivery is considered a premature birth and not a miscarriage.

Unlike the causes of early miscarriages, which are frequently related to the fetus, the causes of second-trimester miscarriages are usually related to either the placenta or the mother.[3] The placenta may separate prematurely from the uterus, be implanted abnormally, or fail to produce adequate hormones to maintain the pregnancy. The mother may have taken certain drugs, or may have undergone surgery that affected her pelvic organs. Or she may suffer from serious infection, uncontrolled chronic illness, severe malnutrition, endocrine dysfunction, myomas (tumors of the uterus), an abnormally shaped uterus, or an incompetent cervix that opens prematurely. Serious physical trauma, such as that sustained in an accident, appears to play only a small role in miscarriage at any stage in pregnancy.

Early symptoms of a midtrimester miscarriage include a pink vaginal discharge for several days, or a scant brown discharge for several weeks. Should you experience such a discharge, don't panic—it could be nothing serious. But do call your practitioner the day you first notice it. If you have heavy bleeding with or without cramping, call your practitioner immediately or go to the hospital. See page 348 for treatment of threatened miscarriage and prevention of future miscarriages.

ABDOMINAL PAIN

"I'm very worried about the pains I've been getting on the sides of my pelvis."

What you are probably feeling is the stretching of muscles and ligaments supporting the uterus—

---

3. Many maternal causes of late miscarriage can be prevented by good medical care.

something most pregnant women experience. The discomfort may be crampy or sharp and stabbing, and often is most noticeable when you are getting up from a bed or chair, or when you cough. It may be brief, or may last for several hours. As long as the pain is occasional and not persistent—and is not accompanied by fever, chills, bleeding, increased vaginal discharge, faintness, or other unusual symptoms—there's no cause for concern. Getting off your feet and resting in a comfortable position should bring some relief. You should, of course, mention the pain to your practitioner at your next visit.

CHANGES IN SKIN PIGMENTATION

"I have a dark line down the center of my abdomen and dark spots on my face. Is this discoloration normal, and will it remain after pregnancy?"

Once again those pregnancy hormones are at work. Just as they caused the darkening of the areolas around your nipples, they are now responsible for the darkening of the *linea alba*—the white line you probably never noticed—which runs down the center of your abdomen to the top of your pubic bone. During pregnancy, it's renamed the *linea nigra,* or black line.

Some women, usually those with darker complexions, also develop discolorations in a mask-like configuration on foreheads, noses, and cheeks. The patches are dark in light-skinned women and light in dark-skinned women. This mask of pregnancy, or chloasma, will gradually fade after delivery. In the meantime, bleaching probably won't lighten chloasma (and is not a good idea anyway), though cover-up makeups may camouflage it.

Sun can intensify the coloration, so use a sun block with a sun protection factor (SPF) of 15 or more when outdoors in sunny weather, or wear a hat that completely shades your face. Since there is some evidence that the excess pigmentation may be related to folic acid deficiency, be sure that your vitamin supplement contains folic acid and that you are eating green leafy vegetables, oranges, and whole-wheat bread or cereal daily.

Hyperpigmentation (darkening of the skin) may occur in high-friction areas, such as between the thighs. This, too, will fade after delivery.

OTHER STRANGE SKIN SYMPTOMS

"My palms seem to be red all the time. Is it my imagination?"

No, and it isn't your dishwashing liquid, either. It's your hormones. Increased levels of pregnancy hormones cause red, itchy palms (and sometimes red, itchy soles of the feet) in two-thirds of white and one-third of black pregnant women. The dishpan look will disappear soon after delivery.

Your nails may not escape pregnancy unscathed either. You may find they are more brittle or soft, and have developed grooves. Nail polish may make them worse. If they show signs of infection, ask your practitioner about treatment.

"My legs and feet turn bluish and blotchy sometimes. Is something wrong with my circulation?"

Due to stepped-up estrogen production, many women experience this kind of transitory, mottled discoloration when they're chilly. It is insignificant, and will disappear post-partum.

"I've developed a tiny, floppy growth of skin under my arm at the bra line. I'm worried that it could be skin cancer."

What you're describing is probably a skin tag, another benign skin problem common in pregnant women and often found in high-friction areas, such as under the arms. Skin tags frequently develop in the second and third trimesters and may regress after delivery. If they don't, they can be easily removed by your physician.

To be sure of the diagnosis, show it to your practitioner at your next visit.

"I seem to have broken out in a heat rash. I thought only babies got that."

Actually, anyone can develop a heat rash. But it is particularly common in pregnant women because of the increase in eccrine perspiration, the kind that comes from sweat glands that are distributed over the entire body surface and that are involved in heat regulation. Patting on some cornstarch after your shower and trying to keep as cool as possible will help minimize discomfort from the rash, as well as help prevent it in the future.

On the plus side, apocrine perspiration, the kind produced by glands under the arms, under the breasts, and in the genital area, diminishes in pregnancy—so though you may have heat rash you are less likely to have body odor.

DENTAL PROBLEMS

"My mouth has suddenly become a disaster area. My gums bleed every time I brush, and I think I have a cavity. But

I'm afraid to go to the dentist because of the anesthesia."

With so much of your attention centered on your abdomen during pregnancy, it's easy to overlook your mouth—until it begins to scream for equal time, which it frequently does because of the heavy toll a normal pregnancy can take on the gums. The gums, like the mucous membranes of the nose, become swollen, inflamed, and tend to bleed easily because of pregnancy hormones.

It's best not to wait until your mouth is hollering for help. If you suspect a cavity or other incipient trouble, make an appointment right away. Sometimes there's actually more risk to the fetus in putting off necessary dental work than there is in having it done. For example, badly decayed teeth that are not taken care of can be a source of infection that spreads throughout the system, putting both mother and fetus in danger. Impacted wisdom teeth that are either infected or causing severe pain should also be attended to promptly.

However, special precautions must be taken when dental work is done during pregnancy to ensure that the supply of oxygen to the fetus is not compromised through the use of general anesthetics, and that no anesthetic is used that is known to cause harm to a fetus. In most cases a local anesthetic will suffice. If a general anesthetic is absolutely required, then it should be administered by an experienced anesthesiologist. Discuss the anesthesia with both your dentist and your physician beforehand to ensure safety. Check with your physician to see if an antibiotic will be needed prior to or at the time of dental work.

If after the dental work you're left with chipmunk cheeks and can't chew solids, you're going to have to make some dietary alterations. On a fluid-only diet you can obtain adequate nutrients temporarily by sipping milkshakes (see Double-the-Milk Shake, page 95). Supplement the shakes with citrus juices (if they don't burn your gums) and homemade "creamed" soups made from cooked vegetables puréed with cottage cheese, yogurt, or skim milk. Once you can manage soft foods, add puréed vegetables and meats, scrambled eggs, unsweetened yogurt, apple sauce, mashed bananas, mashed potatoes, and creamy cooked cereals enriched with nonfat dry milk.

Of course, for all dental difficulties the best treatment is prevention. Following a program of preventive dental care throughout pregnancy—and preferably throughout life—will avert most dental problems:

❖ Make an appointment with your dentist at least once during the nine months for a checkup and cleaning—once each trimester may be even better. The cleaning is important to remove plaque, which can not only increase the risk of cavities but also make your gum problems worse. Avoid x-rays unless they are absolutely necessary, and then take the special precautions suggested on page 66. Routine repair work requiring anesthesia should be postponed, because even a local anesthetic can enter your bloodstream and reach the fetus. If you've had gum problems in the past, you should also see your periodontist during your pregnancy.

❖ Follow the Best-Odds Diet, eating little or no refined sugar, particularly between meals (also avoid dried fruit between meals), and plenty of foods high in vitamin C. Sugar contributes to both decay and gum disease; vitamin C strengthens gums, reducing the possibility of bleeding. Also be sure to fill your calcium requirements daily (see page 85). Calcium is needed throughout life to keep teeth and bones strong and healthy.

❖ Floss and brush regularly, according to your dentist's prescription. (If your dentist does not instruct you in such preventive measures, you are probably going to the wrong dentist.)

❖ To further reduce bacteria in the mouth, brush your tongue when you brush your teeth. This will also help keep your breath fresh.

❖ When you're not near a faucet and a toothbrush after eating, chewing on a stick of sugarless gum or nibbling on a chunk of cheese or a handful of peanuts (all seem to have antibacterial cleansing capabilities) can stand in temporarily for a thorough brushing.

"I found a nodule on the side of my gum that bleeds every time I brush my teeth."

What you discovered is probably a pyogenic granuloma, which can appear on the gum or elsewhere on the body. Though it bleeds easily and is also known by the ominous-sounding term "pregnancy tumor," it is perfectly harmless. If it becomes extremely annoying, it can be removed surgically. If it isn't removed, it usually regresses on its own after delivery.

TRAVEL

"Is it safe for me to go ahead with the vacation my husband and I had planned for this month?"

For most women, travel during the midtrimester is not only safe but the perfect chance to get away with their husbands for a last fling (at least for a while) as a twosome. And with no diapers, no bottles, no jars of messy baby food to worry about, it'll certainly never be as easy to vacation with your baby again.

Of course you will need your doctor's permission; if you have high blood pressure, diabetes, or other medical or obstetrical problems, you may not get the green light. (That doesn't mean you can't vacation at all. If you can't travel, pick a hotel or resort within an hour's drive of your doctor's office—and enjoy!) Even in a low-risk pregnancy, traveling a great distance isn't a terrific idea in the first trimester, when the possibility of miscarriage is greatest and when your body is still making its initial physical and emotional adjustment to pregnancy. Likewise, long-distance travel is usually not recommended in the last trimester because, should labor begin early, you would be far from your doctor and hospital.

Travel to areas at high altitudes isn't recommended at any time during pregnancy, since adjusting to the decrease in oxygen may be too taxing for both mother and fetus. If you must make such a trip, you should plan on limiting exertion for several days after arrival to minimize the risk of developing acute mountain sickness (AMS).[4] If you are in your last trimester, your doctor may recommend you have a nonstress test on arrival at your destination and then daily for the next two days, then semi-weekly. Any signs of fetal distress will probably warrant the administration of oxygen and a return to a lower altitude.

Other inappropriate destinations are developing regions of the world for which vaccinations would be necessary, since some vaccines may be hazardous during pregnancy. Not insignificantly, these same locales may be hotbeds of certain potentially dangerous infections for which there are no vaccines—another reason to avoid them.

Once you have your doctor's permission, you will only need to do a little planning and take a few precautions to ensure a safe and *bon* voyage for you and your baby:

Plan a Trip That's Relaxing. A single destination is preferable to a Grand Tour that takes you to nine cities in six days. A trip on which you set the pace is a lot better than a group tour that sets it for you. A few hours of sightseeing or shopping should be alternated with time spent sitting reading, relaxing, or napping.

Take Your Best-Odds Diet with You. You may be on vacation, but your baby is working as hard as ever at growing and developing, and has the same nutritional requirements he or she always has. Total self-sacrifice isn't required at mealtimes, but prudence is. Order thoughtfully and you will be able to savor the local cuisine while also fulfilling your baby's requirements. (See Eating Out Best-Odds Style, page 184.) Don't skip breakfast or lunch in order to save up for a lavish dinner.

Don't Drink the Water if you're traveling to a foreign country, unless you're certain it's safe. (But do substitute fruit juices and bottled water to get your daily fluids.) In some regions, it may not be safe to eat raw unpeeled fruits or vegetables. For complete information on such restrictions, on other foreign health hazards, and on immunizations for travel, contact the American College of Obstetricians and Gynecologists, One East Wacker Drive, Chicago, IL 60601.

---

4. Symptoms of AMS include: lack of appetite, nausea, vomiting, flatulence, restlessness, headache, lassitude, shortness of breath, scanty urine, and psychological changes.

Pack a Pregnancy Survival Kit. Make sure you take enough vitamins to last the trip; packets of dry skimmed milk if you think you won't be able to find fresh milk; a small jar of wheat germ to enrich white bread or cereal in case whole-grain versions aren't available; medication for traveler's stomach *prescribed by your doctor;* your favorite pregnancy book for reference; comfortable shoes roomy enough to accommodate feet swelled by long hours of sightseeing; and a spray disinfectant in case you have to sanitize a public toilet.

Have the Name of a Local Obstetrician Handy, just in case. Your doctor may be able to provide you with one. If not, contact the local medical association in the city you're traveling to or the International Association for Medical Assistance to Travelers, Suite 5620, Empire State Building, 350 Fifth Avenue, New York, NY 10001—which will, for a small donation, provide you with a directory of English-speaking physicians throughout the world. Some major hotel chains can also provide you with this kind of information. If for any reason you find yourself in need of a doctor in a hurry and can't find one, call the nearest hospital or head for its emergency room.

Carry a Medical History. It is always wise, but particularly when you're pregnant, to travel with a medical information card listing your blood type, medications you're taking and/or are allergic to, and any other pertinent medical data, along with your doctor's name, address, and telephone number. Tuck an extra prescription for each medication you are taking into your passport folder, in case your bags and medication are lost—temporarily or permanently—en route. You may have to have a prescription you've brought from home cosigned by a local doctor; often a doctor at a hospital emergency room will agree to do the honors.

Head Off Traveler's Irregularity. Changes in schedule and diet can compound constipation problems. To avoid this, make sure you get plenty of the three most effective constipation-combators: fiber, fluids, and exercise. (See Constipation, page 135.) It may also help to eat breakfast a little early, so you'll have time to use the bathroom before you set out for the day.

When You've Got to Go, Go. Don't encourage urinary tract infection or constipation by postponing trips to the bathroom. Go as soon as you feel the urge.

Get the Support You Need. Support hose, that is. Particularly if you already suffer from varicose veins—but even if you only suspect you may be predisposed to them—wear support hose when you'll be doing a lot of sitting (in cars, planes, trains, for example) and when you'll be doing a lot of standing (in museums, on lines).

Don't Be Stationary While on the Move. Sitting for long periods can restrict the circulation in your legs, so be sure to get up and walk at least every hour or two when you are on a plane or train. When traveling by automobile, don't go for more than two hours without stopping for a stretch. While you're sitting, do the simple exercises described on page 194.

If You're Traveling by Plane: Check with the airline in advance to see if it has special regulations concerning pregnant women (many airlines do). Arrange ahead of time for a seat in the front of the plane (preferably on the aisle, so you can get up and stretch or use the restroom as needed), or if seating is not reserved, ask for preboarding. *Do not fly in an unpressur-*

ized cabin. All commercial jets are pressurized; but small private or feeder airline planes may not be, and pressure changes at high altitudes may rob you—and your baby—of oxygen.

When booking your flight, ask about the special meals available and order one that provides a good protein serving along with a whole-grain bread, if it's available. On some airlines, low-cholesterol, ovo-lacto vegetarian, or seafood meals provide more of the Daily Dozen than do the regular menu selections. Drink plenty of water, milk, and fruit juice to counter the dehydration caused by air travel, and bring along whole-grain crackers or bread sticks, individually wrapped packets of cheese, raw vegetables, fresh fruit, and other healthful snacks to supplement the airline meal.

Wear your seat belt comfortably fastened below your abdomen. If you're traveling to a different time zone, take jet lag into account. Rest up in advance, and plan on taking it easy for a few days once you arrive. It may also help to try to gradually switch yourself to the time zone you're headed for by moving meal- and bedtimes forward or back, and once you've arrived, by exposing yourself to bright outdoor-like light during the time you would ordinarily be asleep at home.

If You're Traveling by Car: Keep a bagful of nutritious snacks and a thermos of juice or milk handy for when hunger strikes. For long trips, be sure the seat you will occupy is comfortable; if it isn't, consider buying or borrowing a special back-supporting cushion, available in auto supply stores and through some catalogs. A neck support pillow may also add to your comfort. If you aren't behind the wheel, set your seat as far back as possible to give your legs maximum stretching space. And of course keep your seat belt fastened at all times (see page 186).

If You're Traveling by Train: Check to be sure there's a dining car with a full menu. If not, bring adequate meals and snacks along. If you're traveling overnight, arrange for a sleeper. You don't want to start your vacation exhausted.

EATING OUT

"I try hard to stay on a proper diet, but with a business lunch nearly every day, it seems impossible."

For most pregnant women it isn't substituting mineral water for martinis that poses a challenge at business lunches (or when dining out after hours); it's trying to put together a meal that's nutritionally sound from a menu of cream sauces, elegant but empty starches, and tempting sweets. But with the following suggestions, it is possible to take the Best-Odds Diet out to lunch or dinner:

❖ Push away the breadbasket unless it's filled with whole-grain choices (make an exception if you're unhealthily hungry and no other sustenance is on the near horizon). Be aware that "dark" breads, such as pumpernickel or dark rye, may get their wholesome-looking color from caramel color or molasses rather than from whole grains.[5] Be sure that you tally the butter or margarine you spread on your bread into your daily fat allowance;

---

5. The occasional serving of white pasta, white rice, or white bread won't diminish the odds in your Best-Odds Diet, but frequent servings of such foods will. If that's all you can get when eating out, and you eat out frequently, carry a small flask of toasted wheat germ (you *can* develop a taste for it) and sprinkle some on these depleted foods to bring them closer to the way they were meant to be. Or bring along your own whole-grain roll or bread.

Eating Out, Best-Odds Style

❖ **Best** restaurants are seafood, American, continental, and steak houses where broiled, grilled, or poached fish, poultry, and lean cuts of meat are served, along with simply prepared fresh vegetables, salads, and potatoes.

Another excellent choice, if your stomach isn't too out of sorts for spices, is an Indian restaurant, where wholesome, protein-rich baked and roasted entrées (often marinated in yogurt) are served alongside vegetables and salads (also often made with yogurt), whole-grain Indian breads, which are sometimes stuffed with vegetables, and vegetable curries. (Vegetarians can easily make a high-protein meal out of the lentil, pea, chickpea, and cheese vegetarian selections.)

A new entry in the Best category are health food establishments and restaurants of any stripe that, heeding currently accepted dietary guidelines, limit fat, sugar, and excess sodium in some or all of their dishes (or at least are willing to do so on request); offer whole-grain breads, rice, and pasta; use olive oil or polyunsaturated vegetable oil rather than other less healthful shortenings; and emphasize fresh salads and vegetables.

❖ **Next Best** are ethnic restaurants where meats, fish, and poultry are featured. Included in this group are Italian eateries, if cream-based pasta sauces are eschewed for lighter ones (such as marinara or a tomato primavera), or fish, chicken, and veal entrées and fresh vegetables (arugula, spinach, kale, broccoli rabe) are chosen; French nouvelle (lighter than classic French), though sauces should still be ordered on the side; Cajun, or Louisiana-style, if you stick with boiled, steamed, broiled, and grilled fish or seafood and hearty seafood/poultry/vegetable stews such as jambalayas (but easy on the white rice); Jewish, if you avoid fatty meats (and those deli specials laced with nitrates), gravies, superfluous starches, rye bread, and salty pickles; and Greek or Middle Eastern, if you order baked or grilled fish, meats, and poultry accompanied by bulgur wheat or brown rice.

Chinese restaurants are fast securing a Next Best rating, as more and

---

when spreading, keep in mind that there may be other fats in your meal (for example, salad dressing and buttered vegetables).

❖ Order salad as a first course, and ask for the dressing (or plain oil and vinegar) on the side so you can stay within the Best-Odds Diet guidelines for fat intake. Other good first-course choices include fresh mozzarella and tomatoes, shrimp cocktail, and grilled or marinated vegetables.

❖ If you're ordering soup, opt for a clear consommé or broth, or a vegetable-, milk-, or yogurt-based soup. Generally steer clear of cream soups (unless you know they're made with milk).

❖ Select a high-protein, low-fat main course. Fish, chicken, and veal are usually the best bets, as long as they're broiled, grilled, or poached and not fried or bathed in butter or rich sauces. If everything comes with a sauce, ask for yours on the more offer brown rice, "light" or steamed preparations that don't contain whopping amounts of soy sauce, and the option of ordering dishes without MSG (but steer clear of deep-fried and high-sugar sweet-and-sour dishes). An abundance of tofu dishes makes Chinese restaurants a "Best" bet for vegetarians.

Mexican and Spanish restaurants that feature lighter cuisine, prepare foods with vegetable oil rather than lard, and include vegetables on their menus (a bowl of gazpacho can do it all) can also provide a Next-Best meal; they're in the Best category for vegetarians, who can get plenty of protein and calcium from corn enchiladas stuffed with cheese and beans.

Also Next Best, particularly for lunches, are delis (if you avoid cold cuts and stick with a tuna, egg, chicken, or chef's salad, or a tuna, egg, chicken, turkey, or roast beef sandwich on whole-wheat bread with lettuce and tomato and a side of cole slaw); coffee shops, where you can get everything from broiled fish to salads to poached eggs to sandwiches on whole-wheat bread; some fast-food restaurants, specifically those that offer salad bars or other healthier menu selections; and traditional health food and vegetarian restaurants (these are "Best" for vegetarians, of course, and many of the more modern ones fall into the "Best" category for everyone), where you can get a wholesome meal as long as you're careful not to overdose on fat or fall short on protein.

❖ **Least Best** restaurants to frequent during pregnancy include: Japanese, since sushi, like all uncooked fish and meat, is completely taboo, tempura is deep-fried, and sukiyaki and teriyaki dishes are heavy on the soy sauce (which is extremely high in sodium); German, Russian, and Middle European, where empty calories lurk in breading, deep-frying fat, dumplings, and gravies, and excesses of fat and nitrates are found in sausages and wursts; Southern, where vats of deep-frying fat dominate the kitchens, vegetables are overcooked, usually in pork fat, and whole grains are unheard of; and fast-food restaurants that don't offer salad bars or other healthy options (see page 128).

A very occasional dining-out indiscretion won't upset the odds of the Best-Odds Diet. But frequent ones may—so diner beware.

side. Often chefs will accommodate a request for fish broiled with little or no fat. If you're a vegetarian, scan the menu for tofu, beans and peas, cheeses, and combinations of these. A vegetable lasagne, for example, might be a good choice in an Italian restaurant, bean curd and vegetables in a Chinese one.

❖ As side dishes, white or sweet potatoes (in any form but fried, heavily buttered, or candied), brown rice, kasha or groats, pasta, legumes (dried beans and peas), and lightly cooked fresh vegetables are all appropriate.

❖ Desserts should, except on special occasions, be limited to unsweetened and unliqueured fresh or cooked fruits and berries (with a dollop of whipped cream, if you like). An occasional swirl of frozen yogurt or scoop of ice cream is okay, too. If you crave something more, take a couple of bites of a dining companion's dessert. Indulge in juice-sweetened treats when you get home; see pages 93 to 98 for recipes, or try some of the numerous commercially available varieties.

WEARING A SEAT BELT

"Is it safe to fasten my seat belt in the car or on an airplane?"

What's the major cause of death among women of childbearing age? Toxemia? Childbirth? Postpartum infection? Actually, none of the above. The most common way for a young woman to lose her life is in an auto accident. And the best way to avoid such a fatality—as well as serious injury to you and your unborn child—is to always buckle up. Statistics prove conclusively that it is a lot safer to fasten your seat belt than not to fasten it.

For maximum safety and minimum discomfort, fasten the belt below your belly, across your pelvis and upper thighs. If there is a shoulder harness, use it over your shoulder and diagonally across your chest, *not* under your arms. And don't worry that the pressure of the belt in a short stop will hurt the baby—he or she is well cushioned by amniotic fluid.

SPORTS

"I like to play tennis and swim. Is it safe to continue?"

Keeping fit is certainly recommended for anyone; the pregnant woman is no exception. And in most cases, pregnancy doesn't mean giving up the sporting life—just remembering you are carrying a new life and practicing a little extra common sense and moderation. Most practitioners permit patients whose pregnancies are progressing normally to continue participating in sports they are proficient at for as long as is practical—but with several caveats. Among the most important: "Never exercise to the point of fatigue." (See Exercise During Pregnancy, page 189 for more information.)

VISION

"My eyesight seems to be deteriorating since I got pregnant. And my contacts don't seem to fit anymore. Am I imagining it?"

No, chances are you really aren't seeing as well as you were pre-pregnancy. Your eyes are just another of the seemingly unrelated body parts that can fall prey to pregnancy hormones. Not only can your vision seem less sharp, but hard contact lenses, if you wear them, may suddenly no longer feel comfortable. And though these eye effects, which are probably related to fluid retention, are temporary, they can be annoying.

Your vision should clear up after delivery, and your eyes return to normal. Since being refitted for new hard lenses during pregnancy doesn't make financial sense, you might consider switching to glasses or soft contacts, if that's possible, until you deliver.

Though a slight deterioration in visual acuity is not unusual in pregnancy, other symptoms could signal a problem. If you experience blurring, dimming, spots or floaters, or double vision that persists for more than two or three hours, don't wait any further for it to pass; call your practitioner at once.

A LOW-LYING PLACENTA

"The doctor said my sonogram showed that the placenta was down near the cervix. He said that it was too early to worry about it now; when should I start worrying?"

L ike a fetus, a placenta can do a lot of moving around during pregnancy. It doesn't actually pick up and relocate, but it does appear to migrate upward as the lower segment of the uterus stretches and grows. Though an estimated 20% to 30% of placentas are in the lower segment in the second trimester (and an even larger percentage before 20 weeks), the vast majority move into the upper segment by the time delivery nears. If this doesn't happen and the placenta remains low in the uterus, a diagnosis of "placenta previa" is made. This complication occurs in only about 1%, or less, of full-term pregnancies. And in only 1 out of 4 of these cases is the placenta located low enough—partially or completely covering the os, or mouth of the uterus—to cause a serious problem.

So as you can see, your doctor is right. It's too early to worry—and statistically speaking, the chances are slim that you'll ever have to worry. If a sonogram still shows a low-lying placenta once you're well into your eighth month, read about placenta previa on page 356.

OUTSIDE INFLUENCES IN THE WOMB

"I have a friend who insists that taking her unborn baby to concerts will make him a music lover, and another one whose husband reads to her tummy every night to give their baby a love of literature. Isn't this all nonsense?"

I n the study of the unborn, it's getting harder and harder to distinguish between nonsense and fact. And while there's plenty of pure nonsense out there, scientists are coming to believe that some of these apparently outlandish theories may turn out to have a basis in fact. Still, much more research needs to be done before anyone can answer your question with certainty.

Because the ability to hear is quite well developed in the fetus by the end of the second trimester or the beginning of the third, it's true that your friends' babies are hearing the music and the readings. What that will mean in the long run isn't really clear. Some researchers in the field believe that it is actually possible to stimulate the fetus prior to birth to produce, in a sense, a "super baby." At least one has claimed to turn out babies who can speak at six months and read at a year and a half, by exposing the fetus to increasingly complex rhythmic imitations of a mother's heartbeat. Others question the wisdom of tampering with nature in this way, believing that it could, in the long run, be harmful.

Certainly, anyone who understands child development should be very wary of trying to create a super baby, either before birth or after it. It's much more important for a baby to be taught that he or she is loved and wanted than to be taught how to speak and read.

That isn't to say that attempting to make contact with your baby before birth, and even reading to it or playing music for it, is either harmful or a waste of time. Any kind of prenatal communication may give you a head start on the long process of parent-baby bonding. This may not necessarily translate into more closeness as your baby gets older, but it may make those earliest days easier.

Of course, if you feel silly talking to your bloated abdomen, you needn't

Carrying Baby, Fifth Month

Here are just three of the very different ways that a woman may carry near the end of her fifth month. The variations on these are endless. Depending on your size, your shape, the amount of weight you've gained, and the position of your uterus, you may be carrying higher, lower, bigger, smaller, wider, or more compactly.

worry that your baby will miss out on getting to know you. He or she is getting used to the sound of your voice—and probably that of your spouse's, too—every time you talk to each other or someone else. That's why so many newborns seem to recognize their parent's voices. They may even be familiar with other sounds that are common in their mother's surroundings. Whereas a newborn who had little prenatal exposure to a barking dog may startle at hearing the sound, one who's heard a lot of barking won't even blink.

Exposure to music, too, may have some impact on the fetus. There have been reports that some fetuses have shown a preference (by a change in their movements) for certain types of music—usually the gentler kind. And reports that playing a certain piece (in the study, it was one by Debussy) over and over for the fetus at times when both mother and fetus were tranquil has resulted in the baby later seeming to like the piece, and to quiet down and be soothed upon hearing it. Of course, most experts would agree that exposing a baby to good music after he or she is born is probably a lot more significant in the creation of a music lover than exposing a fetus in utero.

It's also been suggested that, since the sense of touch is also already developed in the uterus, stroking your abdomen and "playing" with a little knee or bottom when it's pushed up may also help parent-child bonding— and whether this is true or not, there's certainly no harm in trying. Of course, it's unlikely that you'll need to make a conscious effort to touch your baby more; even strangers can hardly keep their hands off a pregnant belly.

So enjoy making baby contact now, but don't worry about teaching facts or imparting information—there'll be plenty of time for that later. As you'll soon discover, children grow up all too soon anyway. There's no need to rush the process, particularly before birth.

MOTHERHOOD

"Will I be happy with the baby once I have it?"

Most people approach any major change in their lives—marriage, a new career, or an impending birth— wondering whether it will be a change they'll be happy with. And if they start out with unrealistic expectations, they may very well end up disappointed. If your visions of motherhood consist of nothing but leisurely morning walks through the park, sunny days at the zoo, and hours coordinating a wardrobe of miniature, sparkling clean clothes, you're in for a heavy dose of reality shock. There'll be many mornings that will turn into evenings before you and your baby ever have the time to see the light of day, many sunny days that will be spent largely in the laundry room, and few tiny outfits that will escape unstained by spit-up puréed bananas and baby vitamins. And if you have images of bringing a cooing, enchanting Gerber baby home from the hospital, you are headed for certain postpartum disillusionment. Not only won't your newborn be smiling or cooing for many weeks, he or she may hardly communicate with you at all, except to cry—most notably when you're sitting down to dinner or starting to make love, have to go to the bathroom, or are so tired you can't move.

What you *can* expect realistically, however, are some of the most wondrous, miraculous experiences of your life. The fulfillment you will feel when cuddling a warm, sleeping bundle of baby (even if that cherub was a colicky devil moments before) is incomparable. That—along with that first toothless smile meant just for you—will be well worth all the sleepless nights, delayed dinners, mountains of laundry, and frustrated romance.

Can you expect to be happy with your baby? Yes, as long as you expect a real baby and not a fantasy.

WHAT IT'S IMPORTANT TO KNOW: EXERCISE DURING PREGNANCY

Executives do it. Senior citizens do it. Doctors, lawyers, and construction workers do it. If they do it, pregnant women wonder, shouldn't we?

"It," of course, is exercise. And the answer for most women with normal pregnancies seems to be: yes. The

Basic Position and Kegel Exercises

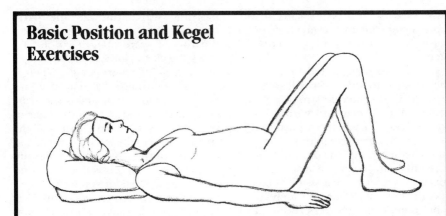

Lie on your back, knees bent, feet about 12 inches apart, soles flat on the floor. Your head and shoulders should be supported by cushions, and your arms resting flat at your sides. To do Kegels, firmly tense the muscles around your vagina and anus. Hold for as long as you can (working up to 8 to 10 seconds), then slowly release the muscles and relax. These also can be done, and after the fourth month should be done, in a standing or sitting position or while urinating. Do at least 25 repetitions at various times during the day. Note: The Basic Position should be used only through the fourth month. After that time exercising flat on one's back is not recommended, since the growing uterus could put excessive weight on major blood vessels.

concept of pregnancy as an illness, and of the pregnant woman as an invalid too delicate to climb a flight of stairs or carry a bag of groceries, is as dated as general anesthesia in routine deliveries. Though there still isn't a vast body of research on the subject of exercise during pregnancy, moderate physical activity is now considered not only thoroughly safe, but extremely beneficial for most expectant mothers and their babies.

As anxious as you might be to hit the jogging trail, however, there is one vitally important stop you must make first—at your doctor's office. Even if you're feeling terrific, you must obtain medical clearance before suiting up in your husband's sweatpants. Pregnant women who are in a high-risk category may have to curb exercise or even eliminate it entirely for now. But if yours is among the great majority of normal pregnancies, and your doctor has given you the go-ahead, suit up and read on.

THE BENEFITS OF EXERCISE

It appears that women who don't get any exercise during pregnancy become progressively less fit as the months pass by—particularly because they are becoming heavier and heavier. A good exercise program (which can be built right into your daily lifestyle) can counteract this trend toward decreasing fitness.

There are four kinds of exercise that can be useful during pregnancy: aerobics, calisthenics specifically designed for pregnancy, relaxation techniques, and Kegel exercises.

Aerobics. These are rhythmic, repetitive activities strenuous enough to demand increased oxygen to the muscles, but not so strenuous that demand exceeds supply (walking, jogging, bicycling, swimming, tennis singles). Aerobic exercises stimulate the heart and lungs, and muscle and joint activity—producing beneficial overall body changes, especially an increase in the ability to process and utilize oxygen, which is a plus for you and your baby. Exercise too strenuous to be sustained for the 20 to 30 minutes necessary to reach this "training effect" (such as sprinting), or not strenuous enough (tennis doubles), is not considered aerobic.

Aerobic exercise improves circulation (enhancing the transport of oxygen and nutrients to your fetus while decreasing the risk of varicose veins, hemorrhoids, and fluid retention); increases muscle tone and strength (often preventing or relieving backache and constipation, making it easier to carry the extra weight of pregnancy, and facilitating delivery); builds endurance (making you better able to cope with a lengthy labor); burns calories (allowing you to eat more of the good food you and your baby need without gaining excessive weight, and promising a better postpartum figure);

lessens fatigue and promotes a better night's sleep; imparts a feeling of well-being and confidence; and in general heightens your ability to cope with the physical and emotional challenges of childbearing.

Calisthenics. These are rhythmic, light gymnastic movements that tone and develop muscles and can improve posture. Calisthenics especially designed for pregnant women can be very useful in relieving backache, in improving physical and mental well-being, and in preparing your body for the arduous task of childbirth. Calisthenics designed for the general population, however, may be unsafe.

Relaxation Techniques. Breathing and concentration exercises relax mind and body, help conserve energy for when it's needed, assist the mind to focus on a task, and increase body awareness—all of which can help a woman better meet the challenges of childbirth. Relaxation techniques are

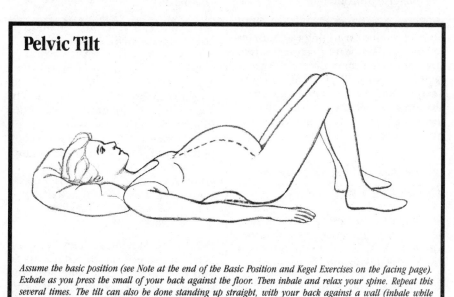

Pelvic Tilt

Assume the basic position (see Note at the end of the Basic Position and Kegel Exercises on the facing page). Exhale as you press the small of your back against the floor. Then inhale and relax your spine. Repeat this several times. The tilt can also be done standing up straight, with your back against a wall (inhale while pressing the small of your back into the wall). The standing version is an excellent way to improve your posture and is preferable after the fourth month.

Dromedary Droop

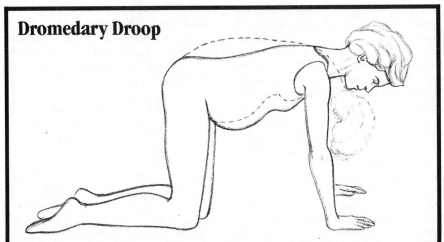

This exercise is useful throughout pregnancy and into labor, to relieve the pressure of the enlarged uterus on your spine. Get down on your hands and knees, with your back in a naturally relaxed position (don't let your spine sag). Keep your head straight, your neck aligned with your spine. Then hump your back, tightening your abdomen and buttocks, and allow your head to drop all the way down. Gradually release your back and raise your head to the original position. Repeat several times.

valuable in combination with more physical routines, or alone—especially in pregnancies when more active exercise is prohibited.

Pelvic Toning. Kegel exercises are simple techniques for toning the muscles in the vaginal and perineal area, strengthening them in preparation for delivery. This will also aid recovery postpartum. This exercise is one virtually every pregnant woman can perform and benefit from, any time, any place.

DEVELOPING A GOOD EXERCISE PROGRAM

Get Started. The best time to get fit is before you get pregnant. But it's never too late to start exercising—even if you're already pushing nine months.

Get Off to a Slow Start. Once you've decided to begin a fitness program, it's tempting to start off with a bang, running 3 miles the first morning or

working out twice the first afternoon. But such enthusiastic beginnings lead not to fitness but to sore muscles, sagging resolve, and abrupt endings. They can also be dangerous.

Of course, if you followed an exercise program before pregnancy, you can probably continue it—though possibly in a modified form (see Playing It Safe, page 195). If you're a fledgling athlete, however, build up slowly. Start with 10 minutes of warm-ups followed by 5 minutes of more strenuous workout and a 5-minute cooldown. Stop strenuous exercise sooner if you begin to tire. After a few days, if your body has adjusted well, increase the period of strenuous activity by a couple of minutes a day up to 15 minutes maximum.

Get Off to a Slow Start Every Time You Start. Warm-ups can be tedious when you're eager to get your workout started (and over with). But as every athlete knows, they're an essential part of any exercise program. They ensure that the heart and circulation aren't taxed suddenly, and reduce the chances of injury to muscles and joints, which are more vulnerable when "cold"—and particularly vulnerable during pregnancy. Walk before you run, stretch before you begin calisthenics, swim slowly before you start your laps. If you do stretching exercises, be sure not to stretch to your limit, since this can damage joints that have been loosened by pregnancy.

Finish as Slowly as You Start. Collapse seems like the logical conclusion to a workout, but it isn't physiologically sound. Stopping abruptly traps blood in the muscles, reducing blood supply to other parts of your body and to your baby. Dizziness, faintness, extra heartbeats, or nausea may result. So finish your exercise with exercise: about 5 minutes of walking after running, paddling after a vigorous swim, light stretching exercises after almost any activity. Top off your cool-down with a few minutes of relaxation.

You can also help avoid dizziness (and a possible fall) if you get up slowly when you've been exercising on the floor.

Watch the Clock. Too little exercise won't be effective; too much can be debilitating. A full workout, from warm-up to cool-down, can take anywhere from 30 minutes to an hour. But the American College of Obstetricians and Gynecology recommends that the period of strenuous exercise—during which the pulse rate should not exceed 140—should be limited to 15 minutes. For healthy women who were sedentary before pregnancy, working up to between 20 and 30 minutes of exercise, including warming up and cooling down, every other day is a realistic and safe goal. The already active woman can, with her doctor's okay, do more.

Keep It Up. Exercising erratically (four

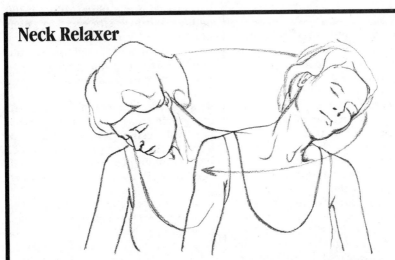

Neck Relaxer

The neck is often a focus of tension, tightening under stress. This exercise can help to relax both your neck and the rest of you: Sit in a comfortable position (Tailor Sit, page 195, might be best) with your eyes closed. Gently roll your head around, making a full circle, and inhaling as you do. Exhale and relax, letting your head drop forward comfortably. Repeat 4 or 5 times, alternating the direction of the roll and relaxing between rolls. Do this exercise several times a day.

Don't Just Sit There . . .

Sitting for an extended period without a break is not a good idea for anyone, but it is particularly unwise when you're pregnant. It causes blood to pool in your leg veins, can cause your feet to swell, and could lead to other problems. If your work entails a lot of sitting, or if you watch TV for hours at a time or travel long distances frequently, be sure to break up every hour or so of sitting with five or ten minutes of walking. And at your seat, periodically do some exercises that enhance circulation, such as taking a few deep breaths; extending your lower legs, flexing your feet, and wiggling your toes; and contracting the muscles in your abdomen and buttocks (a sort of sitting pelvic tilt). If your hands tend to swell, also try stretching your arms above your head and opening and closing your fists.

times one week and none the next) won't get you in shape. Exercising regularly (three or four times a week, every week) will. If you're too tired for a strenuous workout, don't push yourself; but do try to do the warmups so that your muscles will stay limber and your discipline won't dissolve. Many women find that they feel better if they do some exercise every day.

Work Exercise into Your Schedule. The best way to be sure of doing your exercise is to allot a specific time for it: first thing in the morning; before going off to work; during a coffee break; or before dinner. If you have no regular block of free time for an exercise session, you can build exercise into your existing schedule. Walk to work, if you can, or park your car or get off the bus a distance from the job and walk part of the way. Or walk an older child to school (or to a friend's) instead of driving. Do your vacuuming in a steady, 20-minute stretch after a few warm-ups, and you will exercise your body and clean the carpets at the same time. Instead of flopping down in front of the TV with your spouse after the dinner dishes are done, ask him to join you for a walk. No matter how busy your day, if there's the will, there's always a way to fit in some form of exercise.

Compensate for the Calories You Burn. Probably the best part of a pregnancy exercise program is the extra eating you'll have to do. As always, make those calories count. Take this opportunity to add even *more* good-for-baby nutrients to your diet. You'll have to consume about 100 to 200 additional calories for every half hour of strenuous exercising. If you believe you're consuming enough calories but you still are not gaining weight, you may be exercising too much.

Replace the Fluids You Use Up. For every half hour of strenuous activity, you will need at least a full glass of extra liquid to compensate for fluids lost through perspiration. You will need more in warm weather, or when you are perspiring profusely: drink before, during, and after exercising. The scale can give you a clue to how much extra fluid you need to drink: 2 cups for each pound lost during exercise.

If You Choose the Group Approach: take an exercise class that is specifically designed for pregnant women. Since not everyone who claims to be an expert is one, ask for the instructor's credentials before enrolling. Classes are better for some women than solo exercising (particularly when self-discipline is lacking) and provide support and feedback. The best programs maintain moderate intensity; meet at least three times weekly; individualize to each woman's capabilities; don't use fast-tempoed music, which may push participants into working too hard; and have a network of medical specialists available for questions.

PLAYING IT SAFE

Don't Work Out on an Empty Stomach. Mother's rule about not swimming after a meal had some validity. But exercising on an empty stomach can be hazardous too. If you haven't eaten for hours, it's a good idea to have a light snack and a drink 15 to 30 minutes before beginning your warm-ups. If you're uncomfortable eating that close to exercising, have your snack an hour before.

Dress for the Occasion. Wear clothes that are loose or that stretch when you move. Fabrics should let your body breathe—right down to your underwear, which should be cotton. Well-fitting athletic shoes, designed for the appropriate activity, will protect your feet and joints.

Select the Right Surface. Indoors, wood floors or a tightly carpeted surface is better than tile or concrete for your workouts. (If a surface is slippery, don't exercise in socks or footed tights.) Outdoors, soft running tracks and level grassy or dirt trails are better than hard-surfaced roads or sidewalks, avoid surfaces that are uneven.

Do Everything in Moderation. *Never* exercise to the point of exhaustion when you're pregnant; the chemical

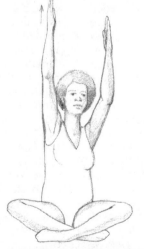

Tailor Sit, Tailor Stretch

Sitting cross-legged is particularly comfortable during pregnancy. Sit this way often and do arm stretches: Place your hands on your shoulders, then lift both arms above your head. Stretch one arm higher than the other, reaching for the ceiling, then relax it and repeat with the other arm. Repeat 10 times on each side. Do not bounce.

Leg Lifts

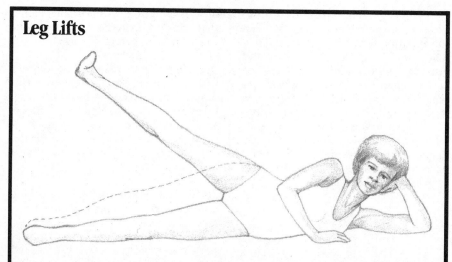

Lie on your left side, with your shoulders, hips, and knees in a straight line. Place your right hand on the floor in front of your chest and support your head with your left. Relax and inhale; then exhale while slowly raising your right leg as high as you can, keeping your foot flexed (pointing up toward your belly) and your inner ankle facing directly down. Inhale while slowly lowering your leg. Repeat 10 times on each side. This exercise can be done with the leg either straight or bent at the knee.

by-products of overexertion are not good for the fetus. (If you're a trained athlete, you still shouldn't exercise to your fullest capacity, whether it exhausts you or not.) There are several ways of checking to see whether you're overdoing it. First, if it feels good, it's probably okay. If there's any pain or strain, it's not. A little perspiration is fine; a drenching sweat is a sign to slow down. So is being unable to carry on a conversation as you go. A pulse that is still over 100 beats per minute five minutes after completing a workout means you've worked too hard. So does needing a nap when you're finished. You should feel exhilarated, not drained.

Know When to Stop. Your body will signal when it's time. Signals include: pain anywhere (hip, back, pelvis, chest, head, and so on); a cramp or stitch; lightheadedness or dizziness; tachycardia, or palpitations; severe breathlessness; difficulty walking or loss of muscle control; headache; increased swelling of your hands, feet, ankles, face; amniotic fluid leakage or vaginal bleeding; or after the 28th week, a slowing down or cessation of fetal movement. If any of these symptoms aren't relieved by a short rest, check with your doctor (but call immediately if you have any bleeding or amniotic fluid leakage). In the second and third trimesters, you may notice a gradual decrease in your performance and efficiency. It's best to slow down.

Stay Cool. Don't exercise in very hot or humid weather; don't use saunas, steam rooms, or hot tubs. Until research shows otherwise, exercise or environments that raise a pregnant woman's temperature more than 1½ to 2 degrees Fahrenheit should be considered dangerous (blood is shunted away from the uterus to the skin as the body attempts to cool off). So don't exercise in the heat of the day or in a warm or stuffy room. And

Choosing the Right Pregnancy Exercise

Select the type of exercise that's right for you. Though you can probably continue a sport or activity you are already proficient at, it's not advisable to take up a new one during pregnancy. Exercises that even a novice can do during pregnancy include:

❖ Walking at a brisk pace

❖ Swimming in shallow water that is neither too hot nor too cold

❖ Cycling on a stationary bike at a comfortable tension and speed

❖ Calisthenics designed especially for pregnant women

❖ Pelvic toning (Kegel exercises)

❖ Relaxation routines

Exercises that only a well-trained, experienced athlete should engage in during pregnancy:

❖ Jogging, up to 2 miles per day*

❖ Doubles tennis (but not singles, which can be too strenuous)

❖ Cross-country skiing below 10,000 feet

❖ Light weight lifting, if Valsalva maneuver (holding your breath and straining) is avoided

❖ Cycling

❖ Ice skating (with extreme caution)

Exercises that even an athlete should avoid, because of their greater risks, include:

❖ Jogging more than 2 miles per day*

❖ Horseback riding

❖ Waterskiing

❖ Diving and jumping into pools

❖ Scuba diving (diving gear may re-

strict circulation; decompression sickness is hazardous to the fetus)

❖ Sprinting (too much oxygen is demanded too quickly)

❖ Downhill skiing (risky because of the possibility of a serious fall)

❖ Cross-country skiing above 10,000 feet (the high altitude deprives both mother and fetus of oxygen)

❖ Bicycling on wet pavement or winding paths (where falls are likely), and cycling leaning forward in racing posture (can cause backache)

❖ Contact sports, such as football (they carry a high risk of injury)

❖ Calisthenics not designed for pregnancy. These include those that pull on the abdomen (such as sit-ups or double leg lifts); that might force air into the vagina (such as upside-down "bicycling," shoulder stands, or exercises where you bring your knee to your chest while kneeling on all fours); that stretch the inner thigh muscles (such as sitting on the floor with the soles of the feet together and pressing down on or bouncing your knees); that cause the small of the back to curve inward; that require "bridging" (bending over backward) or other contortions; or that involve deep flexion or extension of joints (such as deep knee bends), jumping, bouncing, sudden changes in direction, or jerky motions.

---

*Some very fit women have continued more rigorous exercise programs during pregnancy with no negative effects, but it isn't clear that this is always safe. Check with your physician before doing so yourself.

don't wait for your body to tell you when you're overheated—stop before you reach that point.

Proceed with Caution. Even the most skilled sportswoman can lack grace when she's pregnant. As the center of gravity shifts forward with the uterus, a fall becomes an ever-increasing possibility. Be aware, and be careful. Late in pregnancy, avoid sports that require sudden moves or a good sense of balance, such as tennis.

Be Aware of the Added Risk of Injury. For a variety of reasons (an altered center of balance, lax joints, absent-mindedness), women are more subject to injury when they are expecting.

Stay Off Your Back, and Don't Point Your Toes. After the fourth month, don't exercise flat on your back, as the weight of your enlarging uterus could compress major blood vessels, restricting circulation. Pointing, or extending, your toes—at any time in pregnancy—could lead to cramping in your calves. Flex your feet instead, turning them up toward your face.

Taper Off in the Last Trimester. Though everyone has heard stories of pregnant athletes who have stayed in the pool or on the slopes right up until delivery, it is wise for most women to slack off during the last three months. This is especially true during the ninth month, when stretching routines and brisk walking should provide adequate exercise. Serious athletic pursuits can be resumed at about six weeks postpartum.

IF YOU DON'T EXERCISE

E xercising during pregnancy can certainly do you a lot of good. It can relieve backache, prevent constipation and varicose veins, give you a general sense of well-being, make childbirth a little quicker and easier, and leave you in better physical shape postpartum. But sitting it out (whether by choice or on doctor's orders), getting most of your exercise from opening and closing your car door, won't do you or your baby any harm. In fact, if you're abstaining from exercise on doctor's orders, you're helping your baby and yourself. Your doctor will almost certainly restrict exercise if you have a history of three or more spontaneous abortions or of premature labor, or if you have an incompetent cervix, bleeding or periodic spotting, a diagnosis of placenta previa, or heart disease. Your activity may also be limited if you have high blood pressure, diabetes, thyroid disease, anemia or other blood disorders; are seriously over- or underweight; or have had an extremely sedentary lifestyle up until now. A history of precipitous (very brief) labor or of a fetus that didn't thrive in a previous pregnancy might also be a reason for a red light on exercise.

In some cases arm-only exercises may be okayed when other exercises are taboo. Check with your doctor.

10
The Sixth Month

WHAT YOU CAN EXPECT AT THIS MONTH'S CHECKUP

This month you can expect your practitioner to check the following, though there may be variations depending upon your particular needs and upon your practitioner's style of practice:[1]

❖ Weight and blood pressure

❖ Urine, for sugar and protein

❖ Fetal heartbeat

❖ Height of fundus (top of uterus)

❖ Size of uterus and position of fetus, by external palpation

❖ Feet and hands for edema (swelling), and legs for varicose veins

❖ Symptoms you may have been experiencing, especially unusual ones

❖ Questions and problems you want to discuss—have a list ready

WHAT YOU MAY BE FEELING

You may experience all of these symptoms at one time or another, or only a few of them. Some may have continued from last month, others may be new. Still others may hardly be noticed because you've become so used to them. You may also have other, less common, symptoms.

PHYSICALLY:

❖ More definite fetal activity

❖ Whitish vaginal discharge (leukorrhea)

❖ Lower abdominal achiness (from stretching of ligaments supporting the uterus)

❖ Constipation

❖ Heartburn, indigestion, flatulence, bloating

---

1. See Appendix for an explanation of the procedures and tests performed.

❖ Occasional headaches, faintness or dizziness

❖ Nasal congestion and occasional nosebleeds; ear stuffiness

❖ "Pink toothbrush" from bleeding gums

❖ Hearty appetite

❖ Leg cramps

❖ Mild swelling of ankles and feet, and occasionally of hands and face

❖ Varicose veins of legs and/or hemorrhoids

❖ Itchy abdomen

❖ Backache

❖ Skin pigmentation changes on abdomen and/or face

❖ Enlarged breasts

EMOTIONALLY:

❖ Fewer mood swings; continued absentmindedness

❖ A beginning of boredom with the pregnancy ("Can't anyone think about anything else?")

❖ Some anxiety about the future

WHAT YOU MAY LOOK LIKE

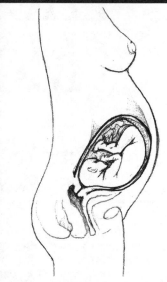

By the end of the sixth month, the fetus is about 13 inches long and weighs about 1¼ pounds. Its skin is thin and shiny, with no underlying fat; its finger and toe prints are visible. Eyelids begin to part, and the eyes open. With intensive care, the fetus may survive if born now.

WHAT YOU MAY BE CONCERNED ABOUT

PAIN AND NUMBNESS IN THE HAND

"I keep waking up in the middle of the night because some of the fingers on my right hand are numb; sometimes they even hurt. Is that related to my pregnancy?"

If the numbness and pain are confined to your thumb, index finger, middle finger, and half of your ring finger, you probably have carpal tunnel syndrome. Though this condition is most common in people who regularly perform tasks that require repetitive motions of the hand (such as meat cutting, piano playing, typing), it is also common in pregnant women. That's because the carpal tunnel in the wrist, through which the nerve to the affected fingers runs, becomes swollen during pregnancy (as do so many other tissues in the body), with the resultant pressure causing numbness, tingling, burning, and/or pain. The symptoms can also affect the hand

and wrist, and can radiate up the arm. Because fluids accumulate in your hands all day thanks to gravity, the swelling and accompanying symptoms may be more severe at night. Try to avoid sleeping on your hands, which can aggravate the problem. When numbness occurs, hanging the affected hand over the side of the bed and shaking it vigorously may relieve it. If it doesn't, and the numbness (with or without pain) is interfering with your sleep, discuss the problem with your doctor. Often wearing a wrist splint and taking vitamin B_6 daily is helpful. Some people have gotten relief from acupuncture. The non-steroidal anti-inflammatory drugs and steroids usually prescribed for carpal tunnel syndrome may not be recommended during pregnancy. If other treatments fail and the condition persists after delivery, simple surgery may be indicated.

PINS AND NEEDLES

"I frequently get a tingling sensation in my hands and feet. Does this indicate a problem with my circulation?"

As if it weren't enough to be on tenterhooks during pregnancy, some women occasionally experience the disconcerting tingling sensation of pins and needles in their extremities. Although it may feel as if your circulation is being cut off, this isn't the case. No one knows why this phenomenon occurs or how to eliminate it, but it is known that it doesn't indicate anything serious. Changing your position may help. If the tingling interferes in any way with your functioning, report it to your practitioner.

BABY KICKING

"Some days the baby is kicking all the
time; other days he seems very quiet. Is this normal?"

Fetuses are only human. Just like us, they have "up" days, when they feel like kicking up their heels (and elbows and knees), and "down" days, when they'd rather lie back and take it easy. Most often, their activity is related to what you've been doing. Like babies out of the womb, fetuses are lulled by rocking. So when you're on the go all day, your baby is likely to be pacified by the rhythm of your routine, and you're likely not to notice much kicking—partly because baby's slowed down, partly because you're so busy. As soon as you slow down, he or she is bound to start acting up. That's why most expectant mothers feel fetal movement more often in bed at night or in the morning. Activity may also increase after the mother has had a meal or snack, perhaps in reaction to the surge of glucose (sugar) in her blood. Some pregnant women also report increased fetal activity when they are excited or nervous; the baby may be stimulated by the mother's adrenalin response.

Babies are actually most active between weeks 24 and 28. But their movements are erratic and usually brief, so though they are visible on ultrasound, they aren't always felt by the busy mother-to-be. Fetal activity usually becomes more organized and consistent, with more clearly defined periods of rest and activity, between 28 and 32 weeks.

Don't be tempted to compare baby-movement notes with other pregnant women. Each fetus, like each newborn, has an individual pattern of activity and development. Some seem always active; others mostly quiet. The kicking of some is regular; that of others may exhibit no discernible pattern. As long as there is no radical slowdown or cessation of activity, all variations are normal.

Recent research suggests that from the 28th week on it may be a good idea for mothers to test for fetal movements twice a day—once in the morning, when activity tends to be sparser, and once in the evening, when most babies tend to be more active. This is how to perform such a test:

Check the clock when you start counting. Count movements of any kind (kicks, flutters, swishes, rolls). Stop counting when you reach ten, and note the time. Often, you will feel ten movements within ten minutes or so. Sometimes it will take longer.

If you haven't counted ten movements by the end of an hour, have some milk or another snack; then lie down, relax, and start counting again. If another hour goes by without ten movements, call your practitioner without delay. Though such an absence of activity doesn't necessarily mean there's a problem, it can occasionally indicate fetal distress. In such cases, quick action may be needed.

The closer you are to your due date, the more important regular checking of fetal movements becomes.

"Sometimes the baby pushes so hard it hurts."

As your baby matures in the uterus, he or she becomes stronger and stronger, and those once butterfly-like fetal movements pack more and more power. Don't be surprised if you get kicked in the ribs or poked in the abdomen or cervix with such force it hurts. When you seem to be under a particularly fierce attack, try changing your position. It may knock your little linebacker off balance and temporarily stem the assault.

"The baby seems to be kicking all over. Could I be carrying twins?"

At some point in her pregnancy, just about every woman begins to think that she's carrying either twins or a human octopus. For most, of course, neither is true. Until a fetus grows to the point that his movements are restricted by the confines of his uterine home (usually at about 34 weeks), he's able to perform numerous acrobatics. So, while it may sometimes feel as if you're being pummeled by a dozen fists, it's more likely to be two fists that really get around—along with tiny knees, elbows, and feet.

For more on twins and how they are diagnosed, see page 143.

LEG CRAMPS

"I have leg cramps at night that interfere with my sleep."

Between your racing mind and your bulging belly, you probably have enough trouble sleeping without having to suffer from leg cramps. Unfortunately, these painful spasms, which occur most often at night, are very common among pregnant women in the second and third trimesters. Fortunately, however, there are ways of both preventing and alleviating them.

Since some leg cramps are believed to be caused by an excess of phosphorus and a shortage of calcium circulating in the blood, taking calcium tablets that do not contain phosphorus (calcium carbonate is most absorbable) may be effective in alleviating them. It may be necessary—but only on your practitioner's advice—to reduce phosphorus intake by cutting down on milk and meat. (But be sure that you are getting your calcium and protein elsewhere. See the Best-Odds Diet, page 80, for substitutes.) Because fatigue and the pressure of the enlarging uterus on certain nerves are also thought to be possible contributing factors, wearing support hose during the day and alternating periods of rest (with your feet up) with periods of physical activity may also be helpful in eliminating the problem of leg cramps.

If you do get a cramp in your calf, straighten your leg and flex your ankle and toes slowly up toward your nose. This should soon lessen the pain. (Doing this several times with each leg before retiring at night may even help ward off the cramps.) Standing on a cold surface sometimes works, too. If either technique reduces the pain, massage or local heat can then be used for added relief. If neither reduces it, don't massage your calves or apply heat. Do contact your doctor if the pain continues, as there is a slight possibility that a blood clot may have developed in a vein, making medical treatment necessary.

RECTAL BLEEDING AND HEMORRHOIDS

"I'm concerned about the rectal bleeding I've been having."

B leeding is always a frightening symptom, especially during pregnancy—and particularly in an area so close to your birth canal. But unlike vaginal bleeding, rectal bleeding is not a sign of a possible threat to your pregnancy. During pregnancy it's frequently caused by external and, less often, internal hemorrhoids. Hemorrhoids, which are varicose veins of the rectum, afflict between 20% and 50% of all pregnant women. Just as the veins of the legs are more susceptible to varicosities at this time, so are the veins of the rectum. Constipation often causes or compounds the problem.

Hemorrhoids (also called piles because of the resemblance these swollen veins sometimes bear to a pile of grapes or marbles) can cause itching and pain as well as bleeding. Rectal bleeding may also stem from fissures—cracks in the anus caused by constipation, which can accompany hemorrhoids or appear independently. Fissures are generally extremely painful.

Don't try to self-diagnose hemorrhoids. Rectal bleeding is occasionally a sign of serious disease and should always be evaluated by a physician. But if you do have hemorrhoids and/ or fissures, your role will be the most important in treating them. Good self-care can usually eliminate the need for more radical medical therapy.

❖ Avoid constipation. It is *not* a necessary component of pregnancy; see page 135. (Preventing constipation from the start is, incidentally, frequently an excellent way to prevent hemorrhoids completely.)

❖ Sleep on your side, not your back, to avoid putting extra pressure on the rectal veins; avoid long hours of standing or sitting.

❖ Don't strain when having a bowel movement. Sitting with your feet on a stepstool may make evacuation easier.

❖ Do Kegel exercises regularly: they improve circulation to the area (see page 190).

❖ Take warm sitz baths twice a day.

❖ Apply witch hazel soaks or ice packs (whichever is more soothing) to the hemorrhoids.

❖ Use topical medications or suppositories *only* if prescribed by a doctor who knows you're pregnant. Do not take mineral oil.

❖ Keep the perineal area (from vagina to rectum) scrupulously clean. Wash the area with warm water after bowel movements, always wiping from front to back. Use only white toilet paper.

❖ If sitting is painful, get a special inflatable seat cushion shaped like an inner tube.

❖ Lie down several times a day—if possible, on your side. Watch TV, read, and talk to your husband in this position.

With good care, hemorrhoids can be kept from becoming chronic. They may be made worse by delivery, especially if the pushing phase is long, but usually disappear postpartum if preventive measures are continued.

ITCHY ABDOMEN

"My belly itches constantly. It's driving me crazy."

Join the club. Pregnant bellies are itchy bellies, and they can become progressively itchier as the months pass. Your skin is stretching, being pulled taut across your abdomen, and the result is dryness (more pronounced in some women than others) and itching. Try not to scratch, or at least keep scratching to a minimum. Lubricating the area with lotion may ease the itch but probably won't cure it. An anti-itching lotion (such as calamine) may provide more relief.

TOXEMIA, OR PREECLAMPSIA

"Recently a friend of mine was hospitalized for toxemia. How can you tell if you have it?"

Fortunately toxemia, also known as preeclampsia/eclampsia or pregnancy-induced hypertension (PIH), is uncommon. Even in its mildest form it occurs in only 5% to 10% of pregnancies—and most of these cases are among women who came into pregnancy with chronic high blood pressure. Toxemia is most common in first pregnancies and beyond the 20th week of gestation. In women who are receiving regular prenatal care, it is diagnosed and treated early, preventing needless complications. Though routine office visits sometimes seem a waste of time in a healthy pregnancy, it is at such visits that the earliest signs of preeclampsia can be picked up.

If you have had a sudden weight gain apparently unrelated to excess food intake, severe swelling of your hands and face, unexplained headaches, and/or vision disturbances, call your practitioner. Otherwise, assuming you are getting regular prenatal care, you needn't worry about toxemia. See page 152 for tips on preventing and dealing with high blood pressure in pregnancy, and page 351 for more information on toxemia.

STAYING ON THE JOB

"I stand a lot on my job. I was planning to work up until I deliver, but is that safe?"

The question of how a mother-to-be's job affects an unborn fetus is an important one, especially these days, when so many expectant mothers are working. The answer at this point, however, isn't all that clear. We all know women who went from the office or the studio or the shop right to the hospital and delivered perfectly healthy babies. And, in fact, one study of pregnant doctors in arduous residency training programs found that although these women were on their feet for 65 hours a week, they didn't seem to have any more pregnancy complications than the male residents' pregnant wives, who worked many fewer usually less stressful hours. Other studies, however, suggest that steady strenuous or stressful activity or long hours of standing during the last half of pregnancy may increase the risk of the mother developing high blood pressure, as well as the risk of a damaged placenta and a low-birthweight baby. Some studies show the risk of complications from standing on the job after 28 weeks increases if the expectant mother has other children at home to care for.

Should women who stand on the job—salespeople, cooks, police officers, waitresses, doctors, nurses, and so on—work past the 28th week? Clearly, more study will need to be done before definitive answers to that question will be available. The American Medical Association, in fact, recommends that women who work at jobs requiring more than four hours a day on their feet should quit by the 24th week, and that those who must stand for 30 minutes out of each hour should quit by the 32nd. But many practitioners feel this recommendation is too strict, and will permit women who feel fine to work longer. Standing on the job all the way to term, however, may not be a good idea, less because of the theoretical risk to the fetus than the real risk that such pregnancy discomforts as backache, varicose veins, and hemorrhoids will be aggravated.

Research shows that underweight women who gain little weight during pregnancy are at a greater risk of having small babies when they have outside employment than when they don't, so it may be wise for such women—if they are really unable to gain adequate weight (gaining should be their first approach to the problem; see page 81)—to temporarily give up employment if they can, or at least to reduce their hours.

Some experts recommend that a woman not stay past the 20th week at a job that requires heavy lifting,[2] pulling, pushing, climbing (stairs, poles, or ladders), or bending below the waist, if this kind of work is intensive, and past the 28th week if it is moderate. It's probably also a good idea to take early leave from a job that requires frequent shift changes (which can upset appetite and sleep routines, and worsen fatigue); one that seems to exacerbate any pregnancy problems, such as headache, backache, or fatigue; or one that increases the risk of falls or other accidental injuries.

On the other hand, you can probably plan on going straight from a desk job to the delivery room without any threat to you or your baby. A sedentary job that isn't particularly stressful may actually be less of a strain on you both than staying at home with a vacuum cleaner and mop. And doing a small amount of walking—up to an hour or two daily—on the job or off, is not only harmless but may be beneficial (assuming you aren't carrying heavy loads as you go).

No matter how long you keep working, there are ways of reducing physical on-the-job stress during pregnancy:

❖ Wear support hose.

❖ If you are standing for long stretches, keep one foot on a low stool, knee bent, to take some of the pressure off your back. (See illustration, page 174.)

---

2. Lifting weights of 25 pounds or less, even repetitively, is usually not a problem, nor is lifting weights of up to 50 pounds intermittently (which should be reassuring to pregnant mothers of babies and preschoolers). But women in jobs requiring repetitive lifting of weights of 25 to 50 pounds should probably quit by the 34th week, by the 20th week if the weights are over 50 pounds. Those in jobs requiring only intermittent lifting of weights over 50 pounds should quit by the 30th week.

❖ Take frequent breaks. Stand up and walk around if you've been sitting; sit down with your feet up if you've been standing. Do some stretching exercises, especially for your back and legs.

❖ Rest a lot when you are not working; cut down on strenuous activities such as running, tennis, climbing, and so on. The more strenuous your job, the more you need to cut down on other strenuous activities.

❖ Rest on your left side during your lunch hour, if possible. Sleep on your left side at night.

❖ At your desk, keep your legs elevated (on a stool or carton) when possible.

❖ Listen to your body. Slow down your pace if you're feeling tired; go home early if you're exhausted.

❖ Stay out of smoke-filled areas; they are not only bad for the baby but can increase your fatigue.

❖ Avoid extremes in temperature.

❖ Avoid noxious fumes and chemicals (see page 67).

❖ Do any necessary lifting properly to avoid strain on your back (see page 174), and reduce the weight you ordinarily lift by at least 25%.

❖ Empty your bladder at least every two hours.

❖ If you must stand or walk on the job, cut down on your hours, if possible, and increase the time you spend napping or resting with your feet up.

❖ Remember that no job is as important as that of nourishing your baby. Don't let your other work interfere with your getting breakfast, lunch, and dinner every day, supplemented by nutritious snacks (keep a plentiful supply at your workplace or bring them in daily.)

CLUMSINESS

"Lately I've been dropping everything I pick up. Why am I so clumsy suddenly?"

L ike the extra inches on your belly, the extra thumbs on your hands are part and parcel of being pregnant. As with so many pregnancy side effects, this temporary clumsiness is caused by the loosening of joints and the retention of water, both of which can make your grasp on objects less firm and sure. Another factor may be a lack of concentration as a result of the scatterbrain syndrome (see page 155).

Besides making a conscious effort to pick up things more carefully, there isn't much you can do about pregnancy "dropsies"—so it might be a good idea to let your husband handle the good china for the next few months.

THE PAIN OF CHILDBIRTH

"Now that pregnancy has become an inescapable reality, I'm worrying about whether I will be able to tolerate the pain of childbirth."

T hough almost every expectant mother eagerly awaits the birth of her child, very few look forward to the labor and delivery that precede it. Especially for those who've never experienced significant discomfort, the fear of this unknown is very real—and very normal. Unhappily, it's often compounded for these women by the horror tales of mothers, aunts, and friends in whose footsteps to the labor room they dread to follow.

There's no point in dreading the pain—which may end up being worse than you bargained for or not so bad after all—but there's a lot to be said for being prepared for it. When women who anticipate that labor will be an incomparably exhilarating and ultimately fulfilling experience end up with 24 hours of excruciating back labor, they suffer as much from disappointment as from pain. And because the pain is unexpected, they have trouble dealing with it.

In general, both women who fear pain the most and those who expect it the least have a harder time during labor and delivery than women who are realistic in their expectations and are prepared for any eventuality.

If you prepare both your mind and your body, you should be able to reduce your anxiety now, and at the same time help make your actual labor more comfortable and tolerable.

Get Educated. One reason earlier generations of women found labor so unbearable was that they didn't understand what was happening to their bodies. Take a good childbirth education class with your husband if at all possible (see Childbirth Education, page 209); otherwise, read as much on the subject of labor and delivery as you can (try to touch on all the major schools of thought), including the descriptions beginning on page 212. What you don't know can hurt you more than it should.

Get Moving. You wouldn't think of running a marathon without the proper physical training. Neither should you consider going into labor (which is a no less Herculean feat) untrained. Work out faithfully with all the breathing and toning-up exercises your practitioner and/or childbirth educator recommends. (If they have not recommended any, see page 189 for several basic exercises.)

Put Pain in Perspective. There are at least two good things to be said about the pain of childbirth, no matter how intense. First, it has a definite time limit. Though it may be difficult to believe at the time, you will not be in labor forever. Average labor with a first child is between 12 and 14 hours—and only a few of those hours are likely to be very uncomfortable. (Many doctors will not allow labor to continue much beyond 24 hours, and will perform a cesarean at that point if adequate progress has not been made.) Second, it's a pain with a very definite positive purpose: Contractions progressively thin and open your cervix, each contraction bringing you closer to the birth of your baby. Don't feel guilty, however, if you lose sight of that purpose during very hard labor and care very little about anything but getting it over with. Your tolerance for pain does not reflect on the depth of your maternal love.

Don't Plan on Going It Alone. Even if you don't feel like holding hands with your mate during labor, it will be comforting to know he (or a close friend or relative) is there to mop your brow, to feed you ice chips, to massage your back or neck, to coach you through contractions, or just for you to curse at. Your coach should go through childbirth classes with you if possible, or if it's not, should read up on the coach's role, starting on page 288.

Be Ready to Accept Pain Relief If It's Needed. Asking for or accepting medication is a sign neither of failure nor of weakness (you don't have to be a martyr to be a mother), and some kind of pain relief is sometimes absolutely necessary to keep a laboring woman at her most effective. See page 226 for more on pain relief during labor and delivery.

LABOR AND DELIVERY

"I'm getting very anxious about labor and delivery. What if I fail?"

The advent of childbirth education probably did as much as any of the miraculous medical advancements in the past decades to improve the experience of women in labor. However, by creating a mystique of the perfect labor and delivery, it sometimes left parents-to-be feeling pressured to achieve that ideal. Couples prepared themselves for childbirth as if for a final exam. It's not surprising that many worried about failing, and of thereby letting down not only themselves and each other but also their doctors, nurse-midwives, and especially their childbirth educators.

But fortunately most childbirth educators have now come to recognize that there isn't just one way to experience childbirth, and that the only goal—which all parents share—is a healthy mother and a healthy baby. They are letting parents know that labor and delivery aren't a test that a mother passes (if she does her breathing exercises, has a vaginal delivery, and takes no medication) or fails (if she neglects her breathing exercises, has a cesarean, or accepts pain relief). That's something you need to recognize, too. Even forgetting, because of pain and excitement, everything you're "supposed" to do won't change the outcome of the delivery or make you a failure.

Learn everything you can in your classes and from your reading, but don't become so obsessed that you forget that childbirth is a natural process—one that women managed to stumble through successfully for thousands of years before Mrs. Lamaze gave birth to her son, the doctor.

"I'm afraid I'll do something embarrassing during labor."

The prospect of screaming or crying out, or of involuntarily emptying your bladder or bowel, might seem embarrassing now. During labor, however, avoiding humiliation will be the farthest thing from your mind. Besides, nothing you can do or say during labor will shock or disgust your birth attendants, who've doubtless seen and heard it all before. The important thing is to be yourself, to do what makes you feel most comfortable. If you are ordinarily a vocal, emotive person, don't try to hold in your moans or hold back your grunts and groans. On the other hand, if you're normally very inhibited and would rather whimper quietly into your pillow, don't feel obligated to out-yell the woman in the next room.

"I dread losing control during labor and delivery."

To members of the take-charge-of-your-life generation, the thought of relinquishing control of your labor and delivery to the medical staff can be a little unnerving. Of course you want the doctors and nurses to take the best possible care of you and your baby. But you'd still like to maintain a modicum of control. And you can—by working hard now at your childbirth preparation exercises, becoming familiar with the birth process (see page 288), and by developing rapport with a practitioner who respects your opinions. Setting up a birthing plan (see page 225) with your practitioner, specifying what you would like and would not like during labor and delivery, also increases your control.

But with that said and done, it's important to understand that you won't necessarily be able to stay in complete control of your labor and to have everything go your way. The best-laid plans of obstetrical patients and their practitioners can give way to a variety of unforeseen circumstances. It's only sensible to be mentally prepared for the more common scenarios that can unfold at a birth, and for the possibility that procedures and interventions that you'd hoped to avoid may become unavoidable at the last minute. For instance, you'd hoped to deliver without an episiotomy but your perineum refuses to budge after three hours of pushing. Or you'd planned to go through labor completely unmedicated, but an extremely long and trying active phase has zapped you of your strength. Learning when relinquishing the reins will be in the best interest of you and your baby is an important part of your childbirth education.

WHAT IT'S IMPORTANT TO KNOW: CHILDBIRTH EDUCATION

When your parents were expecting you, being prepared for childbirth meant that the baby's room was painted, the layette was ordered, and a suitcase packed with pretty nightgowns for the hospital stay was waiting at the door. It was the arrival of the child—not the childbirth experience—that was anticipated, planned for, and looked forward to. Women knew little of what to expect from labor and delivery; husbands knew even less. And since mother was likely to be unconscious during the birth and father was likely to be absently thumbing through *Time* magazines in the waiting room, their ignorance was of little consequence.

Now that general anesthesia is reserved mainly for emergency cesareans, waiting rooms are for nervous grandparents, and mom and dad can go through childbirth together, ignorance is neither wise nor acceptable. Preparing for childbirth has come to mean preparing for the labor and delivery experience as much as for the new baby. Expectant couples devour stacks of books, magazine articles, and pamphlets. They participate fully in their prenatal visits, seeking answers to all their questions, reassurance for all their worries. And more and more often, they attend childbirth education classes.

Just what are these classes about, and why are they proliferating faster than stretch marks in the sixth month? The original, pioneering classes were intended to explain a new approach to childbirth—without medication and without fear—and were commonly known as "natural childbirth" classes. Since then, there has been a shift in emphasis from natural childbirth (though it's still considered the ideal) to education and preparation for many of the possible eventualities of labor and delivery—so that whether the birth turns out to be medicated or unmedicated, vaginal or surgical, with an episiotomy or without one, parents will have an understanding of what is happening and will be able to participate as fully as possible.

Most curricula are based on the following:

❖ The imparting of accurate information, intended to reduce fears, improve the ability to cope with pain, and enhance decision-making skills.

❖ The teaching of specially designed techniques of relaxation, distraction, muscular control, and breathing—all of which can increase a couple's sense of being in control while contributing to the woman's endurance and a reduction in her perception of pain.

❖ The development of a productive working relationship between the laboring mother and her coach, which, if maintained during labor and delivery, may serve to provide a supportive environment that can, in turn, help the mother to minimize her anxieties and maximize her efforts during labor.

BENEFITS OF TAKING A CHILDBIRTH CLASS

Just how much a couple benefits from childbirth education depends on the course they take, on the teacher, and on their own attitudes. These classes work better for some couples than for others. Some thrive in group situations and find sharing feelings natural and helpful; others are uncomfortable in groups and find sharing difficult and unproductive. Some enjoy learning the relaxation and breathing techniques, while others feel that the repetition of such exercises is forced and intrusive, tension-producing rather than tension-alleviating. Some ultimately find these exercises effective in the control of pain during labor; others end up not using them at all. Just about every couple, however, stands to gain something from taking a *good* childbirth class—and certainly has nothing to lose. Some benefits include:

❖ The opportunity to spend time with other expectant couples: to share pregnancy experiences, compare progress, and swap tales of woes, worries, aches and pains. It's also a chance to make friends-with-babies, for later. Many classes hold "reunions" once everyone has delivered.

❖ Increased involvement of the father in the pregnancy, particularly important if he isn't able to attend prenatal visits. Classes will familiarize him with the process of labor and delivery so that he can be a more effective coach, and will allow him to meet other expectant fathers. Some courses even include a special session for fathers only, which gives them the chance to express and find relief for the anxieties they're reluctant to burden their partners with.

❖ A weekly chance to ask questions that come up between prenatal visits, or that you don't feel comfortable asking your practitioner.

❖ An opportunity to get hands-on instruction in breathing, relaxation, and coaching techniques, and to get feedback from an expert.

❖ An opportunity to develop confidence in your ability to meet the strenuous demands of labor and delivery, through increased knowledge (which helps banish fear of the unknown) and the acquisition of coping skills, which may enable you to feel more in control.

❖ A chance to learn coping strategies that may help to decrease your perception of pain and, hopefully, increase your ability to tolerate it during labor and delivery—which may translate into less need for medication.

❖ The possibility of an improved, less stressful labor, thanks to a better understanding of the birthing process and the development of coping skills. Couples who've had childbirth preparation generally rate their childbirth experiences as more satisfying overall than those who haven't.

❖ Possibly, a slightly shorter labor. Studies show that the average labor of women who have had childbirth education is somewhat shorter than that of women who haven't, probably because the training and preparation better enable them to work with, instead of against, the work of the uterus. (There is no guarantee of a short labor, only the possibility of a *shorter* one.)

CHOOSING A CHILDBIRTH CLASS

In some communities where childbirth classes are few and far between, the choice is a relatively simple one. In others, the variety of offerings can be overwhelming and confusing. There are courses run by hospitals, by private instructors, by practitioners through their offices. There are "earlybird" prenatal classes—taken in the first or second trimester—which cover such concerns of pregnancy as nutrition, exercise, fetal development, hygiene, sexuality, dreams and fantasies; and there are down-to-the-wire six- to ten-week childbirth classes, usually begun in the seventh or eighth month, which concentrate on labor, delivery, and postpartum mother and baby care.

If the pickings are slim, taking any childbirth class is probably better than taking none at all—as long as you keep your perspective and don't accept every word spoken in class as gospel. If there is a selection of courses where you live, it may help to consider the following when making your decision:

❖ Taking a class that is run either by your practitioner or under the auspices of your practitioner, or is recommended by him or her, often works out best. If the laboring and delivering philosophies of your childbirth education teacher vary greatly from those of the person who'll be assisting you during labor and delivery, you're bound to run into contradictions and conflicts. If differences of opinion do arise, make sure you address them with your practitioner well before your delivery date.

❖ Small is best. Five or six couples to a class is ideal; more than ten isn't recommended. Not only can a teacher give more time and individual attention to couples in an intimate group—particularly important during the breathing and relaxation technique practice sessions—but the camaraderie in a small group tends to be stronger.

❖ Classes that set up unrealistic expectations can work against you. (If you're guaranteed that taking the class will make labor short or painless or glorious, for instance, beware.) There's no way to know for sure what a teacher's philosophy of childbirth is until you take the class—but sitting in on one or talking to her before signing up can give you some idea.

❖ What is the rate of drug-free labors among class "graduates?" This may be helpful information, but it can also be misleading. Does a low rate indicate that students were so well prepared in the various natural pain-reducing strategies that they rarely needed medication? Or were they so convinced that asking for medication was a sign of failure that they stoically withstood severe pain? Perhaps the best way to find the answer is to talk to some of the graduates.

❖ What is the curriculum like? Ask for a course outline, and if you can,

For Information on Childbirth Classes

Ask your practitioner for information on classes in your area, or call the hospital where you plan to deliver. If you are interested in pregnancy classes, ask at one of your early visits; otherwise the question can wait until the third trimester. You can also obtain referrals on local classes from:

❖ *Gamper Method:* Midwest Parentcraft Center, 627 Beaver Rd., Glenview, IL 60025; 312-248-8100.

❖ The Read Natural Childbirth Foundation, P.O. Box 956, San Rafael, CA 94915; 415-456-3143 (for general information only).

❖ *Lamaze:* American Society for Psychoprophylaxis in Obstetrics, 1840 Wilson Blvd., Suite 204, Arlington, VA 22201; 800-368-4404.

❖ International Childbirth Education Association, P.O. Box 20038, Minneapolis, MN 55420; 612-854-8660 (ICEA provides referrals from other groups as well).

❖ *Bradley:* American Academy of Husband-Coached Childbirth, P.O. Box 5224, Sherman Oaks, CA 91413; 800-423-2397; in California 800-42-BIRTH.

---

sit in on a class. A good course will include a discussion of cesarean section (recognizing that 15% to 25% of students may end up having one) and of medication (recognizing, too, that some will need this). It will deal with the psychological and emotional as well as the technical aspects of childbirth.

❖ How is the class taught? Are films of actual childbirths shown? Will you hear from mothers and fathers who've recently delivered? Is there discussion, or just lecture? Will there be an opportunity for parents-to-be to ask questions? Is adequate time provided during class for practicing the various techniques that are taught? Is one particular philosophy espoused— Lamaze or Bradley, for example?

THE MOST COMMON SCHOOLS OF THOUGHT

There are three major childbirth education philosophies, though many instructors combine elements of each in their classes.

Grantly Dick-Read. Combining relaxation techniques and prenatal education to break the fear-tension-pain cycle of labor and delivery, this psychophysical childbirth philosophy dates back to the '40s and '50s and represents the first organized approach to childbirth preparation in the United States. It was the first to include fathers in the education process and to bring them into the labor room. Programs begin in the fourth month and are conducted by instructors trained and certified in the Gamper method, named for Margaret Gamper, the nurse who inspired Dr. Dick-Read.

Lamaze. Also called the psychoprophylactic method, this approach, pioneered by Dr. Ferdinand Lamaze, is similar in some ways to the psychophysical approach in that its major weapons against pain are knowledge and relaxation techniques. In addition, Dr. Lamaze's approach depends on conditioning, à la Dr. Pavlov, who conditioned dogs to salivate at the sound of a bell. The expectant mother is conditioned, through intensive training and practice, to substitute useful responses to the stimulus of labor contractions in place of counter-productive ones. The father or other coach trains with the mother to assist her during both labor and delivery.

Bradley. This approach, which origi-nated the husband-coached delivery, emphasizes good diet and uses exer-cise to ease the discomforts of preg-nancy and to prepare muscles for birth and breasts for nursing. Women learn to imitate their sleeping position and breathing (which is deep and slow) and to use relaxation to make the first stage of labor more comfort-able. Rather than the usual panting and Lamaze breathing patterns, the Bradley method employs deep ab-dominal breathing; instead of using distraction and a focus of concentra-tion outside the body to take the mind off discomfort, Bradley recommends that the laboring woman concentrate within and work with her body. Medi-cation is reserved for complications and cesareans, and about 94% of Bradley graduates go without it. Bradley-based classes begin as soon as pregnancy is confirmed and continue into the postpartum period in the be-lief that it takes a full nine months to get physically and emotionally pre-pared for labor and delivery.

Other Childbirth Classes. Childbirth educators certified by the Interna-tional Childbirth Education Associa-tion support family-centered mater-nity care and a minimum of medical intervention. There are also childbirth education classes designed to prepare parents to deliver in a particular hos-pital, and classes sponsored by a medi-cal group, health maintenance organi-zation (HMO), or other health-care provider group. Many childbirth classes take no particular party line, selecting the best from what is known about childbirth preparation and changing their curricula as new infor-mation becomes available. In some cities, education for pregnancy as well as childbirth is offered, in classes that usually begin in the first trimester.

11
The Seventh Month

WHAT YOU CAN EXPECT AT THIS MONTH'S CHECKUP

This month you can expect your practitioner to check the following, though there may be variations depending upon your particular needs and upon your practitioner's style of practice:[1]

❖ Weight and blood pressure

❖ Urine, for sugar and protein

❖ Fetal heartbeat

❖ Height of fundus (top of uterus)

❖ Size and position of fetus, by external palpation

❖ Feet and hands for edema (swelling), and legs for varicose veins

❖ Symptoms you have been experiencing, especially unusual ones

❖ Questions and problems you want to discuss—have a list ready

WHAT YOU MAY BE FEELING

You may experience all of these symptoms at one time or another, or only a few of them. Some may have continued from last month, others may be new. Still others may hardly be noticed because you've become so used to them. You may also have other, less common, symptoms.

1. See Appendix for an explanation of the procedures and tests performed during office visits.

PHYSICALLY:

❖ Stronger and more frequent fetal activity

❖ Increasingly heavy whitish vaginal discharge (leukorrhea)

❖ Lower abdominal achiness

❖ Constipation

❖ Heartburn, indigestion, flatulence, bloating

❖ Occasional headaches, faintness, or dizziness

❖ Nasal congestion and occasional nosebleeds; ear stuffiness

❖ Pink toothbrush from bleeding gums

❖ Leg cramps

❖ Backache

❖ Mild swelling of ankles and feet, and occasionally of hands and face

❖ Varicose veins of the legs

❖ Hemorrhoids

❖ Itchy abdomen

❖ Shortness of breath

❖ Difficulty sleeping

❖ Scattered Braxton Hicks contractions, usually painless (the uterus hardens for a minute, then returns to normal)

❖ Clumsiness (which increases the risk of falling)

❖ Colostrum, either leaking or expressed, from enlarged breasts

EMOTIONALLY:

❖ Increasing apprehension about motherhood, baby's health, and about labor and delivery

❖ Continued absentmindedness

❖ Increased dreaming and fantasizing about the baby

❖ Increased boredom and weariness with the pregnancy, the beginning of anxiousness for it to be over

WHAT YOU MAY LOOK LIKE

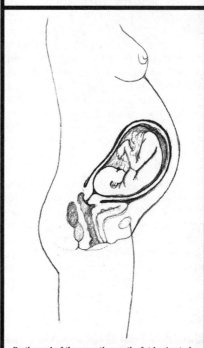

By the end of the seventh month, fat begins to be deposited on the fetus. It may suck its thumb, hiccup, cry; can taste sweet or sour; responds to stimuli, including pain, light, and sound. Placental function begins to diminish, as does the volume of amniotic fluid, as the 3-pounder fills the uterus. Good chance of survival if born now.

WHAT YOU MAY BE CONCERNED ABOUT

INCREASING FATIGUE

'I've heard women are supposed to feel terrific in the last trimester. I feel tired all the time.''

"Supposed to" is a phrase that ought to be stricken from a pregnant woman's vocabulary. There's no one way you're supposed to feel at any time in pregnancy. Though some women feel less tired in the third tri-mester than in the first and second, it can be perfectly normal to continue feeling fatigued or to feel even more fatigued. Actually, there are probably more reasons to feel tired than to feel terrific in the last trimester. First of all, you're carrying around a lot more weight than you were earlier. Second, because of your bulk, you may be having trouble sleeping. You may also be losing sleep because your mind is overloaded with baby concerns, plans, and fantasies. Taking care of other children, a job, or both may be taking a toll on you—and so may pre-paring for the new baby.

Just because fatigue is a normal part of pregnancy doesn't mean you should ignore it. As always, it's a sig-nal from your body that you should slow down. Take the hint: Rest and relax as much as you can. You'll need every bit of strength you can save up for labor, delivery, and—more important—what follows them.

Extreme fatigue that doesn't ease up when you get more rest should be reported to your doctor. Anemia (see page 154) sometimes strikes at the be-ginning of the third trimester, which is why many practitioners do a routine blood test for it in the seventh month.

CONCERN ABOUT THE BABY'S WELL-BEING

"I worry all the time that something is wrong with my baby."

There probably isn't an expectant mother (or father) who hasn't been haunted by this same fear. Some will even put off buying baby clothes and furniture, or choosing the baby's name, until toes and fingers have been counted, the Apgars have been calcu-lated, and the doctor has congratu-lated them on their healthy baby.

But the odds of having a completely normal baby have never been better. The U.S. infant mortality rate is the lowest in history, down to a little over 9 per 1,000 births (and lower than that for middle-class women).[2] Most of these perinatal (around the time of birth) deaths occur in the newborns of women who receive medical care late or not at all and who are inadequately nourished. A majority of the remain-der, occur in infants of high-risk women: those with a family history of genetic disease; with uncontrolled chronic illnesses; who drink heavily and/or smoke or take drugs; or who are carrying multiple fetuses. Even for these women, close medical supervi-sion and improved prenatal care have recently greatly increased the chances of having healthy babies.

Some experts had forecast that as the death rate fell—because more ba-bies with birth defects would be saved by medical miracles—the rate of chil-dren with handicaps would rise. This hasn't happened; the percentage of birth defects, in fact, appears to be declining. And when a child *is* born with a birth defect, he or she isn't necessarily permanently handi-capped. Most minor, and many seri-ous, defects are now correctable. If diagnosed in utero, some can be treated even before birth through sur-gery or medication. Shortly after birth, many heart defects and other internal abnormalities can be repaired with surgery, as can cleft palates and bone or limb abnormalities later on. Children who are intellectually dis-abled can, with early intervention, make remarkable strides.

So when worry strikes, strike

---

2. Estimated by government sources for 1990. Though this is an improvement over the past, it is still much higher than the rates in many other countries. The reason: inade-quate health care for the poor.

back—with the knowledge that your baby couldn't have picked a better time to be born (and to grow up) healthy. And, of course, continue to do all you can to give your baby the best odds possible.

EDEMA (SWELLING) OF THE ANKLES AND FEET

"My ankles seem to be swollen, especially when the weather is warm. Is this a bad sign?"

Any degree of edema (swelling due to excessive accumulation of fluids in the tissues) was once considered a potential danger sign in pregnancy. Now doctors recognize that mild edema is related to the normal and necessary increase in body fluids in pregnancy. Some swelling of the ankles and legs, without accompanying symptoms to suggest the development of preeclampsia (see below), is considered completely normal. In fact, 75% of women develop such edema at some point in their pregnancies.[3] It's particularly common late in the day, in warm weather, or after standing or sitting for a period of time. Most women find that much of the swelling disappears overnight—after several hours spent lying down.

Generally, edema is nothing but a little uncomfortable. To ease the discomfort, elevate your legs or lie down when you can, preferably on your left side; wear comfortable shoes or slippers; avoid elastic-top socks or stockings.

If you find the swelling very bothersome, try support hose. Several types are available for pregnancy wear—

including full pantyhose (with roomy tummy space) and knee highs—so check with your practitioner to see if he or she has a recommendation for you. When shopping, select the size based on your prepregnancy weight. Put the support hose on before you get up in the morning, while the swelling is down.

Help your system to flush out waste products by drinking at least eight to ten 8-ounce glasses of liquid a day. Paradoxically, drinking even greater amounts of liquids—up to a gallon a day—helps many women avoid excess water retention. But don't drink more than 16 ounces (2 glassfuls) at once, and don't fill up with so much liquid that you have no room for the other 11 components of your Daily Dozen. Though it's no longer believed that salt restriction is wise during a normal pregnancy (salt may be restricted for some women with high blood pressure), excessive salt intake isn't any smarter and could increase excess fluid retention.

If your hands and/or face become puffy, or if edema persists for more than 24 hours at a time, you should notify your doctor. Such swelling may be insignificant, or—if accompanied by rapid weight gain, a rise in blood pressure, and protein in the urine—it could signal the beginning of preeclampsia (pregnancy-induced hypertension; see page 204).

OVERHEATING

"I feel so warm most of the time, and I sweat a lot. Is this normal?"

With your basal metabolic rate (the rate at which your body expends energy at total rest) up about 20% during pregnancy, the heat's on. Not only are you likely to feel too warm in warm weather, you may even

---

3. One in 4 pregnant women never experience edema, and this can be completely normal, too. Others may not notice swelling.

feel overheated in the winter—when everyone else is shivering. You will also probably perspire more, especially at night. This is a mixed blessing. While it helps to cool you off and rids your body of waste products, it is admittedly unpleasant.

To minimize discomfort, bathe often; use a good antiperspirant; and dress in layers—especially in the winter—so you can peel down to shirtsleeves when you start heating up. And don't forget to take in extra fluids to replace those lost through your pores.

ORGASM AND THE BABY

"After I have an orgasm my baby usually stops kicking for about half an hour. Is sex harmful to him or her at this stage of pregnancy?"

B abies are individuals, even in the womb. And their responses to their parents' lovemaking vary. Some, perhaps like your baby, are rocked to sleep by the rhythmic motion of coitus and the uterine contractions that follow orgasm. Others, stimulated by the activity, may become more lively. Both responses are normal; neither indicates any awareness of the proceedings on the part of the fetus or that the fetus has been harmed in any way.

Whether sexual intercourse is totally safe during the last two months of pregnancy, even in a normal pregnancy, is a matter of increasing controversy in the obstetrical community. Acquitted several years ago as an accessory to premature labor and perinatal infection, coitus in the final weeks of gestation is once again being implicated in such complications by researchers. To learn what is believed safe in sexual relations for expectant parents, see Making Love During Pregnancy, page 164.

PREMATURE LABOR

"Is there anything I can do to ensure that my baby won't be born prematurely?"

F ar more babies are born late than early. In the U.S., only 7 to 10 in every 100 deliveries are premature or preterm—that is, take place before the 37th week of pregnancy. One-third of preterm births occur because labor begins early; one-third because the membranes rupture prematurely; and one-third because of a maternal or fetal problem. About 3 in 4 occur in women who are known to be at high risk for premature delivery. The rate of premature deliveries is lower for white women (fewer than 6 in 100) and higher for black women (nearly 13 out of 100), at least partly for socioeconomic reasons. Dramatic advances in preventing preterm labor, combined with better and more accessible prenatal care, should go a long way in reducing the incidence of premature births.

There are a wide variety of factors that are believed to be related to increased risk of preterm delivery. The more risk factors in a woman's history, the greater the chance that she will deliver prematurely. The risk factors that follow can often be eliminated, greatly increasing the odds that a woman will carry to term:

Smoking. Quit before conception or as early as possible in pregnancy.

Alcohol Use. Avoid regular consumption of beer, wine, and liquor (no one yet knows how much is too much, so it's safer to abstain).

Drug Abuse. Don't take any medication without the approval of a physician who knows you are pregnant; don't take any other drugs at all.

Inadequate Weight Gain. If your pre-pregnant weight was normal, gain a minimum of 25 pounds; if you were significantly underweight before conceiving, gain closer to 35 pounds. (Overweight women, with excellent nutrition and their doctor's permission, may safely be able to gain less.)

Inadequate Nutrition. Follow a well-balanced diet (See the Best-Odds Diet, page 80) throughout pregnancy. Be sure that your vitamin supplement contains zinc; some recent studies have linked zinc deficiency with preterm labor.

Standing, or Heavy Physical Labor. If your job alone or your job plus housework require you to stand for several hours each day, stop working or cut back.

Sexual Intercourse (for Some Women). Expectant mothers who are at high risk for premature delivery are generally advised to abstain from intercourse and/or orgasm during the final two or three months of pregnancy because, in these women, orgasm might activate uterine contractions.

Hormonal Imbalance. Just as it can trigger late miscarriage, an imbalance of hormones can sometimes trigger premature delivery; hormone replacement may prevent both.

Other risk factors are not always possible to eliminate, but their effects can sometimes be modified:

Infections (such as rubella; certain venereal diseases; and urinary tract, vaginal, and amniotic fluid infections). When there is an infection that could harm the fetus, early labor seems to be the body's way of trying to get the baby out of a dangerous environment. In the case of amniotic fluid infection

(chorioamnionitis), which may be a major cause of preterm labor, the body's immune response apparently triggers production of prostaglandins, which can initiate labor, as well as of substances that can damage the fetal membranes, leading to their premature rupture.

To reduce the risk that you will contract an infection, stay away from people who are ill and make sure you get adequate rest and exercise, optimum nutrition, and regular prenatal care. Some doctors also recommend using a condom during the last months of pregnancy to reduce the risk of amniotic fluid infection.

Incompetent Cervix. This condition, in which a weak cervix opens prematurely, often goes undiagnosed until after at least one instance of late miscarriage or premature labor. Once the condition is diagnosed, premature delivery can be avoided by suturing the cervix closed at about the 14th week. It is also suspected that in some women, for reasons unknown and apparently not related to incompetent cervix, the cervix begins to efface and dilate early, leading to early delivery. Routine examination of the cervix to uncover such changes in the last months of pregnancy in high-risk women is a common and probably useful procedure.

Uterine Irritability. Research suggests that in some women the uterus is particularly irritable, and that this irritability makes it susceptible to untimely contractions. If these women could be identified and monitored in the third trimester, it's possible, some believe, that their premature labor could be prevented by full or partial bed rest and/or the use of medication to quiet the contractions.

Placenta Previa (a low-lying placenta located near or over the cervix). This condition may be discovered in an ultrasound exam, or may not be suspected until bleeding is noted in mid- or late pregnancy. Premature labor may be headed off by complete bed rest.

Chronic Maternal Illness (high blood pressure; heart, liver, or kidney disease; diabetes). Good medical care, sometimes including bed rest, can often prevent premature delivery.

Stress. Sometimes the cause of stress can be eliminated or minimized (by quitting a high-pressure job or getting counseling for a floundering marriage, for example); sometimes eliminating the cause is more difficult (when you lose your job or are pregnant and alone). But all kinds of stress can be reduced through education, relaxation techniques, good nutrition, a balance of exercise and rest, and by talking out the problem—often in a self-help group (see page 113).

Age Under 17. Optimal nutrition and prenatal care can help compensate for the fact that the mother, like her fetus, is still growing.

Age Over 35. Optimal nutrition, good prenatal care, reduction of stress, and prenatal screening for genetic and obstetrical problems specific to older women all reduce risk.

Low Educational or Socioeconomic Level. Again, good nutrition and early access to, and participation in, culturally sensitive prenatal care, as well as the elimination of as many risk factors as possible, can decrease the risk.

Structural Abnormalities of the Uterus. Once the problem has been diagnosed, prepregnancy surgical repair can frequently prevent future preterm births.

Multiple Gestations. Women carrying more than one fetus deliver an average of three weeks early. Meticulous prenatal care, optimal nutrition, the elimination of other risk factors, along with more time spent lying down and resting, and restrictions on activity as needed in the last trimester, may prevent a too-early birth.

Fetal Abnormality. In some instances, prenatal diagnosis may pick up a defect that can be treated while the fetus is still in the uterus; sometimes correcting the problem can allow the pregnancy to continue to term.

History of Premature Deliveries. A diagnosed cause can be corrected; top-notch prenatal care, reduction of other risk factors, and limitations on activities may help to prevent a repeat.

Occasionally none of the above risk factors is present. A healthy woman with a perfectly normal pregnancy suddenly goes into labor early, for no apparent reason. Perhaps someday a cause will be identified for such premature births, but presently they are labeled "cause unknown."

When risk factors are present, research shows that it is possible to reduce the incidence of preterm births through education and home uterine monitoring. It's not clear whether it is the education and contact with a nurse or the monitoring, or both, that helps, but such programs have been found by some researchers to reduce preterm deliveries.

If preterm labor does begin, the delivery can often be held off until the baby is more mature. Even a brief delay can be beneficial; each additional day the baby remains in the uterus until term improves its chances of survival. So you can see that it's important to be familiar with the signs of early labor, and to alert your practitioner if you've the slightest suspicion that labor is beginning. *Don't worry about bothering your doctor*—no matter what the day or hour.

❖ Menstrual-like cramps, with or without diarrhea, nausea, or indigestion.

❖ Lower back pain or pressure, or a change in the nature of lower backache.

❖ An achiness or feeling of pressure in the pelvic floor, the thighs, or the groin.

❖ A change in your vaginal discharge, particularly if it is watery or tinged or streaked pinkish or brownish with blood. The passage of a thick, gelatinous mucous plug may or may not precede this "bloody show."

❖ Rupture of membranes (a trickle or rush of fluid from your vagina).

You can have all these symptoms and not be in labor, but only your practitioner can tell you for sure. If he or she suspects you're in labor, you will probably be examined promptly. For information about how premature labor is treated, see page 361.

If premature labor does occur—despite steps taken to prevent or postpone it—your chances of bringing a healthy, normal baby home from the hospital are excellent. (Of course, that trip home with the baby may have to be delayed days, weeks, or even months to increase those chances.)

APPROACHING RESPONSIBILITY

"I'm beginning to worry that I won't be able to manage my job, my house, my marriage—and the baby too."

You probably won't be able to manage if you attempt to be a full-time career woman, housekeeper, wife, and mother—expecting perfection in each role. Many new mothers have tried to be "superwoman"; few have succeeded without sacrificing their health and sanity.

But it will be possible to survive if you reconcile yourself to the reality that you can't do it all—at least in the beginning. If job, husband, and baby are top priorities, perhaps keeping the house immaculate will have to take a backseat for now. If full-time motherhood appeals to you and you can afford to stay home for a while, maybe you can shelve your career temporarily. Or work part-time, as a compromise. It's just a matter of deciding what your priorities are.

Whatever decision you make, your new life will be easier if you don't have to go it alone. Behind most successful moms there's a cooperative dad, willing to share the workload. Don't feel guilty about asking your husband to change diapers and bathe the baby after a long day at the office. There's probably no better way for him to unwind and at the same time to get to know his child. If Dad isn't available (all or part of the time), then

---

Don't Hold It In

Making a habit of not urinating when you feel the need increases the risk that your inflamed bladder may irritate the uterus and set off contractions, so *don't hold it in.*

you are going to need to consider other sources of assistance: the baby's grandparents or other relatives, child-care or household workers, play-groups, day care centers.

ACCIDENTS

"I missed the curb today when I was out walking and fell belly-first on the pavement. I'm not worried about my skinned knees and elbows, but I'm terrified that I've hurt the baby."

A woman in the last trimester of pregnancy isn't exactly the most graceful creature on earth. A poor sense of balance (because her center of gravity keeps shifting forward) and looser, less stable joints contribute to her awkwardness and make her prone to minor falls—particularly belly-flops. So do her tendency to tire easily, her predisposition to preoccupation and daydreaming, and the difficulty she may be having seeing past her belly to her feet.

But while a curbside spill may leave you with multiple scrapes and bruises (particularly to your ego), it's extremely rare for a fetus to suffer the consequences of its mother's clumsiness. Your baby is protected by the world's most sophisticated shock-absorption system, comprised of amniotic fluid, tough membranes, the elastic, muscular uterus, and the sturdy abdominal cavity girded with muscles and bones. For it to be penetrated, and for your baby to be hurt, you'd have to sustain very serious injuries—the kind that would very likely land you in the hospital.

Even though there's probably no harm done, you should let your practitioner know if you have a fall. You may be asked to come in so that your baby's heartbeat can be checked—mostly to set your mind at ease.

On the rare occasion when damage to a pregnancy does occur as a result of an accident, it's most likely to involve separation (abruption) of the placenta, partially or completely, from the uterine wall—an injury that requires swift action on the part of the physician. If you notice vaginal bleeding, leakage of amniotic fluid, abdominal tenderness, or uterine contractions, or if your baby seems unusually inactive, seek medical attention *immediately.* Have someone take you to the emergency room if you can't reach your doctor.

LOWER BACK AND LEG PAIN (SCIATICA)

"I've been having pain on the right side of my back, running right down my hip and leg. What's happening?"

This sounds like another of the occupational hazards of expectant motherhood. The pressure of the enlarging uterus, which has been responsible for so many other discomforts, can also affect the sciatic nerve—causing lower back, buttock, and leg pain. Rest, and a heating pad applied locally, may help. The pain may pass as your baby's position changes, or it may linger until you've delivered. In severe cases, a few days of bed rest or special exercises may be recommended.

SKIN ERUPTIONS

"It's not bad enough that I have stretch marks, now I seem to have some kind of itchy pimples breaking out in them."

C heer up. You have less than three months left until delivery, when you'll be able to bid a grateful goodbye to most of the unpleasant side effects of pregnancy—among them, these new eruptions. Until then, it may help to know that although they may be uncomfortable, the lesions aren't dangerous to you or your baby. Known medically, and unpronounceably, as pruritic urticarial papules and plaques of pregnancy, or PUPPP, the condition disappears after delivery and doesn't usually recur in subsequent pregnancies. Though PUPPP most often develops in abdominal stretch marks, it sometimes also appears on the thighs, buttocks, or arms of the expectant mother. Show your rash to your practitioner, who may prescribe topical medication, an antihistamine, or a cortico steroid shot to ease any discomfort.

There are a variety of other skin conditions and rashes that can develop during pregnancy. Though they should always be shown to your practitioner, they are rarely serious. Some will need to be treated; others will run a mild course and disappear after delivery.

FETAL HICCUPS

"I sometimes feel regular little spasms in my abdomen. Is this kicking, or a twitch, or what?"

B elieve it or not, your baby's probably got hiccups. This phenomenon is not uncommon in fetuses in the last half of pregnancy. Some get hiccups several times a day, every day. Others never get them at all. The same pattern may continue after birth.

But before you start holding a paper bag over your belly, you should know that hiccups don't cause the same discomfort in babies (in or out of the uterus) as they do in adults—even when they last as long as 20 minutes or more. So just relax and enjoy this little entertainment from within.

DREAMS AND FANTASIES

"I've been having so many vivid dreams about the baby that I'm beginning to think I'm going mad."

T hough the many night- and daydreams (both horrifying and pleasant) a pregnant woman can experience in the last trimester may make her feel as though she's losing her sanity, they're actually helping to keep her sane. Dreams and fantasies are both healthy and normal, and help expectant women to sort out worries and fears in a nonthreatening way.

Each of the dream and fantasy themes commonly reported by pregnant women expresses one or more of the deep-seated feelings and concerns that might otherwise be suppressed:

❖ Being unprepared, losing things, forgetting to feed the baby; missing a doctor's appointment; going out to shop and forgetting the baby; being unprepared for the baby when it arrives; losing car keys, or even the baby—can express the fear of not being adequate to the task of motherhood.

❖ Being attacked or hurt—by intruders, burglars, animals; falling down the stairs after a push or a slip—may represent a sense of vulnerability.

❖ Being enclosed or unable to escape—trapped in a tunnel, a car, a small room; drowning in a pool, a lake of snowy slush, a car wash—can signify the fear of being tied down and deprived of freedom by the baby.

❖ Going off your pregnancy diet—gaining too much weight, or gaining a lot of weight overnight; overeating; eating or drinking the wrong things (two hot fudge sundaes or a bottle of wine) or not eating the right things (forgetting to drink milk for a week)—is a theme common among those trying to adjust to a restricted dietary regimen.

❖ Losing appeal—becoming unattractive or repulsive to her husband; her husband finding another woman—expresses nearly every woman's fear that pregnancy will destroy her looks forever and drive her husband away.

❖ Sexual encounters—either positive or negative, pleasure- or guilt-provoking—may reflect the sexual confusion and ambivalence often experienced during pregnancy.

❖ Death and resurrection—lost parents or other relatives reappearing—may be the subconscious mind's way of linking old and new generations.

❖ Family life with the new baby—getting ready for the baby; loving and playing with the baby—is practice parenting, bonding mother with the baby prior to birth.

❖ What the baby will be like—can represent a wide variety of concerns. Dreams about the baby being deformed or unusual in size express anxiety about its health. Fantasies about the infant having unusual skills (like talking or walking at birth) may indicate concern about the baby's intelligence and ambition for his or her future. Premonitions that the baby will be a boy or a girl could mean your heart's too set on one or the other. So could dreams about the baby's hair or eye color or resemblance to one parent

or the other. Nightmares of the baby being born fully grown could signify another problem—your fear of having to handle a tiny baby.

Though dreams and fantasies can be more anxiety-provoking in pregnancy than they are at other times, they can also be more useful. If you listen to what your motherhood fantasies are telling you about your feelings and deal with them now, you can make the transition into real-life motherhood more easily.

A LOW-BIRTHWEIGHT BABY

"I've been reading a lot about the high incidence of low-birthweight babies. Is there anything I can do to be sure I won't have one?"

Since most cases of low birthweight are preventable, you can do a lot—and inasmuch as you're reading this book, chances are you already are. Nationally, nearly 7 of every 100 newborns are categorized as low birthweight (under 5 pounds 8 ounces, or 2,500 grams), and slightly more than 1 in 100 babies as *very* low birthweight (3 pounds 5 ounces, or 1,500 grams, or less). But among informed women who are conscientious about both medical and self care as well as their lifestyle habits, the rate is much lower. Most of the common causes of low birthweight are preventable (tobacco, alcohol, or drug use by the mother, poor nutrition, inadequate prenatal care, for example); many others (such as chronic maternal illness) can be controlled by a good working partnership between the mother and her practitioner. A major cause—premature labor—can in some instances also be prevented (see page 218).

Of course, sometimes a baby is small at birth for reasons that no one can control—the mother's own low weight when she was born, for example, or an inadequate placenta, or a genetic disorder (see page 354 for more on causes of growth retardation in the fetus). But even in these cases, excellent diet and prenatal care can often compensate. And when a baby does turn out to be small, the top-notch medical care currently available gives even the very smallest an increasingly good chance of surviving and growing up healthy.

If you think you have reason to worry about the possibility of having a low-birthweight baby, you should share your concern with your practitioner. A sonogram will probably be able to determine right now whether or not your fetus is growing at a normal pace. If it isn't, then steps can be taken to uncover the cause of the slow growth and, if possible, correct it (see page 355).

A BIRTHING PLAN

"A friend who recently delivered said she worked out a birthing plan with her doctor before delivery. Is this common?"

Birthing plans are becoming increasingly common as practitioners recognize that more and more women—and their partners—would like to be involved in making as many of the childbirth decisions as they possibly can. Some practitioners routinely ask expectant parents to fill out a birthing plan; most others are willing to discuss such a plan if a patient requests it. The typical plan combines the parents' wishes and preferences with what the practitioner and hospital find acceptable—and what is feasible from a practical point of view. It's not a contract but a written understanding between practitioner and/or

hospital and patient with the goal of bringing childbirth as close as possible to the patient's ideal while heading off unrealistic expectations, minimizing disappointment, and avoiding major conflict during labor and delivery.

A birthing plan may deal with a wide variety of topics; the precise content of each will depend on the parents, practitioner, and hospital involved, as well as on the particular situation. Some of the issues that you may want to express your preferences about include the following (refer to the appropriate pages before making your decision):

❖ How far into your labor you would like to remain at home (see page 270).

❖ Eating and/or drinking during active labor (page 291).

❖ Being out of bed (walking about or sitting up) during labor (page 289).

❖ Wearing contact lenses during labor and delivery (usually not permitted if general anesthesia is required).

❖ The locale of your labor and delivery—birthing room, labor room, delivery room (page 261).

❖ Personalizing the atmosphere (with music, lighting, items from home).

❖ The use of a still camera or videotape.

❖ Administration of enemas (page 277).

❖ Shaving of the pubic area (page 278).

❖ The use of an IV (intravenous fluid administration; page 279).

❖ Routine catheterization (page 378).

❖ The use of pain medication (page 226).

❖ External fetal monitoring (continuous or intermittent); internal fetal monitoring (page 280).

❖ The use of oxytocin (to induce or augment contractions; page 273).

❖ Delivery positions (page 300).

❖ Episiotomy; the use of steps to reduce the need for an episiotomy (page 283).

❖ Forceps use (page 286).

❖ Cesarean section (page 242).

❖ Suctioning of the newborn; suctioning by the father.

❖ The presence of significant others (besides your spouse) during labor and/or at delivery.

❖ The presence of older children at delivery or immediately postpartum.

❖ Holding the baby immediately after birth; breastfeeding immediately.

❖ Postponing weighing the baby and administering eye drops until after you and your baby greet each other.

You may also want to include some postpartum items on your birthing plan, such as:

❖ Your presence at the weighing of the baby, the administration of eye drops, the pediatric exam, and baby's first bath.

❖ Baby feeding in the hospital (whether it will be controlled by the nursery's schedule or your baby's hunger; whether support will be given to breastfeeding; whether supplementary bottles can be avoided).[4]

❖ Management of breast engorgement if you're not breastfeeding (page 382).

❖ Circumcision.

❖ Rooming in.

❖ Other children visiting with you and/or with the new baby.

❖ Postpartum medication or treatments for you or your baby.

❖ The length of the hospital stay, barring complications.

Of course with some of these items, your practitioner's judgment or hospital rules will affect the final plan. And remember that while it is ideal if your plans can be carried through the way you drew them up, it isn't always possible. Since there is no way to predict in advance precisely how labor and delivery will progress, childbirth plans you make before the process begins may not end up being in the best interests of you and your baby, and may have to be changed at the last minute. If this happens, try to keep in mind that the priorities in any birth should be the health and safety of mother and child—and that all other considerations must be secondary.

WHAT IT'S IMPORTANT TO KNOW:
ALL ABOUT CHILDBIRTH MEDICATION

On January 19, 1847, Scottish physician James Young Simpson splashed a half teaspoonful of chloroform on a handkerchief and held it over the nose of a laboring woman. Less than half an hour later,

she became the first woman to deliver while under anesthesia. (There was only one complication: When the

---

4. For more information on these postpartum issues, see *What to Expect the First Year.*

woman—whose first baby had been born after three days of painful labor—awoke, Dr. Simpson was unable to convince her that she'd actually given birth.)

This revolution in obstetrical practice was welcomed by women but fought by both the clergy and some members of the medical profession, who believed that pain in childbirth (woman's punishment for Eve's indiscretions in Eden) was a burden that women were born to carry. Relief of the pain would be immoral.

But opponents didn't stand a chance at halting the revolution. Once word got around that childbirth didn't have to hurt, obstetrical patients wouldn't take "no pain relief" for an answer. No longer was it a question of whether anesthesia had a place in obstetrics, but what kind of anesthesia would fill that place best.

The search for the perfect pain reliever—a drug that would eliminate pain without harming mother or child—was on. Enormous progress was made (and is still being made); analgesics and anesthetics became safer and more effective every year.

And then, during the 1950s and '60s, the love affair between childbirth medication and obstetrical patients began to get shaky. Women wanted to be awake for their deliveries and to experience every sensation, in spite of the discomfort. And they wanted their babies to arrive as alert as they were—not drugged from the effects of anesthesia.

Through the 1970s and into the 1980s, singleminded women waged war against recalcitrant physicians, the battle cry being "natural childbirth for all." Today enlightened practitioners and patients alike recognize that wanting relief from excruciating pain is natural, and that therefore pain relief medication can play a role in natural childbirth. Though an unmedicated birth is still considered the

ideal, it's understood that there are times when it's not in the best interests of mother and/or child. Medication is recommended when:

❖ Labor is long and complicated—since pain stress can lead to chemical imbalances that can interfere with contractions, compromise blood flow to the fetus, and exhaust the mother, reducing her ability to push effectively.

❖ The pain is more than the mother can tolerate, or is interfering with her ability to push.

❖ Outlet forceps (to ease the baby out once its head is visible at the vaginal outlet) are required.

❖ It's necessary to slow down a precipitous (dangerously rapid) labor.

❖ A mother is so agitated that she is hindering the progress of labor.

Prudent use of any type of medication always requires a careful weighing of risk against benefit. In the case of obstetrical drugs used during labor and delivery, risks and benefits must be examined for both mother and baby, making the equation a more complicated one. In some instances, the risks of medications clearly outweigh the benefits they offer—such as when the fetus, because of prematurity or other factors, doesn't appear strong enough to cope with the combined stress of labor *and* drugs.

Most experts agree that when childbirth medication is used, benefits can be increased and risks reduced by:

❖ Selecting a drug that has minimal side effects and presents the least risk to mother and baby while still providing pain relief; giving it in the smallest dose that will be effective; and administering it at the optimum time in the course of labor. Exposure to general anesthetic agents is usually minimized in cesarean deliveries by extracting the fetus within minutes of administering the drug to the mother, before it has a chance to cross the placenta in significant amounts.

❖ Having an expert anesthesiologist or anesthetist administer anesthesia. (You have the right to insist on this if you are having general or regional—spinal, epidural, etc.—anesthesia.)

A major concern of careful medicating in obstetrics is not only the safety of the direct recipient (the mother), but that of the indirect recipient and innocent bystander (the baby). A baby whose mother has been given medication during delivery may be born drowsy, sluggish, unresponsive, and, less often, with breathing and sucking difficulties and an irregular heartbeat. Studies show, however, that when drugs have been properly used, these adverse effects largely disappear soon after birth. A fetus can handle a certain degree of the depression or arrested activity that sometimes results from too much medication in labor or too much anesthesia during delivery; only extreme depression is hazardous. If a baby is so drugged that he doesn't breathe spontaneously at birth, quick resuscitation (a simple procedure) will prevent long-term damage.

Yet another concern in administering pain relief is how it will affect the progress of labor; given at the wrong time, it could slow or even stop it.

WHAT KINDS OF PAIN RELIEF ARE MOST COMMONLY USED?

A variety of analgesics (pain relievers), anesthetics (substances that produce loss of sensation), and ataraxics (tranquilizers) may be given during labor and delivery. Which drug, if any, will be administered will depend on the stage of labor, the patient's preference (except in an emergency), the past health history of the mother, and her present condition as well as that of her baby, as well as upon the obstetrician's and/or anesthesiologist's preference and expertise. The efficacy will depend upon the woman, the dosage, and other factors. (Very rarely, a drug won't produce the desired effect, and will give little or no pain relief.) Obstetrical pain relief is most commonly accomplished with the following drugs:

Analgesics. Meperidine hydrochloride, a powerful pain reliever commonly known under the trade name Demerol, is one of the most frequently used obstetrical analgesics. It is most effectively administered intravenously (injected slowly into an IV apparatus, so that its effects can be gauged) or intramuscularly (one shot, usually in the buttocks, though the medication may be repeated every two to four hours as needed). Demerol does not usually interfere with the contractions or their work, though with larger doses the contractions may become less frequent or weaker. It may actually help normalize contractions in a dysfunctional uterus (one that is functioning abnormally). Like other analgesics, Demerol is not generally administered until labor is well established and false labor has been ruled out, but at least two to three hours before delivery is expected. A mother's reaction to the drug and the degree of pain relief achieved vary widely. Some women find it relaxes them and makes them better able to cope with contractions. Others very much dislike the drowsy feeling and find they are less able to cope. Side effects may, depending on a woman's sensitivity, include nausea, vomiting, depression, and a drop in blood pressure. The effect Demerol will have on the newborn depends on the total dose and how close to delivery it has been administered. If it has been given too close to delivery, the baby may be sleepy and unable to suck; less frequently, respiration may be depressed and supplemental oxygen may be required. These effects are generally short-term and, if necessary, can be counteracted. Demerol may also be given postpartum to relieve the pain of an episiotomy repair or a cesarean.

Tranquilizers. These drugs (such as Phenergan or Vistaril) are used to calm and relax an anxious woman so that she can participate more fully in childbirth. Tranquilizers can also enhance the effectiveness of analgesics, such as Demerol. Like analgesics, tranquilizers are usually administered once labor is well established, and considerably before delivery. But they are occasionally used in early labor if a first-time mother is extremely nervous. Women's reactions to the effects of tranquilizers vary. Some welcome the gentle drowsiness; others find it interferes with their control. A small dose may serve to relieve anxiety without impairing alertness. A larger dose may cause slurring of speech and dozing between contraction peaks— making use of prepared childbirth techniques difficult. Though the risks to a fetus or newborn from tranquilizers are minimal (except in cases of fetal distress), it's a good idea for you and your coach to try nondrug relaxation techniques before asking for medication.

Inhalants. Nitrous oxide is rarely used today, except in combination with other drugs to induce general anesthesia.

Regional Nerve Blocks. Anesthetics injected along the course of a nerve or nerves may be used to deaden sensation in that region. In childbirth, anesthetics may completely numb the area from the waist down for surgical delivery, or numb a smaller area partially or totally for a vaginal one. Regional blocks have an advantage over general anesthesia for surgical delivery, in that the mother is awake during the birth and is alert afterward. In a vaginal delivery, they have the possible disadvantage of inhibiting the urge to push. Occasionally, oxytocin may be administered to rev up contractions that have become sluggish because of the anesthetic effect. Sometimes a catheter (tube) is inserted into the bladder to drain urine (because the urge to urinate is also suppressed). The most frequently used blocks are: pudendal, epidural, spinal, and caudal.

A pudendal block, occasionally used to relieve early second-stage pain, is usually reserved for the vaginal delivery itself. Administered through a needle inserted into the perineal or vaginal area (while the mother lies on her back with her feet in stirrups), it reduces pain in the region, but not uterine discomfort. It is useful when outlet forceps are used, and its effect can last through episiotomy and repair. It is frequently used in combination with Demerol or a tranquilizer to provide excellent pain relief with relative safety—even when an anesthesiologist is not available.

The epidural block (or lumbar epidural) is becoming increasingly popular for both vaginal and cesarean deliveries, as well as for the relief of severe labor pain. The major reason is its relative safety (less drug is needed to achieve the desired effect) and its ease of administration. The drug (usually bupivacaine, lidocaine, or chloroprocaine) is administered as needed during labor and/or delivery, through a fine tube that has been inserted through a needle in the back (after a local anesthetic numbs the area), into the epidural space between the spinal cord and the outer membrane, usually while the mother lies on her left side or sits up and leans over a table to steady herself. The medication can be stopped in time to allow the mother to have full control over pushing and then be restarted after delivery, during the repair of any episiotomy. Blood pressure is checked frequently because the procedure can cause it to drop suddenly. Intravenous fluids, and possibly medication, may be given to counteract this reaction. Leaning the uterus to the left may also help. Because of the risk of a blood pressure drop, an epidural is generally not used when there is a bleeding complication, such as placenta previa, severe preeclampsia or eclampsia, or fetal distress. Because an epidural is sometimes associated with slowing of the fetal heartbeat, continuous fetal monitoring is usually required.

As the epidural becomes more popular, more of its drawbacks become apparent. Since it can block the mother's urge to push, forceps or vacuum extraction are more frequently necessary to complete the delivery when an epidural has been given. There is also some evidence that suggests that in first labors an epidural can increase the need for cesarean section. Therefore, although an epidural is a valuable approach to pain relief in labor, it should not be used routinely.

Spinal blocks (for cesarean) and low spinal, or saddle, blocks (for forceps-assisted vaginal delivery) are administered in a single dose just prior to delivery. The mother lies on her side (back arched, neck and knees flexed) and an anesthetic is injected into the fluid surrounding the spinal cord. There may be some nausea and vomiting while the drug is in effect, about 1 to 1½ hours. As with an epidural, there is a risk of a drop in blood pressure. Elevation of the legs, leaning the uterus to the left, intravenous flu-

ids, and, occasionally, medication may be used to prevent or counteract this complication. After delivery, spinal-block patients must usually remain flat on their backs for about eight hours, and a few may experience post-spinal headache. As with epidurals, spinals are not usually used when there is placenta previa, preeclampsia or eclampsia, or fetal distress.

The caudal block is similar to the epidural, except that it blocks sensation in a more limited area, takes a larger dose to be effective, and requires greater skill on the part of the anesthesiologist. It also inhibits labor. Because of these potential risks, it is used much less frequently today than it was in the past.

General Anesthesia. Once the most popular pain relief for delivery, general anesthesia—which puts the patient to sleep—is used today almost exclusively for surgical births, and occasionally for delivering the head in a vaginal breech. Because of its rapid effect, it is more likely to be used in emergency cesareans, when there is no time for a regional anesthetic to be administered.

Inhalants, such as those used for analgesic effect, are used to induce general anesthesia—often in conjunction with other agents. This is done by an anesthesiologist in an operating/delivery room. The mother is awake during the preparations and unconscious for however long it takes to complete the delivery (usually a matter of minutes). When she comes to she may be groggy, disoriented, and restless. She may also have a cough and sore throat (due to the endotracheal tube), experience nausea and vomiting, and find her bowels and bladder sluggish. A temporary drop in blood pressure is another possible side effect.

The major problem with general anesthesia is that as the mother is sedated, so is the fetus. Sedation of the fetus can be minimized, however, by administering the anesthesia as close to the actual birth as possible. That way the baby can be delivered before the anesthetic has reached him or her in meaningful amounts. Administering oxygen to the mother, and tilting her to the side (usually the left side), can also help get oxygen to the fetus.

The other major risk of general anesthesia is that the mother may vomit and aspirate (inhale) the vomited material, which can cause complications, such as aspiration pneumonia. That's why you are asked not to eat or drink a lot of liquids when in active labor and why, if you do have general anesthesia, an endotracheal tube will be inserted through your mouth into your throat to prevent aspiration. You may be given oral antacids just prior to the procedure to neutralize the acids in your stomach in case you do aspirate.

Hypnosis. Despite the somewhat disreputable image it's developed on the nightclub circuit, hypnosis, in qualified hands, provides a legitimate, medically acceptable route to pain relief. There's really nothing mysterious about hypnosis. Suggestion and the power of mind over matter are taught in every good childbirth preparation class. With hypnosis a very high level of suggestibility is achieved, which (depending on an individual's susceptibility and the type of hypnosis used) can do anything from making the patient more relaxed and comfortable to completely eliminating awareness of pain. Only about 1 in 4 adults is hypnotizable to some degree. (A very small percentage can even go through an unmedicated cesarean section without feeling any pain.)

Training of a subject in hypnosis for childbirth should start weeks or months in advance, under a physician certified in the subject or another practitioner recommended by your physician. You may use auto- or self-hypnosis, or you may depend upon the practitioner to make the suggestions. Either way, use caution—hypnosis can be misused.

Other Methods of Pain Relief. There are several techniques aimed at reducing the perception of pain that do not require the use of drugs, and that are sometimes effective. They are particularly good choices for women who are in drug or alcohol recovery and those who do not want to use drugs for other reasons.

TENS (Transcutaneous Electrical Nerve Stimulation). TENS uses electrodes to stimulate nerve pathways to the uterus and cervix. It's theorized that this stimulation jams other sensory inputs along those pathways, such as pain. The intensity of stimulation is controlled by the patient, allowing her to increase it during a contraction, reduce it in between. More hospitals are making TENS available and it may be worthwhile checking to see if yours is one of them.

Acupuncture. Long popular in China and sometimes used in the U.S., acupuncture probably works according to the same principles as TENS. But the stimulation is supplied by needles inserted and manipulated through the skin.

Alteration of the risk factors for increased pain perception. A number of factors, emotional and physical, can affect how a woman perceives the pain of childbirth. Altering them can often increase comfort during labor (see page 298).

Physical therapy. Massage, heat, pressure, or counterpressure administered by a health professional or a loving spouse or friend often lessens the perception of pain.

Distraction. Anything—watching TV, listening to music, meditating, practicing breathing exercises—that takes your mind off the pain can decrease your perception of it.

MAKING THE DECISION

W omen have more options in childbirth today than ever before. And with the exception of certain emergency situations, the decision of whether or not to have medication during labor and delivery will be largely yours. To try to make the best possible decision, for you and your baby:

❖ Discuss the topic of pain relief and anesthesia with your practitioner long before labor begins. Your practitioner's expertise and experience make him or her an invaluable partner in your decision-making process. Well before your first contraction, find out what kinds of drugs or procedures he or she uses most often and what side effects may be experienced by mother and/or child. Also find out when he or she considers medication absolutely necessary and when he or she considers the option to be yours.

❖ Recognize that, although childbirth is a natural experience that many women can go through without medication, it is not supposed to be a trial by ordeal or a test of bravery, strength, or endurance. The pain of childbirth has been described as the most intense in the human experience. Medical technology has given women the option of relief from this pain through medication. Not only is this an acceptable option, it is, in certain cases, the preferred one.

❖ Keep in mind that taking childbirth medication (or any medication) en-

tails both risks and benefits, and it should be used only when the benefits outweigh the risks.

❖ Don't make up and close your mind in advance. Though it's okay to theorize what might be best for you under certain circumstances, it's impossible to predict what kind of labor and delivery you'll have, how you will respond to the contractions, and whether or not you'll want, need, or have to have medication. Even if you're scheduled for a cesarean, you can plan only tentatively on an epidural; last-minute complications could necessitate general anesthesia.

❖ If during labor you feel you need medication, discuss it with your coach and the nurse or doctor. But don't insist on it immediately. Try holding out 15 minutes or so and putting that time to the best possible use—concentrating extra-hard on your relaxation or breathing techniques and taking in all the comfort your coach can give you. You may find that with a little more support you can handle the pain, or that the progress you make in those 15 minutes gives you the will to go on without help. If after waiting you find that you need the relief as much or even more, ask for it—and don't feel guilty. If, of course, your physician decides that you need medication immediately, for your sake or your baby's, waiting may not be advisable.

❖ Remember that your well-being and that of your baby are your number one priority (as they have been all through pregnancy), not some preconceived, idealized childbirth scenario. All decisions should be made with that priority in mind.

12
The Eighth Month

WHAT YOU CAN EXPECT AT THIS MONTH'S CHECKUPS

After the 32nd week, your practitioner may ask you to come in every two weeks so you and your baby can be more closely monitored. You can expect the following to be checked, depending upon your particular needs and upon your practitioner's style of practice:[1]

❖ Weight and blood pressure

❖ Urine, for sugar and protein

❖ Fetal heartbeat

❖ Height of fundus (top of uterus)

❖ Size (you may get a rough weight estimate) and position of fetus, by palpation

❖ Feet and hands for edema (swelling), and legs for varicose veins

❖ Symptoms you have been experiencing, especially unusual ones

❖ Questions and problems you want to discuss—have a list ready

WHAT YOU MAY BE FEELING

You may experience all of these symptoms at one time or another, or only a few of them. Some may have continued from last month, others may be new or hardly noticeable. You may also have other, less common, symptoms.

1. See Appendix for an explanation of the procedures and tests performed during office visits.

PHYSICALLY:

❖ Strong, regular fetal activity

❖ Increasingly heavy whitish vaginal discharge (leukorrhea)

❖ Increased constipation

❖ Heartburn, indigestion, flatulence, bloating

❖ Occasional headaches, faintness or dizziness

- Nasal congestion and occasional nosebleeds; ear stuffiness
- Bleeding gums
- Leg cramps
- Backache
- Mild swelling of ankles and feet, and occasionally of hands and face
- Varicose veins of legs
- Hemorrhoids
- Itchy abdomen, protruding navel
- Increasing shortness of breath as uterus crowds the lungs, which eases when the baby drops
- Difficulty sleeping
- Increasing Braxton Hicks contractions
- Increasing clumsiness
- Colostrum, either leaking or expressed, from breasts (though this premilk substance may not appear until after delivery)

EMOTIONALLY:

- Increasing eagerness for the pregnancy to be over
- Apprehension about the baby's health, about labor and delivery
- Increasing absentmindedness

WHAT YOU MAY LOOK LIKE

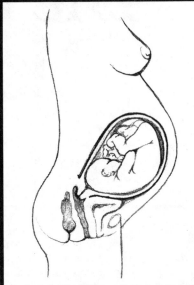

By the end of the eighth month, the baby is about 18 inches long and weighs 5 pounds. Growth, especially of the brain, is great in this period, and the fetus can see and hear. Most systems are well developed, but the lungs may still be immature. Baby has an excellent chance of survival if born now.

- Excitement at the realization that *it* won't be long now

WHAT YOU MAY BE CONCERNED ABOUT

SHORTNESS OF BREATH

"Sometimes I have trouble breathing. Could this mean that my baby isn't getting enough oxygen?"

Shortness of breath doesn't mean you—or your baby—are short of oxygen. Changes in the respiratory system during pregnancy actually allow women to take in *more* oxygen and to use it more efficiently. Still, most women experience varying degrees of difficulty breathing (some describe it as feeling a conscious need to breathe more deeply)—particularly in the last trimester, when the expanding uterus presses against the diaphragm, crowding the lungs. Relief usually arrives when lightening occurs (when the fetus settles back down into the pelvis, in first pregnancies generally two to three weeks before delivery). In the meantime, you may find it easier to breathe if you sit straight up instead of slumped over, sleep in a semi-propped-up position, and avoid overexertion.

Women who carry "low" throughout their pregnancies may never experience such exaggerated shortness of breath, and that's normal too.

Shortness of breath that is severe, however, and is accompanied by rapid breathing, blueness of lips and fingertips, chest pain, and/or rapid pulse isn't normal and requires an immediate call to the doctor or trip to the emergency room.

NOT SO FUNNY RIB TICKLING

"It feels as though my son has his feet jammed up into my rib cage—and it really hurts."

In the later months, when fetuses can't always get comfortable in their cramped quarters, they often do seem to find a snug niche for their feet between their mother's ribs, and that's one kind of rib tickling that doesn't tickle. Changing your own position may convince him to change his. A few Dromedary Droops (page 192) may dislodge him. Or try taking a deep breath while you raise one arm over your head, then exhale while you drop your arm; repeat a few times with each arm.

If none of these tactics work, hang in there. When your little pain-in-the-ribs engages, or drops into your pelvis, which usually happens two or three weeks before delivery in first pregnancies (though not until labor begins in subsequent ones), he probably won't be able to get his toes up quite so high.

STRESS INCONTINENCE

"I've started leaking urine occasionally. Is something wrong?"

In the last trimester, some women start to leak a little urine—usually only when they laugh (or cough, or sneeze). This is called stress incontinence, and in pregnancy is the result of the mounting pressure of the growing uterus on the bladder. Doing Kegel exercises (see page 190), which are also useful for firming up your pelvic muscles for delivery and postpartum recovery, may help. They may also help prevent incontinence postpartum.

YOUR WEIGHT GAIN AND THE BABY'S SIZE

"I've gained so much weight that I'm afraid the baby will be very big and difficult to deliver."

Just because you've gained a lot of weight doesn't necessarily mean your baby has. A 35- to 40-pound weight gain can yield a 6- or 7-pound baby, or an even smaller one if the weight was gained largely on junk food. On the average, however, a larger weight gain produces a larger baby. Your baby's size may also be influenced by your own birthweight (if you were born large or small, your baby will tend to be too) and by your prepregnancy weight (in general, heavier women have heavier babies). By palpating your abdomen and measuring the height of your fundus (the top of the uterus), your practitioner will be able to give you some idea of your baby's size, though such "guess-timates" can be off by a pound or more. A sonogram may more accurately gauge size, but it may be off too.

Even if your baby is large, that doesn't automatically portend a difficult delivery. Though a 6- or 7-pound baby often makes its way out faster than an 8- or 9-pounder, many women are able to deliver a bigger baby vaginally and without complications. The determining factor, as in any delivery, is whether the baby's head (its largest part) can fit through the mother's pelvis. At one time, x-rays were routinely used to try to determine whether or not a mismatch between the fetal head and the mother's pelvis (cephalopelvic disproportion, or CPD) existed. But experience and research have shown that an x-ray is not an accurate predictor of CPD, partly because it can't foresee to what extent the fetal head will mold in order to squeeze through the birth canal. Though the risk of an x-ray is slight, it is recommended only rarely, when benefits outweigh that risk.

More commonly today, when there is some suspicion of cephalopelvic disproportion (sometimes also called fetopelvic disproportion), the practitioner will allow the mother to go into labor naturally. This trial of labor is carefully monitored, and if the fetal head descends and the cervix dilates at a normal rate, then the labor will be permitted to continue. If labor doesn't progress, it may, when appropriate, get a boost with the administration of oxytocin. If no progress is made, a cesarean will usually be required.

HOW YOU'RE CARRYING

"Everyone says I seem to be carrying small and low for the eighth month. Could it be that my baby isn't growing properly?"

It would be a good idea to make earplugs and blinders a part of every pregnant woman's maternity wardrobe. Wearing them for nine months would enable her to avoid the worry generated by the misguided commentary and advice of relatives and friends—even strangers—and prevent invidious comparisons of her belly to those of other pregnant women who are larger, smaller, lower, or higher.

Just as no two prepregnant figures are proportioned in precisely the same fashion, no two pregnant silhouettes are identical. How you carry, both in size and shape, is dependent on whether you started out tall or short, thin or not-so-thin, petite or voluptuous. And it is seldom an indication of the size of the baby you're carrying. A petite woman carrying low and small may give birth to a larger infant than a bigger-boned woman carrying high and wide.

The only accurate assessments of your baby's progress and well-being are likely to come from your practitioner. When you're not in his or her office, keep your earplugs in and your blinders on—and you'll have a lot less to worry about.

PRESENTATION AND POSITION OF THE BABY

"My doctor says the baby is in a breech position. How will this affect my labor and delivery?"

It's never too early to prepare yourself for the possibility of a breech birth, but it's definitely too early now to resign yourself to one. Most babies settle into a head-down position between the 32nd and 36th weeks, but a few keep their parents and doctors guessing until only a few days before delivery.

Some nurse-midwives recommend doing exercises in the last eight weeks, designed to encourage a breech baby to turn. There's no medical proof that these exercises work, but there's also none to suggest that they do any harm.

When a fetus is still in the breech position near term, a physician may attempt external cephalic version (ECV), applying his or her hands to the mother's abdomen and gently, with ultrasound guidance, trying to shift the fetus to the head-down position. The condition of the fetus is monitored continuously to be sure that the umbilical cord isn't accidentally compressed or the placenta disturbed. The procedure is best performed before labor begins or very early in labor, when the uterus is still relatively relaxed. Once turned, most fetuses stay head down, but a few do revert to breech before delivery.

When successful (as it is more than half the time), ECV can reduce the likelihood that a cesarean delivery will be necessary. For this reason ECV has become popular, with a majority of physicians using it at least occasionally. Some, however, hesitate to use it because of the possibility of complica-

Carrying Baby, Eighth Month

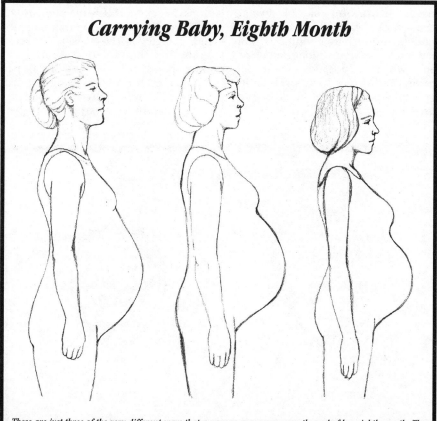

These are just three of the very different ways that a woman may carry near the end of her eighth month. The variations are even greater than before. Depending on the size and position of your baby, as well as your own size and weight gain, you may be carrying higher, lower, bigger, smaller, wider, or more compactly.

tions. Only a physician who has been trained to do ECV—and is prepared to do an emergency c-section if a problem arises—should attempt it.

Breeches are more common when the fetus is smaller than average and not cradled snugly in the uterus, when the uterus is unusually shaped, when there is an excess of amniotic fluid, when there is more than one fetus, and when the uterus is relatively relaxed because of having been stretched during previous pregnancies. If your baby is one of the 3% or 4% in breech position at term, you should discuss the delivery possibilities with your physician (nurse-midwives do not usually handle breech births). You may be able to have a normal vaginal delivery, or, depending on various conditions, you may indeed have to undergo a cesarean. (Which is *not* the end of the world, and for which eventuality every pregnant woman should be prepared anyway. See page 307.)

There appears to be little strong scientific evidence pointing to either vaginal or cesarean as the better way to deliver a breech baby. Vaginal deliveries are believed to be perfectly safe in about one-third to one-half of breech births, but *only* if the doctor is experienced in the proper procedure for such deliveries. Some studies of vaginal breech deliveries show that the potential risk is not always from the delivery itself, but from the reason for the breech: for example, the baby is premature or undersize, there are multiple fetuses, or there is some other congenital problem.

Some physicians routinely perform cesarean sections for breech presentations, believing this is the safest route to follow for the baby (in this malpractice climate, it can also be the best route for the doctors themselves, since they avoid the possibility of being blamed for a baby being harmed because it was delivered vaginally rather than by cesarean). Others, per-

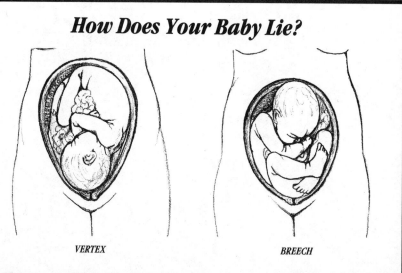

How Does Your Baby Lie?

VERTEX   BREECH

About 96 out of every 100 babies present head first (vertex). The rest are usually in one or another breech position (buttocks first). The complete breech is illustrated here. The frank breech, in which the baby's legs are folded straight up, is the easiest breech to deliver vaginally.

suaded by their own experience or that of others that many breeches can safely be delivered vaginally, permit a trial of labor when all the following conditions are met:

❖ The baby is a frank breech (the legs are folded flat up against the face).

❖ The baby is determined to be small enough (usually under 8½ pounds) for easy passage, but not so small (under 5½ pounds) that a vaginal delivery would be risky. Usually, breech babies under 36 weeks are delivered by cesarean.

❖ There is no evidence of placenta previa, prolapsed umbilical cord, or fetal distress that can't be easily remedied.

❖ The mother has no obstetrical or medical problem that could complicate a vaginal delivery, appears to have an adequate-size pelvis, and has no history of previous difficult or traumatic deliveries. Some physicians add the requirement that the mother be under 35.

❖ The presenting part is engaged (has descended into the pelvis) as labor begins.

❖ The fetal head is not hyperextended, but rather the chin is tucked down toward the chest.

❖ Everything (and everyone) is in readiness for an emergency surgical delivery if one should suddenly become necessary.

When a vaginal delivery is to be attempted, labor is carefully monitored in a surgically equipped delivery suite. If all goes well, it is allowed to continue. If the cervix dilates too slowly or if other problems arise, the doctor and surgical team are ready to perform a cesarean section in a matter of minutes. Continuous electronic fetal monitoring is absolutely essential.

Sometimes an epidural (see page 229) is administered to prevent the mother from bearing down too hard before she is fully dilated (which might lead to the cord being compressed between the baby and the pelvis). Occasionally, general anesthesia is administered to the mother when the baby is halfway delivered, to permit rapid completion of the birth by the physician. Forceps may be used to keep the head properly flexed, and to help deliver the head without pulling too much on the body or neck. A wide episiotomy is often routinely made to facilitate the process.

Sometimes when a cesarean is scheduled, labor progresses so quickly that the baby's buttocks slip into the pelvis before surgery is begun. In that case, most doctors will attempt a vaginal delivery rather than a rushed and difficult cesarean.

"How can I tell if my baby is lying the right way for delivery?"

Playing "name that bump" (trying to figure out which are shoulders, elbows, and bottom) may be better evening entertainment than TV, but it's not the most accurate way of determining your baby's position. Your doctor or nurse-midwife can probably get a better idea than you, by palpating your abdomen with the flat of his or her trained hands for recognizable baby parts. The baby's back, for instance, is usually a smooth, convex contour opposite a bunch of little irregularities which are the "small parts"—hands, feet, elbows. In the eighth month, the head has usually settled near your pelvis; it is round, firm, and—when pushed down—bounces back without the rest of the body moving. The baby's bottom is a less regular shape, and softer, than the head. The location of the baby's heartbeat is another clue to its position—if the presentation is head first, the heartbeat will usually be heard in the lower half of your abdomen; it will be loudest if the baby's back is toward your front. If there's any doubt about the position, a sonogram may be used for verification.

YOUR SAFETY DURING CHILDBIRTH

"I know medical science has taken most of the risk out of giving birth, but I'm still afraid of dying during delivery."

There was a time when mothers routinely risked their lives to have children; they still do in some areas of the world. In the United States today, the risk to maternal life in labor and delivery is virtually non-existent. Fewer than 1 in 10,000 women die in childbirth. And this figure includes not only women with chronic heart conditions and other serious illnesses, but those who give birth in backwoods shacks and dingy tenements, without medical assistance.

In short, even if your pregnancy falls into the highest-risk category—and certainly if it doesn't—you stand a lot better chance of surviving labor and delivery than you do a trip to the supermarket in your car, or a stroll across a busy street.

ADEQUACY FOR DELIVERY

"I'm 5 feet tall and very petite. I'm afraid I'll have trouble delivering a baby."

Fortunately, when it comes to giving birth, it's what's inside, not what's outside, that counts. The size and shape of your pelvis in relation to the size of your baby's head is what determines how difficult your labor will be. And you can't always tell a

pelvis by its cover. A short, slight woman can have a roomier pelvis than a tall, stocky woman. Your practitioner can make an educated guess about its size—usually using measurements taken at your first prenatal exam. If there's some concern that your baby's head is too large to fit through your pelvis while you're in labor, a sonogram may be done.

Of course, in general the overall size of the pelvis, as of all bony structures, is smaller in people of smaller stature. For example, Asian women usually have smaller pelvises than Nordic women. Luckily nature, in its wisdom, rarely presents an Asian woman with a Nordic-size baby—even when the father is a 6-foot fullback. Instead, all things being equal, babies are generally fairly well matched to the size of their mothers.

TWIN LABOR AND DELIVERY

"I'm expecting twins. How will my labor and delivery be different from that of other women?"

There may not be any differences—other than the fact that you'll reap twice the reward for your efforts. Many twin deliveries turn out to be normal, vaginal, and uncomplicated.[2]

However, it's not surprising that there is more potential for complications during the delivery of twins. In most cases the problems don't arise in the first phase of labor, which is actually shorter, on the average, in twin deliveries than in singleton ones. (And though active labor and the pushing

---

2. With each increase in the number of fetuses, however, the likelihood of a surgical delivery increases.

phase are usually longer, the total time from the first contraction to the birth of the babies is generally shorter.) Though most twins can be delivered vaginally (sometimes with the use of forceps to avoid putting the babies through excessive trauma), it is usually recommended that an anesthesiologist be on hand in case a cesarean is needed. A pediatrician or a neonatologist usually stands by too, ready to deal with any immediate problems in the newborns. Often both fetuses are monitored, one externally and the other internally, with scalp electrodes.

With twins, as you will soon find out, you can always expect the unexpected. And this can start at delivery. Because there is more than one baby, and possibly more than one set of circumstances, there may be more than one type of delivery. Perhaps, after the first baby arrives easily via the vaginal route, the second, lying crosswise and unturnable, has to be extracted abdominally. Perhaps though the first infant's amniotic sac ruptures spontaneously, the other twin's has to be ruptured artificially.

In most cases, the second twin comes along within 20 minutes of its sibling. If number two is a slowpoke, the physician may administer oxytocin or use forceps to facilitate delivery, or he or she may perform a cesarean. Once both twins are born, the placenta or placentas usually separate quickly. But sometimes their actual delivery is slow and requires some help from the physician.

BANKING YOUR OWN BLOOD

"I'm worried about the possibility of needing a transfusion during delivery and receiving contaminated blood. Can I store my own blood beforehand?"

First of all, there is very little likelihood you will need a blood transfusion. Only 1% of vaginal deliveries and 2% of cesareans require one. A woman typically loses only 1 to 2 cups of blood (½ to 1 pint) during vaginal childbirth and 2 to 4 cups with a cesarean. This loss presents no problem since in pregnancy the blood volume is up 40% to 50% anyway. Second, the risk of contracting AIDS or hepatitis B or C (the diseases most commonly transmitted through the blood) from a transfusion in the U.S. today is very low (estimated to be anywhere from 1 in 40,000 to 1 in 250,000), since all donated blood is screened by some very accurate (though not foolproof) tests. Third, because facilities for autologous (self) blood donations are limited and priority is given to those about to undergo major high-risk surgery, women who are about to deliver may not even be accepted for such a donation.

If, however, you have reason to believe that you may be at high risk for blood loss during delivery because your blood does not clot normally, because you are scheduled for a cesarean delivery, or for some other reason, speak to your doctor about the possibility of making an autologous blood donation. (Donating the blood late in pregnancy could be a problem because it could lower your blood volume excessively or lead to anemia.) Or plan to have a relative or friend with compatible blood make a directed donation (one to a specific person) just prior to delivery or standing by at the time of delivery just in case. Not every hospital is equipped for or willing to oblige with directed donations, and personnel may point out that the risk of contracting AIDS from a blood transfusion isn't any lower when the donation is from a friend or family member than when it's from the general blood supply.

HAVING A CESAREAN SECTION

"My doctor just told me I will have to have a cesarean. But I'm afraid the surgery will be dangerous."

Though popular lore has it that the cesarean section got its name because Julius Caesar came into the world via abdominal delivery, that's virtually impossible. Julius might have survived such an operation, but his mother wouldn't have—and it is known that Mrs. Caesar lived for many years after his birth.

Today, however, cesareans are nearly as safe as vaginal deliveries for the mother, and in difficult deliveries or when there's fetal distress, they are often the safest delivery mode for the baby. Even though it is technically considered major surgery, a cesarean carries relatively minor risks—much closer to those of a tonsillectomy than of a gall bladder operation, for instance.

Learning all you can about cesarean sections before delivery—from your doctor, in your childbirth class (a special class on cesareans is ideal), and through reading—will help to prepare you and to ease your fears.

"The doctor says I may have to have a cesarean section. I'm worried that this may be dangerous for the baby."

Chances are that if you have a cesarean, your baby will be at least as safe, and possibly safer, than if you had had a vaginal delivery. Every year thousands of babies who might not have survived the perilous journey through the birth canal (or might have survived impaired) are lifted from their mothers' abdomens sound and unscathed.

Though there has been some speculation that cesareans are somehow harmful to babies, there's no hard evidence that this is so. Of course a higher proportion of cesarean babies are found to have medical problems, but these problems are most often due to the distress that necessitated the operation, not to the operation itself. Many of these infants would never have made it at all if left to a natural delivery.

In most ways, babies delivered via cesarean don't differ from those delivered vaginally—though cesarean babies do have the edge in initial appearance. Because they don't have to accommodate to the narrow confines of the pelvis, they usually have nicely rounded, not pointy, heads.

Apgar scores, which rate an infant's condition one and five minutes after birth, are comparable in babies born vaginally and those born by cesarean. Cesarean-born babies do have the slight disadvantage of not having some of the excess mucus squeezed out of their respiratory tracts in the birthing process, but this mucus can be easily suctioned after delivery. Very, very rarely is any serious damage sustained by a baby during cesarean delivery—much more rarely than during vaginal deliveries.

The most likely kind of damage a baby delivered abdominally might suffer is psychological—not from the delivery itself, but because of the mother's attitude toward it. Occasionally a mother who has had a cesarean will subconsciously harbor resentment toward the baby who she feels deprived her of her finest hour and brought such insult to her body.[3] She may allow the jealousy she feels toward mothers who've delivered vaginally, and the guilt she feels about "failing," interfere with the establishment of a

---

3. Women who deliver vaginally may also resent their babies, almost always temporarily, because of the pain of delivery.

good relationship with her baby. Or she may incorrectly assume that the cesarean-born infant is unusually fragile (few are) and become overprotective. If she develops such feelings, the mother should try to confront and resolve them, seeking professional help if necessary.

But often, destructive attitudes can be avoided right from the start. First, by recognizing that the method by which a baby is delivered in no way reflects on either the mother or the child; a woman is no less a mother and her baby is no less the fruit of her womb when there is a cesarean birth rather than a vaginal one. Second, by making sure there is an opportunity for you and your baby to have time together as early as possible. Long before you go into labor, let your doctor know that if you have a cesarean you would like to be able to hold or even nurse the baby on the operating table, or if that's not possible, in the recovery room. If you wait until delivery day to state your case, you may not have the strength or opportunity to make it. Planning ahead also gives you the chance to question contrary hospital rules, such as those requiring every cesarean-delivered newborn, even healthy ones, to spend some time in the neonatal intensive care unit. If you present a strong argument in a rational, nonhysterical way, you may be able to effect a change in, or an exception to, the rules.

If, good intentions notwithstanding, you turn out to be too weak to participate in any serious mother-baby bonding (and many women are, whether they've had abdominal or vaginal deliveries), or if your baby needs to be observed or cared for in the neonatal intensive care unit for a while, don't panic. There is no evidence, despite the hoopla the concept has aroused in the past, that bonding *must* begin immediately after birth (see page 382).

"I so much want a natural birth; but it seems like everybody is having a cesarean these days and I'm terrified I'll have to have one too."

Not quite "everybody" is having a cesarean these days—but far more women are than ever before. In the early 1960s your chances of having a cesarean would have been 1 in 20. Today they are nearly 1 in 4 (higher in some hospitals, lower in others), and if your pregnancy is in a high-risk category, as high as 1 in 3.

Why such a substantial increase? Many point an accusing finger at the medical community: at the occasional doctor who schedules a cesarean during office hours rather than be awakened at 3 A.M. or who, at the slightest medical pretext, jumps at the chance to collect the higher fee a cesarean commands. (The fact that insurance carriers usually pick up the tab assuages any guilt.) And at the malpractice-shy physician, who performs a cesarean to cover him- or herself when a vaginal delivery shows even the slightest potential for problems. (More suits against obstetricians are instituted for *not* performing a cesarean—and consequently getting a bad result—than for performing one.) Add the physicians who decide to do a cesarean the instant a negative reading is picked up on the fetal monitor (without double-checking to be sure the baby, and not the fetal monitor, is in trouble), and it would appear that bad medicine is to blame.

But the major reason for the increase in the cesarean rate is not bad medicine, but *good* medicine: Cesareans save the lives of babies who might not or cannot safely be delivered vaginally. Most doctors perform cesareans not for convenience, or for the money, or for fear of malpractice, but because they believe that in certain circumstances this surgery is the best way to protect the baby.

Several changes in obstetrical practice have also contributed to the increase in cesareans. First of all, mid-forceps delivery (see page 286) is used less frequently than in the past because of doubts about the safety of reaching up into the vaginal canal with a metal implement to extract a recalcitrant fetus by the head.[4] Second, cesarean delivery has become an extremely quick and safe option—and in most instances mothers can be awake to see their babies born. Third, the fetal monitor, and a variety of tests, can more accurately (though not infallibly) indicate when a fetus is in trouble and needs to be delivered in a hurry. Fourth, the current trend among expectant mothers toward higher than recommended weight gains (over 35 pounds) has led to a greater number of large babies, who are sometimes more difficult to deliver vaginally. Then there is the trend toward noninterventionist obstetrics—letting nature set its own pace, rather than hurrying it by rupturing membranes, using oxytocin, or employing forceps—with the result that labors have more of a chance of stalling. In addition, there are the increasing ranks of women with chronic medical problems who are able to have successful pregnancies but require cesarean deliveries. Finally, a major, and now recognized as largely unnecessary, factor in the burgeoning c-section rate is the repeat cesarean.

In spite of many legitimate reasons for c-sections, there is general agreement in the medical community that a significant number of unnecessary cesareans are presently being performed. In order to reverse this trend, many insurers, hospitals, medical groups, and other individuals and agencies are requiring or encouraging second opinions, when feasible, before a cesarean is performed; a trial of labor for all women who have previously had cesareans to see if they can deliver vaginally (see page 23); better training of physicians in interpretation of fetal monitor readings, so that surgery won't be performed unnecessarily; vaginal deliveries for many breech babies; greater patience with slow labor and with the pushing phase, assuming mother and baby are doing well, before resorting to surgery; the judicious use of oxytocin to get arrested labor moving again; and the use of a variety of more reliable fetal assessment techniques (such as fetal scalp blood sampling, biophysical profile, or acoustical stimulation) to confirm fetal distress that may be suspected from readings on a fetal monitor. Some hospitals now fax ambiguous fetal monitor strips to consultants to get an immediate expert opinion on the condition of the fetus. Others have found that instituting a peer review system—wherein all first-time cesareans are carefully studied on a case-by-case basis and doctors found to be doing unnecessary cesareans face disciplinary action—greatly reduces the cesarean rate. It is also generally agreed that better training of residents in vaginal birth after cesarean (VBAC), external cephalic version (ECV), and the vaginal delivery of breech babies would help reduce the number of cesareans done in this country. But in the case of VBAC, physicians will need the cooperation of mothers as well. Some women who've had one or more cesareans refuse to go through a trial labor again—either because they're concerned about the risks of a vaginal delivery or because they just don't want to have to face another long and painful labor.

---

4. That the rate of mid-forceps deliveries and cesareans are linked is clear in comparing rates of each in the U.S. (where cesarean rates are high and mid-forceps rates low) and Great Britain (where mid-forceps rates are high and cesareans lower).

Most women won't know whether or not they will have a cesarean until they are well into labor. There are, however, several advance indications that point to the possibility:

❖ Cephalopelvic disproportion (when a fetus's head is too large to pass through its mother's pelvis; see page 240), suggested either by the size of the baby on ultrasound examination or by a previous difficult delivery.

❖ A fetal illness or abnormality that makes labor and vaginal delivery unacceptably risky or traumatic.

❖ A previous cesarean (see page 22), if the reason for it still exists (maternal disease or an abnormal pelvis, for example) or a vertical incision was made in the uterus.

❖ Maternal hypertension (page 330) or kidney disease, because the mother may be unable to tolerate the stress of labor.

Cesarean Questions to Discuss With Your Doctor

❖ Will it be possible, assuming it isn't an emergency situation, to try other alternatives before a cesarean is resorted to? For example, oxytocin to stimulate contractions, or squatting to make pushing more effective?

❖ If the reason for the proposed c-section is a breech presentation, will trying to turn the baby in the uterus (external cephalic version) be tried first?

❖ What kinds of anesthesia might be used? A general anesthesia, which puts you to sleep, is usually necessary when time is of the essence, but spinal or epidural anesthesia will allow you to remain awake during a nonemergency abdominal delivery. (See All About Childbirth Medication, page 226.)

❖ Does he or she routinely use a low transverse incision in the uterus whenever possible, so that a vaginal delivery can be attempted next time around? You may also want to know, for cosmetic reasons, if the abdominal incision (which is unrelated to that in the uterus) is usually low, or "bikini."

❖ Can your coach be present if you are awake? If you are asleep?

❖ Can your nurse-midwife (if you have one) be with you too?

❖ Will you and your husband be able to hold the baby immediately after birth (if you are awake and all is well), and will you be able to nurse in the recovery room? If you're asleep, will your husband be able to hold the baby?

❖ If the baby doesn't need special care, can he or she room-in with you? Can your husband stay overnight to help you out?

❖ After an uncomplicated cesarean birth, how much recovery time will you need both in and out of the hospital? What physical discomforts and limitations can you expect to experience?

❖ If the fetal monitor suggests the baby may be in trouble, will other tests (such as checking a fetal scalp blood sample, or evaluating the fetal response to sound or pressure; see page 263) be used to verify the monitor readings before a cesarean is decided upon? Will it be possible to get a second opinion?

Hospitals and Cesarean Rates

Cesarean rates vary from hospital to hospital. Many major medical centers have very high rates because they do a lot of high-risk deliveries. But some small community hospitals also have high rates because they don't have the staff on hand at all hours to do an emergency cesarean; if there's some question that a vaginal delivery might not succeed, the anesthesiologist and others needed for the surgery are called in and a cesarean is performed before an emergency arises. A larger hospital can take a wait-and-see attitude. Discuss the cesarean rate at your hospital with your practitioner, and ask whether there are any special procedures in place to discourage unnecessary cesarean deliveries.

❖ Unusual fetal presentation, such as breech (buttocks or feet first) or transverse (crosswise, with the shoulder first), which can make a vaginal delivery difficult or impossible (see page 236).

A cesarean may be scheduled before labor begins for a variety of reasons, including:

❖ Maternal diabetes, in cases where preterm delivery is deemed necessary and it is found that the cervix is not ripe enough for the induction of labor.

❖ Active maternal herpes infection (page 35) is present as labor begins, to prevent the infection being passed to the fetus during a vaginal birth.

❖ Placenta previa (when the placenta partially or completely blocks the cervical opening) to head off labor, which can result in hemorrhage if the placenta detaches prematurely (see page 356).

❖ Abruptio placenta (page 358), when there is an extensive separation of the placenta from the uterine wall and the fetus is in danger.

Cesareans may also be scheduled before labor when prompt delivery is necessary and either there is no time to induce labor or it is believed that mother and/or baby will be unable to tolerate its stresses. Any of the following might necessitate such a delivery:

❖ Preeclampsia or eclampsia (page 351) that doesn't respond to treatment.

❖ A postmature fetus (two or more weeks overdue; see page 262), when the uterine environment has begun to deteriorate.

❖ Fetal or maternal distress, due to any cause.

In most cases, however, it isn't until active labor that the possible need for a cesarean becomes apparent. Then the most likely reasons include:

❖ Failure of labor to progress (the cervix hasn't dilated quickly enough) after 16 to 18 hours (some physicians will wait longer).[5]

❖ Fetal distress, signaled by the fetal monitor or other tests of fetal well-being (see page 263).

❖ A prolapsed umbilical cord (page 360), which if compressed could cut off oxygen to the fetus, causing fetal distress.

---

5. In such cases, some physicians will try to give sluggish contractions a boost with oxytocin before resorting to a cesarean.

❖ Previously undiagnosed cases of placenta previa or abruptio placenta, particularly if there is a risk of hemorrhage.

If cesareans are so safe, and sometimes lifesaving, why do most of us dread the prospect of having one? Partly because major surgery, even when it's routine and almost risk-free, is still a little scary; but mostly because we spend months preparing ourselves for natural childbirth, and we usually enter the labor room utterly unprepared for the very real possibility that we'll have a cesarean instead. For nine months we block that unpleasant possibility out of our minds. We devour childbirth primers, but we bypass the chapters on cesarean section. We ask dozens of questions about natural delivery in childbirth class, but not one about surgical birth. We look forward to holding our husband's hand as we pant and push our baby into the world—not to lying passively, and possibly unconscious, as sterile instruments slice into our abdomen to extract the baby like a hot appendix. When suddenly faced with a cesarean, we feel deprived of control over the birth of our baby. As we see it, medical technology has taken over, ushering in frustration, disap-

pointment, anger, and guilt.

But that's not how it has to be. Not if you are as prepared for an abdominal delivery as for a vaginal one, if you recognize that both can be beautiful, and if you focus on the product of childbirth rather than the process.

Several steps taken now can make the prospect of a cesarean less ominous and the reality more fulfilling. Even if you have no reason to believe that you might end up needing a cesarean, be sure that at least one session on the subject is included in your childbirth preparation course. If you do have some reason to believe a cesarean section might be necessary, try to take a full preparatory course. Do some reading on your own, too.

If your obstetrician decides in advance that a cesarean will be necessary, be sure to ask for a detailed explanation of the reasons. Ask if there are any alternatives, such as a trial of labor—in which, once labor begins spontaneously, you would be allowed to continue as long as it progressed normally. (This option may not be available in a small hospital that doesn't have the facilities for an emergency c-section should it be needed; some have suggested such hospitals shouldn't do deliveries at all.) If you come away from your consultation

Making the Cesarean Birth a Family Affair

Family-centered cesarean birth is becoming more commonplace across the country, with the vast majority of practitioners and hospitals relaxing the usual surgical rules for cesarean deliveries. During a nonemergency cesarean, most now make it possible for the mother to be awake, the father to be in attendance, and the new family to get to know each other in the period just after birth, just as they would after an uncomplicated vaginal delivery. Studies show that this "normalizing" of surgical delivery helps couples feel better about the experience, reduces the possibility of postpartum depression and low self-esteem in the mother (both of which are more likely to be a problem after cesarean delivery), and allows the bonding process to begin sooner.

wondering whether the major reason a cesarean has been recommended is physician convenience, you should ask for, and get, another opinion.

Whether you're preparing for a scheduled cesarean or just for the possibility of one, there are a number of issues you might want to talk over with your doctor or the on-call physician your nurse-midwife uses (see page 245). Don't be put off by assurances that you aren't likely to need one; explain that you want to be prepared, just in case. Let the doctor know if you would like to be part of the decision-making team should a cesarean seem necessary.

Of course most pregnant women would not select a cesarean as their delivery of choice, and better than 3 out of 4 will end up delivering vaginally. But for those who don't, there's no reason for disappointment or feelings of guilt or failure. Any delivery (vaginal or abdominal, medicated or unmedicated) that yields a healthy mother and baby is an unqualified success.

TRAVEL SAFETY

"I've got an important business trip scheduled this month. Is it safe for me to travel, or should I cancel?"

If you can possibly avoid traveling in the last trimester, do. Not only is traveling in late pregnancy uncomfortable, it can be hazardous—since you could suddenly go into labor (premature labor can't always be predicted) hundreds or thousands of miles from your doctor. The threat of labor occurring thousands of feet in the air (and hours away from landing) is enough to keep airlines from allowing pregnant women in their ninth month to fly without a doctor's letter of permission. And such a letter may prove difficult to obtain, since most physicians don't recommend travel in the last trimester, particularly in the eighth and ninth months. If you must travel, refer to the tips on page 180. It's particularly important to secure the name of a reputable obstetrician at your destination.

DRIVING

"Should I still drive?"

Long car trips (lasting more than an hour) are probably too exhausting late in pregnancy, no matter who's driving. If you must take a longer trip, however, and have your practitioner's okay, be sure to stop every hour or two to get up and walk around. Driving shorter distances is fine up until delivery day, as long as you're not experiencing any dizzy spells and as long as you can still fit behind the wheel. Don't, however, try to drive yourself to the hospital while in labor. And don't forget—on any car trip, whether you are driver or passenger— fasten your seat belt.

BRAXTON HICKS CONTRACTIONS

"Every once in a while my uterus seems to bunch up and harden. What's going on?"

These are probably Braxton Hicks contractions, which usually begin to rehearse the pregnant uterus for labor sometime after the 20th week of pregnancy. These contractions are felt earlier and are more intense in women who have had a previous pregnancy. In effect, your uterus is flexing its muscles, warming up in preparation for the real contractions, which will normally push your baby out at term.

You'll feel these practice contractions as a painless (but possibly uncomfortable) tightening of your uterus, beginning at the top and gradually spreading downward before relaxing. They usually last about 30 seconds (ample time to practice your breathing exercises), but may last as long as 2 minutes or more.

As pregnancy draws to a close in the ninth month, Braxton Hicks contractions may become more frequent, intense—sometimes even painful—and thus more difficult to distinguish from true labor contractions (see Prelabor, False Labor, Real Labor, page 268). Though they're not efficient enough to deliver your baby, Braxton Hicks contractions may get the prebirth processes of effacement and early dilatation started, thereby giving you a leg up on labor before it even begins.

To relieve any discomfort you may feel during these contractions, try lying down and relaxing, or getting up and walking around. Changing your position may stop the contractions completely.

Though Braxton Hicks contractions are not true labor, they may be difficult for you to differentiate from preterm uterine activity of the kind that precedes premature labor. So be sure to describe the contractions to your practitioner at your next visit. Report them immediately if they are very frequent (more than 4 per hour) and/or are accompanied by pain (back, abdominal, or pelvic) or by any kind of unusual vaginal discharge, or if you are at high risk for premature labor (see page 218).

BATHING

"My mother says I shouldn't take a bath after the 34th week. My doctor says it's okay. Who's right?"

This is one case where mother doesn't know best. Though well intentioned, she is misinformed. It's likely that she is basing her warning on the orders she got from her doctor when she was pregnant with you. Most doctors 20 or 30 years ago believed that dirty bath water could travel up the vagina to the cervix in pregnancy and cause an infection. But while further research remains to be done, doctors today believe that water does not enter the vagina unless it is forced, as in douching; thus, worry about infection from bathwater is not justified. Even if water does enter the vagina, the cervical mucous plug that seals the entrance to the uterus effectively protects the membranes that surround the fetus, the amniotic fluid, and the fetus itself from invading infectious organisms. Therefore, most doctors permit tub baths in normal pregnancies up until the membranes rupture or the mucous plug has been expelled. Showers are usually permitted right up to delivery.

Baths and showers, however, aren't totally risk free, particularly in the last trimester when ungainliness can lead to slips and falls. To avoid such mishaps, bathe with care; be sure your tub or shower has a nonslip surface or use a slip-resistant mat; and have someone nearby, if possible, to help you in and out of the tub.

RELATIONSHIP WITH YOUR SPOUSE

"The baby isn't even born yet, and already my relationship with my husband seems to be changing. We're both so wrapped up in the upcoming birth and the baby—instead of in each other, the way we used to be."

All marriages, to differing degrees, undergo some alterations in dynamics and a reshuffling of priorities after baby makes three, but studies show that the shock of this upheaval is usually less stressful if the couple begins the process during pregnancy. So, though the change you're noticing in your relationship may not seem like a change for the better, it's one you're better off experiencing now, rather than after your baby is born. Couples who romanticize the notion of a cozy threesome, and who don't anticipate at least some disintegration or disruption of their romance, often find the reality of life with a demanding newborn harder to deal with.

But while it's very normal—and healthy—to be wrapped up in the pregnancy and your expected extraspecial delivery, you shouldn't let this new facet of your life completely block out the others, especially your relationship. Now is the time to learn to combine the care and feeding of your baby with the care and feeding of your marriage. Regularly reinforce romance. Once a week, do something together—see a movie, have dinner out, visit a museum—that has nothing to do with childbirth or babies. While you're layette shopping, stop in the men's department and buy a little something special (and unexpected) for your husband. When you leave the practitioner's office after your next visit, surprise him with a pair of tickets for his favorite opera or sports event. At dinner now and then, ask about his day, talk about yours, discuss the day's headlines—all without indulging in baby talk even once. None of this will make the wonderful event any less special, but it will remind you both that there's more to life than Lamaze and layettes.

Keeping this in mind now will make it easier to keep the love light burning later, when you're taking turns walking the floor at 2 A.M. (Tips to fan the flame can be found in *What to Expect the First Year.*) And that love light is,

after all, what will make the cozy nest you're busily preparing for your baby a bright, happy, and secure one.

MAKING LOVE NOW

"I'm confused. I hear a lot of conflicting information about sexual intercourse in the last weeks of pregnancy."

The problem is that existing medical evidence on the subject is confusing and conflicting. It is widely believed that neither intercourse nor orgasm alone precipitates labor unless conditions are ripe (though many impatient-to-deliver couples have enjoyed trying to prove otherwise). For that reason, many physicians and midwives allow patients with normal pregnancies to make love—assuming they're still interested—right up until delivery day. And most couples apparently can do so without any problems arising.

There does, however, seem to be some risk of sexual intercourse triggering premature labor, at least in women at high risk for preterm delivery (such as those carrying multiple fetuses, those who start effacing and dilating early, and those with a history of premature labor). Intercourse also seems to be related to premature rupture of the amniotic membranes, particularly when they are already inflamed, and to infection, both prenatal (of the amniotic sac or amniotic fluid) and postpartum. To help prevent possible infection, as well as possible premature contractions produced by exposure of the cervix to the irritant prostaglandins in semen, many physicians recommend the use of condoms during intercourse in the last eight weeks of pregnancy.

Ease your confusion by checking with your practitioner to see what the latest medical consensus is. If you get a green light, then by all means make love—if you want to and feel comfortable about it. If the light is red (and it will be if you are at high risk for premature delivery, have placenta previa or abruptio, are experiencing unexplained bleeding, or if your membranes have ruptured), then foster intimacy in other ways. Try a romantic rendezvous at a candlelit restaurant or walking hand-in-hand under the stars. Or an evening at home snuggling in bed or under an afghan in front of the TV, hugging and kissing on the sofa, or soaping each other in the shower. Or use massage—of the neck, back, feet, and of course belly and genitals—as the medium.

What It's Important to Know:
FACTS ABOUT BREASTFEEDING

At the turn of the century, nearly every baby was fed at the breast; there was no other choice. But in the early 1900s, women began to demand rights they'd never had—to vote, to work, to smoke cigarettes, to let down or bob their hair, to peel off confining undergarments, and to set their sights outside the kitchen and the nursery. Breastfeeding was old-fashioned, it was restricting, and it represented all that women sought freedom from. To be a modern woman was to bottle-feed. And by the 1950s, the only remaining breastfeeders (besides our senior author and an assortment of bohemian stragglers) were those with whom emancipation hadn't yet caught up.

Ironically, it was the revitalized women's movement of the 1960s and '70s that brought breastfeeding back into vogue. Women wanted not only freedom but control—control of their lives, control of their bodies. They knew that control was gained with knowledge, and knowledge told them that breastfeeding was best—for their babies and, on the whole, for themselves. Today there is clearly a back-to-breast trend.

WHY BREAST IS BEST

There is no question but that given normal circumstances, breast-feeding provides the perfect food and food delivery system for human infants:

❖ Human breast milk contains at least 100 ingredients that are not found in cow's milk and that cannot be exactly duplicated in commercial formulas. Breast milk is individualized for each infant; raw materials are selected from the mother's bloodstream as needed, altering the milk's composition from day to day, feeding to feeding, as the baby grows and changes. The nutrients are matched to infant needs. Variations from breast milk in homemade cow's milk formulas can lead to nutritional deficiencies.

❖ Breast milk is more digestible than cow's milk. The proportion of protein in mother's milk is lower (1.5%) than in cow's milk (3.5%), making it easier for the infant to handle. The protein itself is mostly lactalbumin, which is more nutritious and digestible than the major protein component of cow's milk, caseinogen. The fat content of both milks are similar, but the fat in mother's milk is more easily digested by the baby.

❖ Breast milk is less likely to cause overweight in infants, and obesity later in life.

❖ Virtually no baby is allergic to breast milk (though some can have allergic reactions to a certain food or foods in their mothers' diets, including milk). Beta-lactoglobulin, a substance contained in cow's milk, can trigger an allergic response and, following the formation of antibodies, can even cause anaphylactic shock (a life-threatening allergic reaction) in infants—which some suspect could be a contributing factor in some cases of sudden infant death syndrome (or crib death). Soy milk formulas, which are often substituted when an infant is allergic to cow's milk, stray even farther in composition from what nature intended.

❖ Nursed babies are almost never constipated, because of the easier digestibility of breast milk. They also rarely have diarrhea—since breast milk seems both to destroy some diarrhea-causing organisms and to encourage the growth of beneficial flora in the digestive tract, which further discourage digestive upset. On a purely esthetic note, the bowel movements of a breastfed baby are sweeter-smelling (at least until solids are introduced) and less apt to cause diaper rash.

❖ Breast milk contains one-third the mineral salts of cow's milk. The extra sodium in cow's milk is difficult for baby's kidneys to handle.

❖ Breast milk contains less phosphorus. The higher phosphorus content of cow's milk is linked to a decreased calcium level in the formula-fed infant's blood.

❖ Breastfed babies are less subject to illness in the first year of life. Protection is partially provided by the transfer of immune factors in breast milk and in the premilk substance, colostrum.

❖ Nursing at the breast, because it requires more effort than sucking on a bottle, encourages optimum development of jaws, teeth, and palate.

❖ Breast milk is safe. There is no risk of contamination or spoilage.

❖ Breastfeeding is convenient. It requires no advance planning or packing, no equipment; it is always available (in the car, on an airplane, in the middle of the night) and at just the right temperature. When mother and baby aren't together (if the mother works outside the home, for instance), milk may be expressed in advance and stored in the freezer for bottle feedings as needed.

❖ Breastfeeding is economical. There are no bottles, sterilizers, or formula to buy; there are no half-emptied bottles or opened cans of formula to waste. And the nutritious diet needed for nursing (see page 392) probably costs less than a typical American diet saturated with empty but expensive fast-food calories.

❖ It's been suggested, though not proven, that breastfeeding decreases a woman's risk of developing breast cancer later in life.

❖ Nursing helps speed the shrinking of the uterus back to its prepregnant size and decreases the flow of lochia (the postpartum vaginal discharge).

❖ Lactation suppresses ovulation and menstruation, at least to some degree. Though it shouldn't be relied on for birth control, it may postpone resumption of a woman's periods for months, or at least for as long as she nurses.

❖ Nursing can help burn off the fat accumulated during pregnancy. If a woman is careful to consume only enough calories to keep her milk supply and energy up (see page 392), and makes certain that all those calories come from nutritious foods, she can fill all of her infant's nutritional needs while recovering her own figure.

❖ Breastfeeding enforces rest periods for the new mother—particularly important during the first six postpartum weeks.

❖ Nursing in public is becoming more acceptable. With a little discretion and a big napkin, both mother and baby can dine at the same restaurant table.

❖ Breastfeeding brings mother and baby together, skin to skin, at least six to eight times a day. The emotional gratification, the intimacy, the sharing of love and pleasure, can be very fulfilling.

(A note to mothers of twins: All the advantages of breastfeeding are doubled for you. See page 395 for tips that can make breastfeeding easier.)

WHY SOME PREFER THE BOTTLE

Just as there were holdouts against bottle-feeding 30 years ago, there are women today who choose not to nurse. And though the advantages of bottle-feeding seem to be dwarfed by those of breastfeeding, they can be real and convincing for some women.

❖ Bottle-feeding doesn't tie the mother down to her baby. She's able to work outside the home, shop, go out in the evening, even sleep through the night—because someone else can feed the baby.

❖ Bottle-feeding allows the father to share the feeding responsibilities and its bonding benefits more easily. (Although the father of a breastfed baby can derive the same benefits, assuming his baby will take a bottle at all, by feeding a bottle of expressed mother's milk.)

❖ Bottle-feeding doesn't interfere with a couple's sex life (except when baby wakes up for a feeding at the wrong time). Breastfeeding, on the other hand, can. First, because lactation hormones can keep the vagina relatively dry; and second, because leaky breasts during lovemaking are a turn-off to some couples. For bottle-feeding couples, the breasts can play their sensual role rather than their utilitarian one.

❖ Bottle-feeding doesn't dictate your diet or cramp your eating style. You can eat all the garlic, spicy foods, and cabbage you want, and you don't have to drink even one glass of milk.

❖ Bottle-feeding may be preferable for a woman who is squeamish about having such intimate contact with her infant and uncomfortable about the possibility of nursing in public. Or for a woman who feels she is too high-strung or impatient to breastfeed.

MAKING THE CHOICE

For more and more women today, the choice is clear. Some know they will opt for breast over bottle long before they even decide to become pregnant. Others, who never gave it much thought before pregnancy, choose breastfeeding once they've read up on its many benefits. Some women teeter on the brink of indecision right through pregnancy and even delivery. A few women, convinced that nursing isn't for them, still can't shake the nagging feeling that they ought to do it anyway.

For all undecided women, we have one suggestion: Try it—you may like it. You can always quit if you don't, but at least you will have eased those nagging doubts. Best of all, you and your baby will have reaped some of the most important benefits of breastfeeding, if just for a brief time.

Give breastfeeding a fair trial, though. The first few weeks are always difficult, even for the most ardent breastfeeders. Some experts suggest that a full month, or even 6 weeks, of nursing is needed to establish a successful feeding relationship and to give a mother time to decide whether she likes it or not.

WHEN YOU CAN'T OR SHOULDN'T BREASTFEED

Unfortunately, the option of breastfeeding isn't open to every new mother. Some women can't or shouldn't nurse their newborns. The reasons may be emotional or physical, due to mother's health or the baby's, temporary or long-term.[6] The most

common maternal factors making breastfeeding ill-advised include:

❖ Serious debilitating illness (such as cardiac or kidney impairment, or severe anemia) or extreme underweight.

❖ Serious infection, such as tuberculosis.

❖ Conditions that require medications that pass into the breast milk and might be harmful to the baby, such as antithyroid, anticancer, or antihypertensive drugs; lithium, tranquilizers, or sedatives. If you take any kind of medication, check with your physician before beginning breastfeeding.[7]

❖ AIDS, which can be transmitted via body fluids, including breast milk.

❖ Drug abuse—including the use of tranquilizers, cocaine, heroin, methadone, marijuana, and heavy use of caffeine or alcohol.[8]

❖ A deep-seated aversion to the idea of breastfeeding.

Conditions in the newborn that interfere with breastfeeding include:

❖ Disorders, such as lactose intolerance or phenylketonuria (PKU), in which neither human *nor* cow's milk can be digested.

---

6. There have been some suggestions that, in families with a history of premenopausal breast cancer, the condition might be passed on from mother to daughter through a virus in the breast milk. This theory is unsubstantiated, and it appears that women with such family histories, and even those who have had cancer in one breast, can safely and successfully breastfeed their babies.

7. A temporary need for medication, such as penicillin, even at the time you begin nursing, need not necessarily eliminate the chances of your breastfeeding. It may be possible to start the baby on formula temporarily, express milk to get your milk supply going, and as soon as the medication is discontinued, switch to breastfeeding.

8. Smokers who nurse will pass nicotine along to their babies, and should quit. If they don't quit, they should try to cut back—but they should not use smoking as an excuse not to breastfeed.

❖ Cleft lip and/or cleft palate, and other mouth deformities that make sucking at the breast difficult.

MAKING BOTTLE-FEEDING WORK

Though breastfeeding is a good experience for both mother and child, there is no reason why bottle-feeding can't be too. Millions of happy, healthy babies have been raised on the bottle. When you can't, or don't wish to, breastfeed, the danger lies not in the bottle, but in the possibility that you might communicate any frustration or guilt you feel to your baby. Know that, with but a little extra effort, love can be passed from mother to child through the bottle as well as through the breast. Make every feeding a time to cuddle your baby, just as you would if you were nursing (don't prop the bottle). And when it's practical, make skin-to-skin contact by opening your shirt and letting the baby rest against your bare breast while feeding.

13
The Ninth Month

WHAT YOU CAN EXPECT AT THIS MONTH'S CHECKUPS

After about the 36th week, you will see your practitioner weekly. Both the tenor and the content of these examinations will be reminders that you are getting closer to D-day. In general, you can expect your practitioner to check the following, though there may be variations depending upon your particular needs and upon your practitioner's style of practice:[1]

❖ Weight (gain generally slows down or ceases) and blood pressure (it may be slightly higher than it was at mid-pregnancy)

❖ Urine, for sugar and protein

❖ Fetal heartbeat

❖ Height of fundus

❖ Fetal size (you may get a rough weight estimate), presentation (head or buttocks first?), position

(facing to the front or to the back?), and descent (is presenting part engaged?)

❖ Feet and hands for edema (swelling), and legs for varicose veins

❖ Cervix (by internal examination, usually sometime after the 38th week) for effacement and dilatation, or where appropriate, for repeat cultures of the cervix

❖ Symptoms you have been experiencing, especially unusual ones

❖ Frequency and duration of Braxton Hicks contractions, as reported by you

❖ Questions and problems you want to discuss, particularly those related to labor and delivery—have a list ready

❖ You can also expect to receive instructions from your practitioner as to when to call if you think you are in labor; if you don't, ask for them.

---

1. See Appendix for an explanation of the procedures and tests performed.

WHAT YOU MAY BE FEELING

Y ou may experience all of these symptoms at one time or another, or only a few of them. Some may have continued from last month, others may be new. Still others may hardly be noticed because you are used to them and/or because they are eclipsed by new and more exciting signs indicating that labor may not be far off.

PHYSICALLY:

❖ Changes in fetal activity (more squirming and less kicking, as the fetus has progressively less room to move around in)

❖ Vaginal discharge (leukorrhea) becomes heavier and contains more mucus, which may be streaked red with blood or tinged brown or pink after intercourse or a pelvic exam

❖ Constipation

❖ Heartburn, indigestion, flatulence, bloating

❖ Occasional headaches, faintness, dizziness

❖ Nasal congestion and occasional nosebleeds; ear stuffiness

❖ Bleeding gums

❖ Leg cramps during sleep

❖ Increased backache and heaviness

❖ Buttock and pelvic discomfort and achiness

❖ Increased swelling of ankles and feet, and occasionally of hands and face

❖ Itchy abdomen, protruding navel

❖ Varicose veins of the legs

WHAT YOU MAY LOOK LIKE

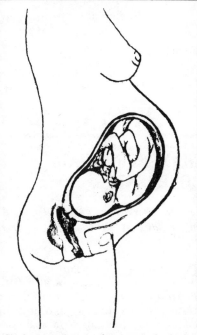

Final preparations are being made for birth, which can safely take place any time now. Lungs are mature. About 2 inches and 2½ pounds are added to baby's length and weight (the average baby will be 20 inches, 7½ pounds at term). More confined, and possibly engaged in the pelvis, the fetus may seem less active.

❖ Hemorrhoids

❖ Easier breathing after the baby drops

❖ More frequent urination after the baby drops

❖ Increased difficulty sleeping

❖ More frequent and more intense Braxton Hicks contractions (some may be painful)

❖ Increasing clumsiness and difficulty getting around

❖ Colostrum, either leaking or expressable from breasts (though this premilk substance may not appear until after delivery)

❖ Fatigue or extra energy, or alternate periods of each

❖ Increase in appetite, or loss of appetite

EMOTIONALLY:

❖ More excitement, more anxiety, more apprehension, more absent-mindedness

❖ Relief that you're almost there

❖ Irritability and oversensitivity (especially with people who keep saying: "Are *you* still around?")

❖ Impatience and restlessness

❖ Dreaming and fantasizing about the baby

WHAT YOU MAY BE CONCERNED ABOUT

CHANGES IN FETAL MOVEMENTS

"My baby, who used to kick so vigorously, isn't kicking at all now—just squirming."

When you first heard from your baby, way back in the fifth month, there was ample room in the uterus for acrobatics—and lots of kicking and punching. Now that conditions are getting a little cramped, gymnastics are curtailed. In this uterine straightjacket, there is room for little more than turning, twisting, and wiggling. And once the head is firmly engaged in the pelvis, baby will be even less mobile.

It's not important what kind of fetal movement you feel at this stage, as long as you're conscious of activity every day.

"I've hardly felt the baby kick at all this afternoon. Should I be alarmed?"

It could be that your baby has settled down for a nap, or that you've been too busy or too active to notice his or her movements. For reassurance, check for activity in a more formal way, by performing the test on page 202. It's a good idea to repeat this test routinely a couple of times each day throughout the last trimester. Ten or more movements during each test period mean that your baby's activity level is normal. Fewer suggests that medical evaluation might be necessary to determine the cause of the inactivity—so contact your practitioner at once. Though a baby who is relatively inactive in the womb can be perfectly healthy, inactivity sometimes indicates fetal distress. Picking up this distress early through fetal movement testing and intervening medically can often prevent serious consequences.

"I've read that fetal movements are supposed to slow down as delivery approaches. My baby seems more active than ever. Could that mean he's going to be hyperactive?"

Before birth is too soon to start worrying about hyperactivity. Studies show that fetuses who are very active in the womb are no more likely than quieter fetuses to be hyperactive in childhood, though they may well turn out to be very active children.

Recent research also contradicts the notion that the average fetus becomes lazy just before delivery. In late pregnancy, there is generally a gradual decline in the number of movements (from about 25 to 40 an hour at 30 weeks to 20 to 30 at term), probably related to tighter quarters, a decrease in amniotic fluid, and improved fetal coordination. But unless you're counting, you're not likely to notice a significant difference.

FEAR OF ANOTHER LONG LABOR

"I had a 48-hour labor my first time around, and finally delivered after 4½ hours of pushing. Though we both came out of it okay, I dread going through that torture again."

Anyone brave enough to go back into the ring after such a challenging first round deserves a break. And chances are good that you'll get one. Second and subsequent labors and deliveries are usually easier and shorter than first ones—often dramatically so. Less resistance will be met from your now roomier birth canal and your laxer musculature, and, though the process won't be effortless (it rarely is), it may well be less of an ordeal. The most marked difference may be in the amount of pushing you have to do; second babies often pop out in a matter of minutes rather than hours.

Of course, though your odds of an easier childbirth are significantly improved the second time around, there are no sure bets in the labor and delivery rooms. Short of a crystal ball, there's no way to predict precisely what each labor will bring.

BLEEDING OR SPOTTING

"Right after my husband and I made love this morning, I began to bleed. Does this mean that labor is beginning—or is the baby in some kind of danger?"

Any new symptom in the ninth month immediately raises one of two questions—or both: Is it time? Is something wrong? Bleeding and spotting are two such anxiety-provoking events. What they indicate depends on the type of bleeding and the circumstances that surround it:

❖ Pinkish-stained or red-streaked mucus appearing soon after intercourse or a vaginal examination, or brownish-tinged mucus or brownish spotting appearing within 48 hours after the same, is probably just a result of the sensitive cervix being bruised or manipulated. This is normal and not a danger sign—although it should be reported to your practitioner. He or she may advise abstinence from intercourse until delivery.

❖ Bright red bleeding or persistent spotting could be originating at the placenta and requires immediate medical evaluation. Call your practitioner at once. If he or she can't be reached, have someone take you to the hospital.

❖ Pinkish- or brownish-tinged or bloody mucus accompanied by contractions or other signs of oncoming labor (see Prelabor, False Labor, Real Labor, page 268), whether it follows intercourse or not, could be signaling the start of labor. Put in a call to your practitioner.

LIGHTENING AND ENGAGEMENT

"If I'm past my 38th week and haven't dropped, does it mean I'm going to be late?"

"**D**ropping," also called "lightening," occurs when the fetus descends into the pelvic cavity. In first pregnancies, this lightening generally takes place two to four weeks before delivery. In women who have had children previously, it rarely occurs until they go into labor. But as with almost every aspect of pregnancy, exceptions to the rules are the rule. A first-time mother can drop four weeks before her due date and deliver two weeks "late," or she can go into labor without having dropped at all.

Often, lightening is quite apparent. The pregnant woman notes that her belly seems to be lower and tilted farther forward. The happy consequences: as the upward pressure of the uterus on the diaphragm is relieved, taking a deep breath becomes easier, and with the stomach less crowded, eating a full meal becomes more comfortable. These welcome changes are offset by the discomforts caused by pressure on the bladder, the pelvic joints, and the perineal area: increased frequency of urination, difficult mobility, a sensation of increased perineal pressure, and sometimes pain. Sharp little shocks or twinges may be felt when the fetal head presses on the pelvic floor. Some women sense a rolling in the pelvis when the baby's head turns. And often, because her center of gravity has again shifted, a pregnant woman feels more off balance once lightening has occurred.

It is possible, however, for lightening to occur without your realizing it.

If, for instance, you were carrying low to begin with, your pregnant silhouette might not alter noticeably. Or if you never experienced difficulty breathing or getting a full meal down, you might not notice any obvious change.

Lightening is a sign that the presenting part, usually the fetal head, is engaged in the upper portion of the bony pelvis. Your practitioner will rely on two basic indicators to determine whether or not your baby's head is engaged: on internal examination, the presenting part is felt in the pelvis; on palpating the head externally, it is found to be fixed in position, no longer "floating."

How far the presenting part has progressed through the pelvis is measured in "stations," each a centimeter long. A fully engaged baby is said to be at "zero (or 0) station"—that is, the fetal head has descended to the level of the ischial spines (prominent bony landmarks on either side of the midpelvis). A baby who has just begun to descend may be at -4 or -5 station. Once delivery begins, the head continues on through the pelvis past 0 to $+1$, $+2$, and so on, until it begins to "crown" at the external vaginal opening at $+5$. Though a woman who goes into labor at 0 station probably has less pushing ahead than the woman at -3, this isn't invariably true, since station isn't the only factor affecting the progression of labor.

Though the engagement of the fetal head strongly suggests that the baby can get through the pelvis without difficulty, it's no guarantee; conversely, a fetus that is still floating going into labor is not necessarily going to have trouble. And in fact, the majority of fetuses that haven't yet engaged when labor begins come through the pelvis smoothly. This is particularly true in women who have already delivered one or more babies previously.

WHEN YOU WILL DELIVER

"Can the doctor tell exactly how close I am to going into labor?"

N o. And don't you believe it if he or she tells you otherwise. There are clues that labor may soon begin, which your practitioner begins to look for in the ninth month. Has lightening or engagement taken place? What level, or station, in the pelvis has the baby's presenting part descended to? Have effacement (thinning of the cervix) and dilatation (opening of the cervix) begun?

But "soon" can mean anywhere from an hour to three weeks or more. Ask the woman whose euphoria at being told by her practitioner, "You'll be in labor by this evening," dissolves into depression as weeks more of pregnancy pass with nary a contraction.

A practitioner's prognostication that, since effacement and dilatation haven't yet begun, labor is weeks away can be equally unreliable—as women will testify who, upon hearing such a prediction, have dragged home from the doctor's office resigned to another long month of pregnancy, only to give birth by the following morning.

The fact is that engagement, effacement, and dilatation can occur gradually, over a period of weeks or even a month or more in some women. In others they can occur in a matter of hours. No one, no matter how well trained, can accurately predict the onset of labor—because no one knows exactly what triggers it. (That's why most practitioners are as loath to venture guesses on when you will deliver as on whether it's going to be a girl or a boy.)

So like every pregnant woman before you, you'll just have to play the waiting game, knowing for certain only that your day, or night, will come—sometime.

LABOR AND DELIVERY ROOMS

"I'm very uneasy about going into the hospital and having my baby in unfamiliar surroundings."

T he labor and delivery floor is by far the happiest in the hospital. Still, if you don't know what to expect, you can arrive filled with trepidation. Most hospitals allow—in fact, encourage—advance tours of the labor and delivery suite by expectant

---

Do-It-Yourself Labor Induction?

One study showed that women who, from 39 weeks on, stimulated their nipples for three hours or more daily were much less likely to carry past their due dates. In the study women stimulated the nipple, areola, and breast with the balls of their fingertips, 15 minutes a breast, alternating breasts, for one hour three times a day. Creams or lotions were optional as was a husband's help. The problem is that not only is this technique time- and energy-consuming, but without careful medical supervision, it can be risky. It can produce very strong contractions (much as oxytocin can), which could lead to trouble. So *do not try this technique unless your practitioner recommends it.*

couples. Inquire when you make your reservation. If tours aren't routine, ask your practitioner if he or she can arrange a visit for you. Some hospitals have video tapes of the labor and delivery areas that you can borrow. You can also stop in during visiting hours, and though you won't see the actual labor and delivery area, you can see what patient rooms look like in the postpartum section, and also take a good look at the nursery. Besides making you feel more comfortable, this will give you the opportunity to see what a newborn looks like before you hold your own in your arms.

Labor and delivery rooms vary from hospital to hospital. Some are very sterile and businesslike; others are more homey. Birthing rooms are becoming more and more common and boast the at-home look, with rocking chairs, bright pictures on the walls, curtains on the windows, and birthing beds that look more as if they came out of an Ethan Allen showroom than a hospital supply catalogue.

But although it's nice to be in pleasant surroundings, in the long run it won't be the artistic flair of the hospital's interior decorator but the skill and caring of the medical personnel that will be important to your well-being and that of your baby.

THE OVERDUE BABY

"I'm a week overdue and my doctor's arranged to give me a non-stress test. Is it possible that I might never go into labor on my own?"

The magic date is circled in red on the calendar; every day of the 40 weeks that precede it is crossed off with great anticipation. Then, at long last, the big day arrives—and, as in about half of all pregnancies, the baby doesn't. Anticipation dissolves into discouragement. The baby carriage and crib sit empty for yet another day. And then a week. And then, in 10% of pregnancies, most often those of first-time mothers, two weeks. Will this pregnancy never end?

Though women who have reached the 42nd week might find it hard to believe, no pregnancy on record ever went on forever—even before the advent of labor induction. (It's true an occasional pregnancy progresses to the 44th week or even slightly beyond, but today a large majority are induced before they go much past the 42nd.)

Studies show that about 70% of apparent post-term pregnancies aren't post-term at all. They are only believed to be late because of a miscalculation of the time of conception, usually thanks to faulty recollection of the exact date of the last menstrual period. And in fact, when ultrasound examination is used to confirm the due date, diagnoses of post-term pregnancy drop dramatically from the long-held estimate of 10% to about 2%.

When a pregnant woman appears to be post-term (technically 42 weeks or more, though some doctors will take action sooner), the practitioner, in evaluating the situation, considers two major factors: One, is the estimated due date accurate? He or she can be reasonably sure that it is if throughout the pregnancy the dating correlated with such physical findings as the size of the uterus and the height of the fundus (the top of the uterus), and with the timing of the first fetal movements felt by the mother and the first fetal heartbeats detected by the examiner. Early pregnancy ultrasound or blood tests for hCG levels (see page 5) may be looked at to further confirm the correct gestational age.

The second factor usually considered is whether the fetus is continuing to thrive. Many babies continue to grow and thrive well into the tenth

How Is Baby Doing?

Doctors are daily discovering new ways of determining how the unborn baby is faring in the uterus. These tests may be performed at any time in pregnancy when there is some concern, or at 41 or 42 weeks when the baby is presumed overdue. The most common are:

At-Home Fetal Movement Assessment. A mother's record of fetal movements (see page 280), though not foolproof, can furnish some indication of her baby's condition and can be used to screen for possible problems. If the mother fails to note adequate activity, other tests are then performed.

The Non-Stress Test (NST). The mother is hooked up to the fetal monitor just as she would be if she were in labor, and the response of the fetal heart to fetal movements can be observed. If, during the non-stress test, the heart rate doesn't react to movement or the baby doesn't move at all, or if other abnormalities are noted, fetal distress may be present. A weakness of the NST (and of electronic fetal monitoring) is that the accuracy of the test depends on the skill of the person interpreting it.

Fetal Acoustical Stimulation (FAS), or Vibroacoustic Stimulation. This non-stress test evaluates the reaction of the fetus to sound or vibrations and has been found to be more accurate than the traditional non-stress tests.

The Stress Test, or Oxytocin Challenge Test (OCT). A test used to evaluate the reactivity of the fetal heart to uterine contractions. In this somewhat more complex and time-consuming test (it may take up to three hours), the mother is hooked up to a fetal monitor. If contractions are not occurring frequently enough on their own, they are given a push via the intravenous administration of oxytocin, or by stimulation of the mother's nipples (with hot towels and, if necessary, manually by the mother). Fetal response to contractions indicates the probable condition of fetus and placenta. This rough simulation of the conditions of labor allows a prediction to be made about whether or not the fetus can safely remain in the uterus or, if necessary, meet the strenuous demands of true labor.

A Biophysical Profile (BPP). A BPP is compiled by means of ultrasound and evaluates fetal movement, fetal breathing, and the quantity of amniotic fluid. Normal movements, breathing, and adequate amniotic fluid are a sign that baby is probably okay. When combined with an assessment of the fetal heart rate, the BPP provides a very clear picture of the baby's condition.

The "Modified" Biophysical Profile. This combination of the results of a biophysical profile (above) with a non-stress test (see below) provides an accurate assessment of fetal well-being.

Other Tests of Fetal Well-Being. These include: serial ultrasound to document fetal growth; amniotic fluid volume check by ultrasound (decreased volume may signal placental insufficiency); amniotic fluid sampling (through amniocentesis; page 44); Doppler velocimetry (which measures the velocity of blood flow through the umbilical cord); the "fetal admissions test" (combining FAS with an assessment of the amniotic fluid volume), used early in labor to predict potential fetal problems; fetal electrocardiography (to assess the fetal heart, usually via an electrode attached to the scalp); fetal scalp stimulation (which tests fetal reaction to pressure on or pinching of the scalp); and fetal scalp blood sampling.

month (although this can be a problem if the baby becomes too large during this time to pass easily through the mother's pelvis). Occasionally, however, the once ideal environment in the uterus begins to deteriorate. The aging placenta fails to supply adequate nutrition and oxygen, and production of amniotic fluid drops, dangerously reducing levels of fluid in the uterus. Under these conditions, it becomes difficult for the fetus to continue to do well.

Babies born after spending time in such an environment are called postmature. They are thin, with skin that is dry, cracked, peeling, loose, and wrinkled and has lost the cheesy vernix coating common in term newborns. Being "older" than other new arrivals, they have longer nails and more abundant hair, and are generally open-eyed and alert. Those with longer stays in a deteriorating uterus may have greenish (meconium) staining of the skin and umbilical cord. Those who have been in the post-term uterus the longest display yellow staining, and are the most at risk during labor or even before.

Both because they are usually larger than 40-week babies, with wider head circumferences, and because they may be somewhat compromised by insufficient oxygen and nutrition or by possibly having inhaled meconium, postmature babies are at increased risk of having a difficult labor and are more likely to be delivered by cesarean. They may also need some special care in the neonatal intensive care nursery for a short time after birth. Still, those born at 42 weeks after uncomplicated pregnancies are at no greater risk of permanent problems than babies born at 40 weeks.

When it has been determined with certainty that a pregnancy is past 41 weeks, and on examination the cervix is found to be ripe (soft), many practitioners will choose to induce labor (see page 273). Delivery by induction or cesarean will also be initiated, whether the cervix is ripe or not, if complications such as hypertension (chronic or pregnancy-induced) or diabetes threaten the mother, or if meconium staining, suspected inadequate fetal growth, or other problems threaten the fetus. If the cervix is not ripe, the practitioner may choose to try to ripen it by administering a drug, such as prostaglandin E_2 (usually via vaginal suppositories or gel), before inducing. Or he or she may choose to wait it out a little longer, performing one or more tests (see page 263) to see if the fetus is still doing okay in the uterus, and repeating these tests once or twice a week until labor begins.

Some practitioners will wait until 42 weeks or even a bit more before deciding to circumvent Mother Nature—assuming the fetus continues to pass its tests and the mother is doing well. If at any point test results indicate placental insufficiency or inadequate levels of amniotic fluid, or if there are any other signs that either mother or baby is in trouble, the practitioner will take action and, depending upon the situation, induce labor or perform a cesarean section. Fortunately for anxious expectant mothers, few pregnancies are allowed to go more than a matter of days beyond 42 confirmed weeks.

A couple of ways of reducing the likelihood of having a post-term baby are sometimes recommended, but both have their drawbacks. One—daily nipple stimulation—can be handled by the mother at home (see page 261), but is risky because it could trigger overly strong contractions. The other—stripping of the fetal membranes—calls for the manual separating of the chorionic membranes surrounding the fetus from the lower section of the uterus and must be performed by the practitioner. Many physicians believe stripping the mem-

What to Take to the Hospital

For the Labor or Birthing Room

❖ This book.

❖ A watch or clock with a second hand for timing contractions.

❖ A radio or a cassette player equipped with your favorite tapes, if music soothes and relaxes you.

❖ A camera, tape recorder, and/or video equipment, if you don't trust your memory to capture the moment (and if the hospital rules allow media coverage of births).

❖ Powder, lotions, oils, or anything else you'd like to be massaged with.

❖ A small paper bag, to breathe into in case you begin to hyperventilate during your breathing exercises.

❖ A tennis ball or plastic rolling pin, for firm counter-massage should lower backache be a problem.

❖ Sugarless lollipops to keep your mouth moist (though sugar-full candies are usually recommended, they will only make you thirstier and more dehydrated).

❖ Heavy socks, in case your feet become cold.

❖ A hairbrush, if having someone brush your hair is comforting.

❖ A washcloth for sponging down with, though the hospital may provide this (don't bring a white one, which might accidentally end up in the hospital laundry).

❖ A sandwich or other snack for Dad (a coach who faints from hunger can't be very useful).

❖ A bottle of champagne or bubbly cider labeled with your name, for celebrating (your coach can ask the nurse to put it in the fridge), though depending on the hour you deliver, you may be more in the mood for an orange juice toast.

For the Hospital Room

❖ A robe and/or nightgowns, if you'd rather wear your own than the hospital's. Be forewarned, however, that though pretty nightgowns can boost your spirits, they may get bled on and permanently stained. Ditto bathrobes. A good compromise might be a favorite bedjacket to wear over the hospital gown.

❖ Perfume, powder, or whatever else makes you feel fresh.

❖ Toiletries, including shampoo, toothbrush, toothpaste, lotion (your skin may be dry from a loss of fluids), a bar of soap in a carrying case, deodorant, hairbrush, hand mirror, makeup, and any other essentials of beauty and hygiene.

❖ Sanitary napkins, preferably the adhesive variety, though pads are usually provided by the hospital.

❖ Playing cards, books (including what-to-name-your-baby books if you're leaving that decision for the last minute), and other distractions.

❖ Packs of raisins, nuts, whole-wheat crackers, and other healthy snacks to keep you healthy and regular in spite of a hospital diet.

❖ A going-home outfit for you, keeping in mind that you'll still be sporting a sizable abdomen.

❖ A going-home outfit for baby—a kimono or stretch suit, T-shirt, booties, a receiving blanket, and a heavy bunting or blanket if it's cold; diapers will probably be provided by the hospital, but take along an extra, just in case.

❖ A copy of *What to Expect the First Year.*

branes is not advisable because of the risks of rupturing them or causing infection.

MEMBRANES RUPTURING IN PUBLIC

"I live in fear of my membranes rupturing in public."

You're not alone in your fear. The idea of the "bag of waters" breaking on a bus or in a crowded department store is as mortifying to most pregnant women as that of losing bladder control in public. One woman reportedly became so obsessed with her worry that she began carrying a jar of pickles in her handbag, ready to be dropped at the first telltale trickle of amniotic fluid.

But before you start rummaging through your cupboards for the garlic dills, there are two things you should know. First, the rupture of membranes before labor begins is uncommon—occurring in less than 15% of pregnancies. And once they do break, the flow of amniotic fluid is unlikely to be heavy except when you are lying down (something you aren't likely to do in public). When you are walking or sitting, the fetal head tends to block the opening of the uterus like a cork in a wine bottle.

And second, should your membranes rupture and the amniotic fluid gush suddenly, you can be sure that those around you will not point, shake disapproving heads, or—worse—chuckle. Instead they will (as you would if you were a bystander) either offer you assistance or discreetly ignore you. Keep in mind, after all, that no one is likely to overlook the fact that you're pregnant and therefore to mistake amniotic fluid for anything else.

Some women whose membranes rupture prior to labor never experience a gushing of amniotic fluid when their membranes rupture—partly because of the cork effect, partly because there are no contractions to force the fluid out. All they notice is a trickle, either constant or intermittent.

Wearing a panty liner in the last weeks may give you a sense of security, as well as keeping you fresher as your vaginal discharge (leukorrhea) increases.

BREASTFEEDING

"My breasts are very small and my nipples are flat. Will I be able to breastfeed?"

As far as hungry babies are concerned, satisfaction comes in all kinds of packages. Breasts don't have to be centerfold-shaped or -sized, and they can come equipped with almost any kind of nipple—small and flat, large and pointy, even inverted. All combinations of breasts and nipples have the capacity to produce and dispense milk—the quantity and quality of which are not in the least dependent on outward appearance. Unfortunately, because so many fallacies and old wives' tales exist about what kinds of breasts can and cannot satisfy a baby, many women are unnecessarily discouraged from breastfeeding.

Inverted nipples that don't become erect with sexual stimulation generally need some special priming prior to childbirth. The use of breast shells, available in many maternity and infant supply shops, which provide a gentle suction, is the best way to "pull out" inverted nipples. At first they should be worn for only short intervals morning and evening; gradually the time they are worn can be extended to a full day. A manual breast pump used several times a day can also help to correct inverted nipples, but do not use a pump if it stimulates uterine contractions or if you are at high risk for premature delivery.

Some experts recommend that all women who expect to nurse try to prepare their breasts in advance by expressing a small amount of colostrum from the nipples daily from the eighth month on (though not every woman will be able to do this) and by pulling, twisting, or rolling the nipples between forefinger and thumb— also daily—to toughen them. Others say that nursing comes naturally to nipples, without special preparation.

"My mother says she had milk leaking from her breasts by this time; I don't. Does this mean I won't have any milk?"

The thin, yellowish discharge that some pregnant women can express, or may notice leaking from their breasts, is not milk. It is a premilk called colostrum. Richer in protein and lower in fat and milk sugar than the breast milk that comes three or four days after delivery, it contains antibodies that may be important in protecting the baby against disease.

Many women, however, don't have any noticeable colostrum until after delivery. (Even then, they may not be aware of it.) This in no way predicts a lack of milk or difficulty in nursing.

MOTHERING

"Now that the baby's arrival is so close, I'm beginning to worry about taking care of it. I've never even held a newborn before."

Women are not born mothers, instinctively knowing how to rock a crying baby to sleep, change a diaper, or give a bath. Motherhood— parenthood, for that matter—is a learned art, one that requires plenty of practice to make perfect (or even near-perfect). A hundred years ago, that practice commonly took place at an early age, when female children learned to care for younger siblings— much as they learned to bake bread and mend socks.

Today, a high percentage of fully grown women have never kneaded bread dough, taken a needle to a worn sock, or held—let alone taken care of—an infant. Their training for motherhood comes on the job, with a little help from books, magazines, and, if they're lucky enough to find one at their local hospital, a baby-care class. Which means that for the first week or two, the baby may do more crying than sleeping, the diapers may leak, and many a tear may be shed over the "no-more-tears" lather. Slowly but surely, however, the new mother begins to feel like an old pro. Her trepidation turns to assurance. The baby she was afraid to hold (won't it break?) is now cradled casually in her left arm while her right sets the table or pushes the vacuum cleaner. Dispensing vitamin drops, giving baths, slipping squirming arms and legs into sleepers, have ceased to be dreaded ordeals. They, like all the daily tasks of parenting, have become second nature. She's a mother, and—difficult though it may be to imagine—you will be one, too.

Though nothing can make those first days with a first baby easy, starting the learning process before delivery can make them seem a little less overwhelming. Any of the following should help: visit a newborn nursery and view the most recent arrivals; hold, diaper, and soothe a friend's new baby; read up on a baby's first year; and take a class in parenting a newborn.

WHAT IT'S IMPORTANT TO KNOW:
PRELABOR, FALSE LABOR, REAL LABOR

It always seems so simple on TV. Somewhere around 3 A.M., the pregnant woman sits up in bed, puts a knowing hand on her belly, and reaches over to rouse her sleeping husband with a calm, almost serene, "It's time, honey."

But how, we wonder, does this woman know it's time? How does she recognize labor with such cool, clinical confidence when she's never *been* in labor before? What makes her so sure she's not going to get to the hospital, be examined by the resident, and be found to be uneffaced, undilated, and nowhere near her time? That she won't be sent home—amid snickers from the night shift—just as pregnant as when she arrived?

On our side of the screen, we're more likely to awaken at 3 A.M. with complete uncertainty. Are these really labor pains, or just more Braxton Hicks? Should I turn on the light and start timing? Should I bother to wake my husband? Do I call the doctor in the middle of the night to report what might really be false labor? If I do and it isn't time, will I turn out to be the pregnant woman who cried "labor" once too often, and will anybody take me seriously when it's for real? Or will I be the only woman in my childbirth class not to recognize labor? Will I leave for the hospital too late, maybe giving birth in a taxicab? The questions multiply faster than the contractions.

The fact is that most women, worry though they might, *don't* end up misjudging the onset of their labor. The vast majority, thanks to instinct, luck, or no-doubt-about-it killer contractions, show up at the hospital neither too early nor too late, but at just about the right time. Still, there's no reason to leave your deliberations up to chance. Becoming familiar in advance with the signs of prelabor, false labor, and real labor will help to allay the concerns and clear up the confusion when those contractions (or are they?) begin.

No one knows exactly what triggers labor. A group of natural substances produced by the body, called prostaglandins (PGs), are believed to be very important in the process. PGs produced by the uterus during pregnancy are known to increase during spontaneous term labor; they stimulate uterine muscle activity and trigger oxytocin release by the pituitary gland, both important factors in the initiation of labor. And prostaglandin inhibitors, such as aspirin, can delay the onset of labor. Probably a combination of fetal, placental, and maternal factors are responsible for setting labor into motion.

PRELABOR SYMPTOMS

The physical changes of prelabor can precede real labor by a full month or more—or by only an hour or so. Prelabor is characterized by the beginning of cervical effacement and dilatation, which your practitioner can confirm, as well as by a wide variety of related signs that you may notice yourself:

Lightening and Engagement. Usually somewhere between two and four weeks before the onset of labor in first-time mothers, the fetus begins to descend into the pelvis. This milestone is rarely reached in second or later births until labor has actually commenced.

Sensations of Increasing Pressure in the Pelvis and Rectum. Crampiness and groin pain are particularly common in second and later pregnancies. Persistent low backache may also be present.

Loss of Weight or Cessation of Weight Gain. In general, weight gain slows in the ninth month; as labor approaches, some women lose up to 2 or 3 pounds.

A Change in Energy Levels. Some ninth-monthers find that they are increasingly fatigued. Others experience energy spurts. An uncontrollable urge to scrub floors and wash woodwork has been related to the "nesting instinct"—in which the female of the species prepares the nest for the impending arrival.

A Change in Vaginal Discharge. You may find that your discharge increases and thickens.

Loss of Mucous Plug. As the cervix begins to thin and open, the "cork" of mucus that seals the opening of the uterus becomes dislodged. This gelatinous chunk of mucus can be passed through the vagina a week or two before the first real contractions, or just as labor begins.

Pink, or Bloody, Show. As the cervix effaces and dilates, capillaries frequently rupture, tinting the mucus pink or streaking it with blood. This "show" usually means labor will start within 24 hours—but it could be as much as several days away.

Intensification of Braxton Hicks Contractions. These practice contractions may become more frequent and stronger, even painful.

Diarrhea. Some women experience loose bowel movements just prior to the onset of labor.

FALSE LABOR SYMPTOMS

Real labor probably has not begun if:

❖ Contractions are not regular and don't increase in frequency or severity.

❖ Pain is in the lower abdomen rather than the lower back.

❖ Contractions subside if you walk around or change your position.

❖ Show, if any, is brownish.[2] (Often the result of an internal exam or intercourse within the past 48 hours.)

❖ Fetal movements intensify briefly with contractions. (A lot of activity could signal fetal distress.)

REAL LABOR SYMPTOMS

When contractions of prelabor are replaced by stronger, more painful, and more frequent ones, the question arises: "Is this the real thing or false labor?" It is probably real if:

❖ The contractions intensify, rather than ease up, with activity and aren't relieved by a change in position.

❖ Pain begins in the lower back and spreads to the lower abdomen; it may also radiate to the legs. Contractions may feel like gastrointestinal upset and be accompanied by diarrhea.

2. Bright red blood requires immediate consultation with your practitioner.

❖ Contractions become progressively more frequent and painful, and generally (but not always) more regular. (This progression isn't absolute—not every contraction will necessarily be more painful or longer than the previous one, but their general intensity does build up as real labor progresses. Nor does frequency always increase in regular, perfectly even intervals—but it does increase.)

❖ Show is present and pinkish or blood-streaked.

❖ Membranes rupture. In 15% of labors the waters break—in a gush or a trickle—before labor begins.

WHEN TO CALL THE DOCTOR

When in doubt, call. Even if you've checked and rechecked the above lists, you may still be unsure whether you're really in labor. Don't wait to find out for sure—unless you're planning a home birth. Call your practitioner. He or she will probably be able to tell from the sound of your voice, as you talk through a contraction, whether it's the real thing. (But only if you don't try to cover up the pain in the name of stoicism or good manners.) Fear of embarrassment if it turns out not to be labor shouldn't prevent your calling your practitioner. If it does turn out to be a false alarm, nobody's going to snicker. You wouldn't be the first patient to misjudge her labor signs—and you certainly won't be the last.

❖ Call anytime, night or day, if all signs indicate that you're ready to go to the hospital. Don't let an overdeveloped sense of guilt or politeness keep you from waking your practitioner up in the middle of the night, or disturbing his or her weekend at home. People who deliver babies for a living don't expect to work only 9 to 5.

❖ Your practitioner has probably specified that you should call when your contractions have reached a particular frequency—say 5, 8, or 10 minutes apart. Call when at least some are that frequent. Don't wait for perfectly even intervals; they may never come.

❖ Your practitioner has probably also instructed you about when to call if your membranes rupture, or if you think they have ruptured, but labor has not begun. Follow these instructions unless: your due date is still several weeks away; you know your baby is small or is not engaged in the pelvis; or the amniotic fluid is stained greenish brown. In these cases, call immediately.

❖ Don't assume that if you're not sure it's real labor, it isn't. Err on the side of caution; call.

Best Medicine for Labor?

Recent studies show that when a woman in labor is supported, encouraged, touched, soothed, and kept abreast of what is happening by an experienced mother, or "doula," the number of cesarean and forceps deliveries, the need for anesthesia, the rate of complications, and even the length of labor can be reduced.

14
Labor and Delivery

It takes nine months to make a baby, and only a matter of hours to bring one out into the world. Yet it's those hours that seem to occupy the minds of expectant women most—more questions, fears, and concerns revolve around the processes of labor and delivery than around any other aspect of pregnancy. When will it start? More important, when will it end? Will I be able to tolerate the pain? Will I have to have an enema? A fetal monitor? An episiotomy? What if I don't make any pro-

gress? What if I progress so quickly that I don't even have time to get to the hospital?

You'll find answers to your questions and reassurance for your fears and concerns in the following chapter. These, teamed with a lot of support from your partner and your birth attendants, and the knowledge that labor and delivery have never been safer and more manageable than they are today, should help prepare you for most anything that labor and delivery might bring your way.

WHAT YOU MAY BE CONCERNED ABOUT

BLOODY SHOW

'I have a pink mucous discharge. Does it mean labor's about to start?''

Don't send your husband out for the cigars yet. Passage of a "bloody show," a mucous discharge tinged pink or brown with blood, is often a sign that your cervix is effacing and/or dilating and that the process that leads to delivery is beginning. But it's a process with an erratic timetable that will keep you in suspense until the first contractions. Labor could be one, two, or even three

weeks away, with your cervix continuing to dilate gradually over that time. Or it could be less than an hour away.

If your discharge should suddenly become bright red or seems to amount to more than an ounce of blood, contact your practitioner immediately. Bleeding could indicate premature separation of the placenta or placenta previa, which require prompt medical attention.

RUPTURE OF MEMBRANES

"I woke up in the middle of the night with

a wet bed. Did I lose control of my bladder, or did my membranes rupture?"

A sniff of your sheets will probably clue you in. If the wet spot smells sort of sweet and not like ammonia, it's likely to be amniotic fluid. Another clue: You'll probably still be leaking the pale, straw-colored amniotic fluid (which won't run dry because it continues to be produced until delivery, replacing itself every three hours). When you stand up or sit down, however, the baby's head may act like a cork and stop up the leak temporarily.

Whether or not there continues to be leakage, if you suspect your membranes have ruptured, you should call your practitioner. Until you've contacted him or her, act as though your membranes have indeed ruptured (see below).

"My water just broke, but I haven't had any contractions. When is labor going to start, and what should I do in the meantime?"

The majority of pregnant women whose membranes rupture prior to labor feel their first contractions within 12 hours; most others feel them within 24 hours. About 1 in 10, however, take longer to go into labor. Because, as time passes, the risk of infection to baby and/or mother through the ruptured amniotic sac increases, most physicians will induce labor with oxytocin within 24 hours of the rupture if a woman is at or near her due date, though a few wait as little as 6 hours to induce. Recent studies show that, when the pregnancy reaches this point, there is no advantage in delaying induction beyond 24 hours, and a definite disadvantage: an increased risk of infection (see page 359).

If you experience a trickle or flow of fluid from your vagina, call your doctor or nurse-midwife. In the meantime, keep the vaginal area as clean as possible, to avoid infection. Don't take a bath or have sexual relations; use sanitary napkins (not a tampon) to absorb the flow of amniotic fluid; don't try to do your own internal exam; and wipe front to back at the toilet.

Rarely, in premature rupture of the membranes (most often when the baby is breech or premature), when the presenting part is not yet engaged in the pelvis, the umbilical cord becomes "prolapsed"—it is swept into the neck of the uterus (the cervix), or even into the vagina, with the gush of amniotic fluid. If you can see a loop of umbilical cord showing at your vaginal opening, or think you feel something inside your vagina, see page 360 and get immediate medical attention.

DARKENED AMNIOTIC FLUID (MECONIUM STAINING)

"My membranes ruptured, and the fluid is greenish-brown. What does this mean?"

Your amniotic fluid is probably stained with meconium, which is a greenish-brown substance that comes from your baby's digestive tract. Ordinarily, meconium is passed after birth as the baby's first stool. But sometimes—particularly when the fetus has been under stress in the womb, and very often when the baby is postmature—it is passed prior to birth into the amniotic fluid.

Meconium staining alone is not a sure sign of fetal distress, but because it suggests the possibility, notify your practitioner immediately.

INDUCTION OF LABOR

"My doctor wants to induce labor. I'm upset because I had wanted a natural delivery."

Though some doctors 20 years ago believed it was safe to routinely induce labor in their patients so that birth would come at a convenient time, doctors today rarely induce without good cause. This has come about partly because the FDA has withdrawn approval of elective (not absolutely necessary) use of the drug oxytocin, with which labor is induced, and partly for fear of malpractice suits should something go wrong. But it has come about mostly because they recognize that, when possible, it's best to let nature take its time taking its course.

In close to 1 in 3 deliveries, however, nature may need a little prodding. There are a variety of situations in which it is necessary to deliver a baby before nature appears ready and willing to do so. In some cases, a cesarean section is the best way to do this. In others, when time is not of the essence, both mother and baby are deemed able to tolerate the stresses of labor, and the practitioner has reason to believe that a normal vaginal delivery is possible, induction is usually the first choice. For example:

❖ When labor is weak or erratic, or has stalled.

❖ When a fetus isn't thriving (because of inadequate nourishment, poor placental function, postmaturity, or any other reason) and is mature enough to do well outside the uterus.

❖ When a stress or non-stress test suggests that the placenta is no longer functioning optimally and the uterine environment is no longer healthy.

❖ When there is premature rupture of the membranes at term (see page 359).

❖ When a pregnancy has gone two or more weeks past a due date that is considered accurate (see page 262).

❖ When the mother has diabetes and the placenta is deteriorating prematurely, or when it's feared her baby will be very large—and thus difficult to deliver—if carried to term.

❖ When the mother has preeclampsia (toxemia) that cannot be controlled with bed rest and medication, and delivery is necessary for her sake and/or her baby's.

❖ When the mother has a chronic or acute illness, such as high blood pressure or kidney disease, that threatens her well-being or that of her baby if the pregnancy continues.

❖ When the fetus is afflicted with severe Rh disease which necessitates early delivery.

Occasionally, all that's required to induce labor is for the physician to artificially rupture the membranes (bag of waters) that surround the fetus. If the cervix is not ripe, pain relief medication may be given during this procedure. Some practitioners will give the mother a dose of mineral oil and/or have her attempt nipple self-stimulation to get contractions going. Prostaglandin E_2 suppositories or gel may be used to help ripen the cervix. But in most cases, the administration of oxytocin turns out to be necessary to consistently activate the uterus.

Oxytocin is a hormone produced naturally by the maternal pituitary gland throughout pregnancy. As pregnancy progresses, the uterus becomes more and more sensitive to the hormone, although it isn't clear whether it plays a significant role in the triggering of natural labor. It is known that the hormone may be released by the pregnant woman when her nipples are stimulated, causing the uterus to contract—which is why nipple stimulation sometimes works to trigger labor. The administration of oxytocin (trade name, Pitocin), however, is a more reliable method of induction. When the cervix is ripe, oxytocin is capable of initiating a labor that closely mimics one that occurs naturally. When the cervix isn't ripe, induction may be carried out (assuming there is time) over a two- or three-day course, to allow gradual ripening. Or efforts may be made to ripen the cervix by using prostaglandin E_2 or to open it manually by using graduated dilators before induction is begun. These procedures can improve the chances for a spontaneous vaginal delivery within 24 hours.

To induce labor, oxytocin is administered through an intravenous IV drip with an infusion pump. This is the safest and easiest route to controlling the rate of administration. The IV is introduced via a needle in the arm or the back of the hand, and connected by tubing to two bottles. One bottle contains unmedicated intravenous fluid, and the other contains the oxytocin. By routing the oxytocin into the primary tubing through an infusion pump, it is possible to precisely control the dosage. Usually the induction begins slowly, with very little oxytocin being infused into the mother, and the reactions of the uterus and the fetus carefully monitored. (A doctor or nurse must be in attendance at all times during induction.) The rate of infusion is increased gradually until effective contractions are established. Should the woman's uterus prove extremely sensitive to the drug and be overstimulated into either too long or too powerful contractions, this method allows the infusion rate to be reduced or discontin-

ued entirely by switching the IV to the primary tubing bottle of unmedicated solution.

Contractions usually begin after 30 minutes in women who are at or close to term, and they're generally more regular and more frequent than those of a naturally occurring labor, right from the start. If, after six to eight hours of oxytocin administration, labor hasn't begun or progressed, the procedure will probably be terminated in favor of an alternative approach, usually a cesarean section. Treatment may also be terminated if contractions become well established and continue on their own.

Induction of labor is inappropriate when immediate delivery is necessary or when there is any doubt that the fetus can fit through the mother's pelvis; the procedure also is avoided when the placenta is near or covering the opening of the uterus (placenta previa), when the woman is judged to be in false labor, and, generally, in women who have had five or more previous births or who have a vertical scar from a past cesarean section, since they are at greater risk for uterine rupture. Some physicians will also not attempt induction when a woman is carrying multiple fetuses or when a baby is in the breech position. The American College of Obstetricians and Gynecologists recommends that when labor is induced with oxytocin the physician be ready and available to perform an emergency cesarean, if one is needed.

Some women find the sudden onset of hard labor that usually occurs with induction unpleasant; some even feel cheated by the artificially shortened duration of their laboring experience. Others enjoy such down-to-business births. With their coach at their side, they go through their induced labor otherwise naturally, using all the breathing exercises and other coping mechanisms learned in childbirth classes. And so can anyone who keeps in mind that labor, no matter how it's triggered, is labor.

HAVING A SHORT LABOR

"Can a short labor actually be harmful to the baby?"

S hort labor isn't always as short as it seems. Often the expectant mother has been having painless contractions for hours, days, even weeks, which have been dilating her cervix gradually. By the time she feels the first contraction, she is well into the transition stage of labor (see the stages of childbirth, beginning on page 288). This slow-buildup, quick-resolution labor places no extra strain on the fetus, and may be even less stressful than the average 12-hour labor.

Occasionally the cervix dilates very rapidly, accomplishing in a matter of minutes what most cervixes (particularly those of first-time mothers) take hours to do. But even with this abrupt, or precipitous, kind of labor (one that takes three hours or less from start to finish), there is rarely any threat to the baby. There is no evidence to support the notion that an infant must go through a minimum amount of labor in order to arrive in good condition.

Once in a great while, however, an extremely rapid labor does deprive the fetus of oxygen or other needed gases, or results in tearing or other damage to cervix, vagina, or perineum in the mother. So, if your labor seems to start with a bang—with contractions strong and close together—get to the hospital quickly. Medication may be helpful in slowing contractions a bit and easing the pressure on the fetus and on your own body.

CALLING YOUR PRACTITIONER DURING LABOR

"I just started getting contractions and they're coming every three or four minutes. I feel silly calling the doctor, who said we should spend the first several hours of labor at home."

M ost first-time mothers-to-be (whose labors often begin slowly, with a gradual buildup of contractions) *can* safely count on spending the first several hours at home. But if your contractions start off strong— lasting at least 45 seconds and coming more often than every five minutes— and/or you've delivered a baby before, your first several hours of labor may very well be your last. Chances are that much of the first stage of labor has passed painlessly, and that your cervix has dilated significantly during that time. This would mean that not calling your doctor—and chancing a dramatic dash to the hospital at the last minute—would be considerably sillier than picking up the phone now.

Before you do, however, it is best to have timed several consecutive contractions. Be clear and specific about their frequency, duration, and strength when you report them. Don't try to minimize your discomfort when you describe it by trying to maintain a calm voice. (Your practitioner is used to judging the phase of labor in part by the sound of a woman's voice as she talks through a contraction.)

If you feel you're ready but your practitioner doesn't seem to think so, don't take "wait" for an answer. Ask if you can go to the hospital and have your progress checked. (See When to Call the Doctor in Prelabor, False Labor, Real Labor, page 268.) You can take your suitcase along "just in case," but be ready to turn around and go home if you've only just begun to dilate.

BACK LABOR

"The pain in my back since my labor began is so bad that I don't see how I'll be able to make it through delivery."

Technically, "back labor" occurs when the fetus is in a posterior (or occipitoposterior) position, with the back of its head pressing against the mother's sacrum—the rear boundary of the pelvis. It's possible, however, to experience back labor when the baby is not in this position, or to continue to experience it after the baby has turned from a posterior to an anterior position—possibly because the area has become a focus of tension.

When you're having this kind of pain—which often doesn't let up between contractions and becomes excruciating during them—the cause is not a crucial consideration. How to relieve it, even slightly, is. There are several measures that may help; all are at least worth trying:

❖ Taking the pressure off your back. Try changing your position—walk around (though this may not be humanly possible once contractions are coming fast and furiously), crouch or squat, get down on all fours, or do whatever is most comfortable and least painful for you. If you feel you can't move and would prefer to be lying down, lie on your side, with your back well rounded.

❖ Heat or cold, applied by your coach or attendant. Use a hot-water bottle wrapped in a towel, warm compresses, a heating pad, or ice packs or cold compresses—whichever soothes best.

❖ Counterpressure. Have your coach experiment with different ways of applying pressure to the area of greatest pain, or to adjacent areas, to find one or more that seem to help. He can try his knuckles, or the heel of one hand reinforced by pressure from the other hand on top of it, using direct pressure or a firm circular motion. Pressure can be applied while you are sitting or while you are lying on your side. The relief you may get from really intense counterpressure will be well worth any black-and-blue marks you find the morning after.

❖ Acupressure. This is probably the oldest form of pain relief—and you don't have to be Chinese to try it. In the case of back labor, it involves applying strong finger pressure just below the center of the ball of the foot.

❖ Aggressive massage to the area may spell relief either in place of counterpressure or alternated with it. A rolling pin or a tennis ball can be used for especially firm massage (although you will probably be a little sore afterward). Oil or powder can be applied periodically to avoid irritation.

IRREGULAR CONTRACTIONS

"In class we were told not to go to the hospital until the contractions were regular and five minutes apart. Mine are less than five minutes apart, but they aren't at all regular. I don't know what to do."

Just as no two women have exactly the same fingerprints, no two women have exactly the same labors. The labor often described in books, in childbirth education classes, and by practitioners is what is typical—and close to what many women can expect. But far from every labor is true-to-textbook, with contractions regularly spaced and predictably progressive.

If you are having strong, long (40 to 60 seconds), frequent (five minutes apart or less) contractions, even if they vary considerably in length and time elapsed between them, do not wait for them to become "regular" before calling your practitioner or heading for the hospital—no matter what you've heard or read. It's possible that your contractions are about as regular as they are going to get, and that you are well into the active phase of your labor. Waste no time in calling your practitioner and getting to the hospital; she who hesitates in a case like this could end up with an unscheduled home birth.

NOT GETTING TO THE HOSPITAL IN TIME

"I'm afraid that I won't get to the hospital in time."

Fortunately, most surprise deliveries take place in the movies and on television. In real life, deliveries, especially those of first-time mothers,

rarely occur without ample warning. But once in a great while, a woman who has had no labor pains, or just erratic ones, suddenly feels an overwhelming urge to bear down; often she mistakes it for a need to go to the bathroom.

Just in case you might turn out to be one of these women, it's a good idea for both you and your husband to become familiar with the basics of an emergency home delivery (see pages 279 and 281). But don't spend a lot of time worrying about this very remote possibility.

ENEMAS

"I've heard that enemas early in labor aren't really necessary, and that they interfere with natural birth."

Enemas were, until fairly recently, not a matter of patient choice. They were administered routinely in early labor, as part of the hospital admissions procedure. The theory was, and still is in some hospitals, that emptying the bowels before delivery eliminates the possibility of fecal matter in the rectum hindering the baby's descent through the birth canal, and prevents contamination of the sterile birthing setup by involuntary evacuation of feces during the pushing stage

---

Emergency Delivery En Route to the Hospital

1. If you're in your own car and delivery is imminent, pull over. If you have a CB or car phone, call for help. If not, turn on your hazard warning lights or turning signal. If someone stops to help, ask him or her to get to a phone and call 911 or the local emergency medical squad. If you're in a cab, ask the driver to radio for help.

2. If possible, you should help the mother into the back of the car. Place a coat, jacket, or blanket under her. Then proceed as on page 281. As soon as delivery is completed, continue to the nearest hospital in a hurry.

of labor. In addition, this precaution may spare the laboring woman "embarrassment" and lessen her inhibitions about pushing.

This way of thinking is less in favor today. It is recognized that compression of the birth canal is not likely to be a problem if a woman has had a bowel movement in the past 24 hours, or if no hard fecal mass is felt in her rectum on internal examination. And the use during delivery of disposable sterile gauze pads to whisk away any fecal matter that is expelled virtually eliminates the threat of fecal contamination. According to some studies, the possibility of neonatal infection from bowel organisms is highly remote to begin with; others suggest that enemas themselves can actually increase the risk of infection. For these reasons, most hospitals have abandoned the routine enema; others are certain to follow.

If your hospital isn't among these and if the prospect of an enema is one you don't relish, discuss the subject with your practitioner in advance of labor. If you feel strongly that you don't want an enema, he or she may agree to skip it. (But be sure that the decision is relayed to hospital staff.) On the other hand, if you're more uncomfortable with the prospect of moving your bowels on the delivery table (though an enema doesn't guarantee you won't), don't let anyone bully you into accepting the idea that enemas are unnatural and unnecessary. Include your preferences in your birthing plan, if you draw one up (see page 225).

You may be more comfortable taking care of the enema yourself at home, while you're in early labor. But whether it's given at home or in the hospital, a warm water enema may provide the added benefit of boosting sluggish contractions and giving labor a little push.

The entire issue may be academic, however, if your labor begins, as many do, with loose or frequent bowel movements, which may effectively empty the colon; or if you arrive at the hospital in active labor, with contractions so close together that it's barely possible for hospital personnel to get you into a gown, much less give you an enema.

SHAVING THE PUBIC AREA

"I don't like the idea of having my pubic hair shaved. Is it obligatory?"

Though shaving of the pubic area is still a routine "prepping" procedure in some hospitals, it is being utilized less and less. It is most often done simply because it's always been done, not because it is necessary. It was once believed that pubic hair harbored bacteria that could infect the baby as it passed through the vaginal outlet. But since the entire area surrounding the vagina is swabbed with an antiseptic solution prior to delivery, infection of this type is not likely. And in fact, some studies have shown a *higher* rate of infection among women who are shaved prior to delivery than among those who aren't, probably because the small—sometimes microscopic—nicks that even very careful shaving can produce may serve as excellent breeding grounds for bacteria. From the woman's point of view, the humiliation of the shaving itself and the postpartum burning and itching as the hair grows back are additional reasons to object to the procedure.

Some doctors feel that shaving facilitates performing and repairing an episiotomy, by providing a clearer area in which to work. But for them, too, shaving is more likely a matter of habit than conviction. An increasing number of physicians are performing and repairing episiotomies without shav-

---

Emergency Delivery If You're Alone

1. Try to remain calm.

2. Call 911 (or your local emergency number) for the emergency medical squad. Ask them to call your practitioner.

3. Find a neighbor or someone else to help, if possible.

4. Start panting to keep from bearing down.

5. Wash your hands and the vaginal area, if you can.

6. Spread some clean towels, newspapers, or sheets on a bed, sofa, or the floor, and lie down to await help.

7. If despite your panting the baby starts to arrive before help does, gently ease it out by pushing each time you feel the urge, catching it with your hands.

8. Proceed with steps 10 to 14 on page 281 as best you can.

---

ing the surrounding area—either clipping the hair with scissors or pushing it back as they work.

Whether or not you will be shaved may depend on the practices of your practitioner and the hospital you are delivering at. Increasingly, it is one of the decisions of childbirth that you can, at the very least, be instrumental in making. Don't wait until you arrive at the hospital, however, to make your feelings about shaving known. Discuss them in advance of labor with your practitioner. Include your preferences in your birthing plan (see page 225).

If your practitioner or the hospital insists on your being shaved, ask that they not shave any more than is absolutely necessary. A "mini-prep," which shaves only the hair in the area of any possible incision or tear, is usually sufficient. An alternative to being shaved at the hospital, which you may also want to discuss with your practitioner, is having your mate shave or clip you at home.

ROUTINE IVs

"When we had our visit to the hospital, I saw a woman being wheeled from the delivery room with an IV attached. Is that necessary with a normal labor and delivery?"

Thanks to reruns of *M*A*S*H* and edge-of-your-seat soap operas, we readily associate IVs (intravenous setups) with wounded GIs, rapidly fading heroines with fatal illnesses, and heros soundly thrashed by jealous lovers. But it's hard to associate an IV with normal childbirth.

Yet in many American hospitals, it is routine to administer an IV containing a simple solution of nutrients and fluid to a woman in labor. This is done partly to be certain that the woman does not become dehydrated from lack of fluids or weak from lack of food during labor, partly to provide ready access for medication should the need arise (it can be injected right into the IV bottle or line, instead of into the patient). In these instances, the IV is precautionary.

Some doctors and midwives, on the other hand, prefer to wait until there is a clear need for an IV—for instance, because the labor has been lengthy and the laboring woman is weakening. Check your practitioner's policy in advance, and if you strongly object to having an IV, say so. It may be possible to hold off until the need, if any, arises.

If it's your practitioner's policy to give IVs routinely and there's no room for discussion, or if you end up needing one, don't despair. The IV is only slightly uncomfortable as the needle is inserted and thereafter should barely be noticed. When it's hung on a movable stand, you can take it with you to the bathroom or on a brief constitutional. (If at any point the area becomes sore or painful, inform your practitioner or nurse.)

Though you can't always make the decision about whether or not you should have an IV, you do have a right to know what the IV is infusing into your veins. Ask the nurse or doctor who inserts it. Or have your labor partner read the label on the bottle. Occasionally medication may be ordered without your being consulted. If this happens, ask to speak to your practitioner as soon as possible.

FETAL MONITORING

"My doctor believes in fetal monitoring at all births. I've heard that monitoring can lead to unnecessary cesareans and also makes labor more uncomfortable."

For someone who's spent the first nine months of his or her life floating peacefully in a warm and comforting amniotic bath, the trip through the narrow confines of the maternal pelvis will be no joy ride. Your baby will be squeezed, compressed, pushed, and molded with every contraction.

It is because there is an element of risk in this stressful journey—not to promote maternal discomfort or unnecessary cesareans—that fetal monitors have come into such common use. In some hospitals, all labor and delivery patients are electronically monitored. In virtually every hospital, at least half of the patients— particularly those in high-risk categories, who have meconium-stained amniotic fluid, who are receiving oxytocin, or who are having a difficult labor—are monitored electronically.

A fetal monitor gauges the response of the baby's heartbeat to the contractions of the uterus. The reader of the monitor printout may be able to pick up signs of possible fetal stress and distress through variations from the normal reactions to labor. Sometimes an alarm is preset to go off if such variations occur. Fetal monitoring can be external or internal:

External Monitoring. In this type of monitoring, used most frequently, two devices are strapped to the abdomen. One, an ultrasound transducer, picks up the fetal heartbeat. The other, a pressure-sensitive gauge, measures the intensity and duration of uterine contractions. Both are connected to a monitor, which displays or prints out the readings. This doesn't mean the laboring woman must be confined to bed, hooked up to a machine like Frankenstein's monster, for hours on end. In most cases, monitoring is required only intermittently, and the laboring woman can walk around between readings. Some hospitals may be equipped with portable monitors that can be hooked up to the patient's clothing, allowing her complete freedom to go for a stroll down hospital corridors while it sends data on her baby's well-being back to her bedside or a nursing station.

During the second (pushing) stage of labor, when contractions may come so fast and furiously that it's hard to know when to push and when to hold back, the monitor is able to accurately signal the beginning and end of each contraction. Or the use of the monitor

Emergency Home (or Office) Delivery

1. Try to remain calm. Remember, even if you don't know the first thing about delivering a baby, a mother's body and her baby can do most of the job on their own.

2. Call 911 (or your local emergency number) for the emergency medical squad; ask them to call the doctor or nurse-midwife.

3. The mother should start panting to keep from bearing down.

4. During all the preparations and during the delivery, comfort and reassure the mother.

5. If there's time, wash the vaginal area and your hands with detergent or soap and water.

6. If there's no time to get to a bed or table, place newspapers or clean towels or folded clothing under the buttocks, to provide some height for delivering the baby's shoulders.

7. If there is time, place the mother onto the bed (or desk or table) so that her buttocks are slightly hanging off, her hands under her thighs to keep them elevated. If available, a couple of chairs can support her feet.

8. Protect delivery surfaces, if possible, with a plastic tablecloth, shower curtain, newspapers, towels, and so on. A dishpan or basin can be used to catch the amniotic fluid and blood.

9. As the top of the baby's head begins to appear, instruct the mother to pant or blow (not push), and apply very gentle counterpressure to the head to keep it from popping out suddenly. Let the head emerge gradually—*never* pull it out. If there is a loop of umbilical cord around the baby's neck, hook a

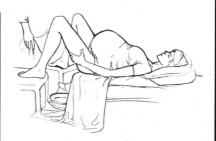

finger under it and gently work it over the baby's head.

10. When the head has been delivered, gently stroke the sides of the nose downward, the neck and under the chin upward, to help expel mucus and amniotic fluid from the nose and mouth.

11. Next take the head gently in two hands and press it very slightly downward (do not pull), asking the mother to push at the same time, to deliver the front shoulder. As the upper arm appears, lift the head carefully, watching for the rear shoulder to deliver. Once the shoulders are free, the rest of the baby should slip out easily.

12. Quickly wrap the baby in blankets, towels, or anything else that is available (preferably something clean; something recently ironed is relatively sterile). Place the baby on the mother's abdomen, or if the cord is long enough (don't tug at it), at her breast.

13. Don't try to pull the placenta out. But if it arrives on its own before the ambulance comes, wrap it in towels or· newspaper, and keep it elevated above the level of the baby, if possible. There is no need to try to cut the cord.

14. Keep both mother and baby warm and comfortable until help arrives.

may be all but abandoned during this stage, so as not to interfere with the mother's concentration. In this case, the fetal heart rate is checked periodically with a stethoscope.

Internal Monitoring. When more accurate results are required—such as when fetal distress is suspected—an internal monitor may be used. Since the electrode that transmits a reading of the fetal heartbeat is attached to the fetus's scalp through the cervix, internal monitoring is possible only once the cervix is dilated to at least 1 or 2 centimeters and the membranes have ruptured. Contractions can be measured either with the pressure gauge strapped to the maternal abdomen or with a fluid-filled catheter (tube) inserted into the uterus. Because an internal monitor can't be periodically disconnected and reconnected, it limits mobility somewhat—but changes in position are possible.

Sometimes internal monitoring employs telemetry, which reads and transmits vital signs via radio waves. This technique, pioneered in the space program, allows the patient to be monitored without being confined by equipment. She is totally mobile—able to strike any position she finds comfortable, to go to the bathroom, or even to take a stroll.

Like any invasive medical procedure (one that enters or intrudes upon the body), internal fetal monitoring entails some risk—mostly of infection. In some instances the fetus later develops a rash, or occasionally an abscess, on the site where the electrode was placed, and, very rarely, may even have a permanent bald spot. It may also be possible that the insertion of the electrode causes momentary pain or discomfort to the baby. Because of the risks, though they are slight, internal fetal monitoring is best used when its benefits are significant.

If your fetal monitor signals trouble, don't panic. The technology is far from perfect and the machine can produce false readings. Sometimes it isn't working right; sometimes it is misread. Frequently the abnormal heart rate reading is a result of the mother's position putting pressure on her vena cava or her baby's cord, interfering with blood flow to the fetus. A change in position (to lying on the left side) often rectifies the problem. If administration of oxytocin is causing the problem, reducing the dosage or terminating the infusion completely will generally eliminate it. Oxygen to the mother may also do the trick.

If the abnormal readings continue, several possible steps can be taken. If the danger to the fetus seems great, the physician may opt for an immediate abdominal delivery. Otherwise, some speedy testing will be done to confirm the diagnosis of fetal distress: the amniotic fluid will be checked for meconium; pH levels in a fetal blood sample, taken from the scalp, will be assessed; and/or the response of the fetal heart to sound stimulation, or to pressure on or pinching of the fetal scalp will be evaluated. Since direct access to the fetus is necessary in order for some of these determinations to be made, the membranes must be ruptured artificially at this point, if they haven't already ruptured spontaneously. In addition, the mother's medical and obstetrical history may be reviewed to determine if the fetal heart rate abnormalities are related to maternal infection or chronic disease or to medication the mother is taking, rather than to actual fetal distress. An experienced and knowledgeable obstetrician will take many factors into account before concluding that a baby is actually in trouble. In some cases, the monitor printout may be faxed to an expert for a second opinion. If fetal distress is confirmed, then an immediate cesarean is usually called for. In some cases, the physician may use drugs to try to improve the condition of the fetus in the uterus. When successful, this approach allows additional time for preparing for a cesarean delivery, enhances the chances of delivering an alert baby, and in some cases may even allow a vaginal delivery to continue.

It isn't clear whether fetal monitoring saves more newborn lives than the old-fashioned nurse-with-a-stethoscope method (checking every 15 minutes during labor and every 5 during delivery), but many physicians think it likely that some cases of fetal distress are detected with a monitor that might be missed otherwise. Still, because electronic monitoring is expensive, because it is believed to have led to an increase in unnecessary cesareans in some hospitals (largely through misreadings), because some view it as just another technological intrusion into the natural birthing process, and because the impersonal machine replaces the personal ministrations of a nurse, its use remains controversial. The American College of Obstetricians and Gynecologists seems to be leaning toward a position that monitoring need only be used in high-risk deliveries, but apparently the very doctors who are making this pronouncement plan on continuing to monitor all their own patients. So clearly, the issues aren't yet all clear.

How expectant parents respond to electronic fetal monitoring depends a great deal on their attitudes. If they come into the labor or birthing room resentful or fearful of all that isn't "natural," they will probably find the fetal monitor objectionable. If they want the best of both worlds—the natural and the scientific—they will feel reassured and more in control at seeing their baby's heartbeats registering rhythmically on the monitor.

THE SIGHT OF BLOOD

"The sight of blood makes me feel faint. What if I pass out while I'm watching my delivery?"

The sight of blood makes many people feel weak-kneed. But remarkably, though they might faint while watching a film of someone else's delivery, even the most squeamish women manage to get through their own without smelling salts.

First of all, there isn't all that much blood—not much more than you see when you're menstruating (a little more with an episiotomy or a tear). Second, you won't be a spectator at your delivery—you'll be a very active participant, putting every ounce of your concentration and energy into pushing your baby those last few inches. Caught up in the excitement and anticipation (and, let's face it, the pain and fatigue), you are unlikely to notice, much less be unsettled by, any bleeding. Few new mothers would be able to tell you just how much blood, if any, there was at their deliveries.

If you feel strongly that you don't want to see any blood, simply avert your eyes from the mirror (if one has been provided for you) during the episiotomy and at the moment of birth. Instead, just look down past your belly for a good view of your baby as it emerges. From this vantage point, virtually no blood will be visible.

EPISIOTOMY

"My childbirth educator says we shouldn't have episiotomies—they aren't natural. My doctor says that's ridiculous. I don't know whether to have one or not."

To have or not to have an episiotomy? That is the question that has some obstetricians shooting it out with some childbirth educators and nurse-midwives, catching pregnant women in the crossfire.

The minor surgical procedure that is at the center of this heated controversy was originated in Ireland in 1742 to help facilitate difficult births, but it wasn't widely performed until the middle part of this century. Today, the episiotomy (a surgical incision made in the perineum to enlarge the vaginal opening just before the birth of the baby's head) is performed in 80% to 90% of first births, and in about 50% of subsequent deliveries.

There are two basic types of episiotomies: the median and the medio-lateral. The median incision is made directly back toward the rectum. In spite of its advantages (it provides more exit space per inch of incision, heals well and is easier to repair, causes less blood loss, and results in less postpartum discomfort or infection), it is less frequently used in the United States because it has a greater risk of tearing completely through to the rectum. To avoid this tearing, most physicians prefer the medio-lateral incision, which slants away from the rectum, especially in first births.

Traditional medical wisdom supports the use of episiotomy for several reasons: Its straight edges are easier to repair than a ragged tear; timed well, it can prevent injury to the muscles of the perineum and vagina; it spares the fetal head from battering against the perineum; and it can shorten the pushing stage of labor by 15 to 30 minutes—particularly advantageous when there is prolonged labor, fetal distress, and/or maternal exhaustion.

Opponents counter that episiotomies are an unnatural, largely unnecessary, technological intrusion into the birth process. They claim that the incision made is often more extensive than tearing would be, and that it results in excessive bleeding, immediate postpartum discomfort, painful intercourse for months afterward, and (sometimes) infection. Instead, they support the use of Kegel exercises (page 190) and local massage for four to six weeks before delivery to prepare and strengthen the perineum for delivery. During labor they recommend warm compresses to lessen perineal discomfort; massage; a standing or squatting position, and exhaling or grunting while pushing to facilitate stretching of the perineum; and avoidance of regional anesthesia, which makes the perineal muscles flaccid. Although all of these measures can improve the odds of a birth occurring without episiotomy, and sometimes without tearing, they don't guarantee such a birth. At birthing centers where they are employed regularly, between 15% and 25% of women have episiotomies, and 25% to 30% of the others tear badly enough to need repair. Another 3% or 4% end up with serious lacerations extending to the rectum.

What hard-liners (those who routinely perform episiotomies, even when they're not needed, and those who routinely refrain from performing them, even when they are needed) fail to recognize is that "to have or not to have an episiotomy" is a question that shouldn't be answered in the classroom or the office—but in the delivery or birthing room, as the baby's head crowns. It is only then that a realistic judgment can be made as to whether or not the perineum can stretch sufficiently to accommodate the baby's head without tearing, and whether not doing an episiotomy will jeopardize fetal or maternal well-being by prolonging labor. The prudent physician or nurse-midwife who has some doubt will generally opt for the episiotomy rather than risk an uncontrolled and difficult-to-repair tear.

If you feel, after reading this, discussing the issue with your practitioner, and weighing the evidence, that you would prefer not to have an episiotomy if at all possible, say so in your birthing plan (page 225) or otherwise make your preference known. But remember that the final decision should be made in the delivery or birthing room, with your well-being and the speedy and safe delivery of your baby the prime considerations.

BEING STRETCHED BY CHILDBIRTH

"The thing that frightens me most is my vagina stretching and tearing. Will I ever be the same again?"

The vagina is a remarkably elastic organ whose accordion-like folds open for childbirth. It is normally so narrow that inserting a tampon may be difficult, yet it can expand to allow the passage of a 7- or 8-pound baby. After birth, over a period of weeks, it returns to almost its original size. For most women the slight increase in roominess is imperceptible and does not interfere with sexual enjoyment. For those who were unusually small before conception, it can be a real plus, as intercourse may become more pleasurable.

The perineum, the area between the vagina and the rectum, is also elastic, but less so than the vagina. In some women, the perineum will stretch enough without tearing to allow the birth of a baby. But in others, it will tear unless an episiotomy is performed by the birth attendant. Stretching may leave the muscles a little slacker than will a carefully timed episiotomy, one in which the perineum wasn't allowed to stretch excessively before the incision was made.

But exercising the muscles of childbirth long before you get to the delivery room may enhance elasticity and certainly will hasten their return to normal tone. Kegel exercises, which strengthen the muscles in the perineal area (see page 190), should be done regularly during pregnancy and for at least six months following childbirth.

Many couples report that sex after delivery is even more satisfying than it was before, thanks to the increased muscular awareness and control the woman has developed as a result of prepared childbirth training. In other words, you may not be the same after childbirth—you may be even better!

Very occasionally, however, in a woman who "just right" before, childbirth does stretch the vagina enough to reduce sexual enjoyment. Often the vaginal muscles tighten up again with the passage of time. Faithfully doing Kegels at frequent intervals during the day—while showering, urinating, washing the dishes, walking the baby, driving the car, sitting at your desk—may help speed the process. If after six months the vagina still seems too slack, medical advice should be sought.

BEING STRAPPED TO THE DELIVERY TABLE

"The idea of being strapped to a table like my mother was terrifies me. Is this really necessary?"

The prospect of being bound, hand and foot, to a delivery table is an appalling one—particularly to women who wish to participate fully in childbirth. Fortunately, though it was once routine procedure, it is virtually unheard of today. Most birthing attendants will simply ask the woman to keep her hands above her waist, away from the area that should remain sterile during the delivery; if she should forget in the middle of a particularly consuming contraction, her coach and the nurse are there to remind her.

Whether or not the woman's feet are up in stirrups during delivery (there's no need for this during labor), and whether her legs are strapped to the stirrups, depends on hospital policy, practitioner preference, and, most of all, the patient's wishes.

The use of stirrups in delivery evolved for several reasons. One, they kept the woman's legs elevated and out of the way so that the doctor had adequate work space. Two, they kept her from involuntarily kicking during a powerful contraction (possibly interfering with the delivery). Finally, they kept her feet out of the area that should remain as sterile as possible.

One reason that stirrups are now used less often in many hospitals—and hardly at all in birthing rooms, where special birthing beds have taken the place of delivery tables—is that a variety of birthing positions have replaced the standard woman-on-her-back-legs-up-and-spread attitude. Another is strong opposition from women who want to retain as much dignity and control as possible during their deliveries. In addition, because woman are now generally better prepared for childbirth, they aren't as likely to thrash around in pain and fear of the unknown. Still many physicians continue to ask their patients to use the stirrups during delivery because they believe this allows room for maneuvering and therefore for a safer delivery.

Discuss this issue with your practitioner in advance, sharing your feelings and listening to his or hers. It is very likely that your wishes will prevail or that, at the very least, a compromise can be reached.

THE USE OF FORCEPS

"I've heard all kinds of horror stories about forceps. What if my doctor wants to use them?"

It was in 1598 that British surgeon Peter Chamberlen the Elder designed the first pair of forceps and used the tong-shaped instrument to ease babies out of the birth canal when a difficult delivery might otherwise cost both mother and infant their lives. Instead of writing himself up in the latest obstetrical journal, however, Dr. Chamberlen kept his discovery a secret—privy only to four generations of Chamberlen medical men and their patients, many of them royalty. Indeed, the use of forceps might have ended forever with the career of the last Chamberlen doctor, had a hidden box of instruments not been uncovered beneath a floorboard in the family's ancestral home in the mid-1800s.

To the minds of some today, the use of forceps should have died with the Chamberlens. But that's not quite a fair assessment. Before cesarean sections became commonplace and safe, forceps delivery was the only way out for a baby stuck in the birth canal. The occasional serious damage caused by the use of forceps was considered a small price to pay for the countless lives saved. The risks were clearly outweighed by the benefits.

But the picture is more complicated. Today, the high-forceps procedure, in which the doctor reaches up into the maternal pelvis to extract a stuck baby, and to which most of the horror stories you've heard are probably attributable, has been totally abandoned in favor of cesarean delivery. But the American College of Obstetricians and Gynecologists and most physicians still see a role for mid-, low-, and outlet forceps deliveries. Such deliveries, the most recent studies show, pose no more risk to mother and baby than cesareans *when carried out properly by someone experienced in forceps use*. Before resorting to a cesarean, many physicians will try the judicious use of forceps when a baby's head is engaged and labor has stalled.

In countries such as Great Britain where this is routine, the rate of cesarean deliveries is, as a consequence, relatively low.

Forceps should be used only when valid indications exist (fetal distress, maternal distress, prolonged labor, prolonged second stage). And all should be in readiness for a cesarean section should a trial of forceps fail.

When forceps are used, a local anesthetic (see page 229) is administered to the mother. Then the curved blunt blades are cradled one at a time around the crowning head, at the temples, and the baby is gently delivered.

The vacuum extractor, an alternative to outlet forceps that suctions the infant out of the birth canal via a metal or plastic cup (less traumatic) applied to the head, is popular in Europe but is used less often in the U.S.

If you have any concerns about the possible use of forceps or vacuum extraction during your delivery, discuss them with your practitioner now, before you go into labor. He or she should be able to allay your fears.

THE BABY'S CONDITION

"The doctor said the baby is okay, but her Apgar score was only 7. Is she really all right?"

Your doctor is right. Any Apgar score of 7 or over indicates a baby in good condition. However, most babies with lower scores also turn out to be normal and healthy.

The Apgar test was developed by Dr. Virginia Apgar, a noted anesthesiologist, to enable medical personnel

APGAR TABLE

SIGN	POINTS		
	0	1	2
Appearance (color)*	Pale or blue	Body pink, extremities blue	Pink
Pulse (heartbeat)	Not detectible	Below 100	Over 100
Grimace (reflex irritability)	No response to stimulation	Grimace	Lusty cry
Activity (muscle tone)	Flaccid (no or weak activity)	Some movement of extremities	A lot of activity
Respiration (breathing)	None	Slow, irregular	Good (crying)

*In non-Caucasian children, the color of mucous membranes of the mouth, of the whites of the eyes, and of the lips, palms, hands, and soles of feet will be examined.

to quickly evaluate the condition of a newborn. At 60 seconds after birth, a nurse or doctor checks the infant's *A*ppearance (color), *P*ulse (heartbeat), *G*rimace (reflex), *A*ctivity (muscle tone), and *R*espiration. Hence the acronym APGAR. (See Apgar Table, below.) Those who score between 4 and 6 often need resuscitation—which generally includes suctioning their airways and administering oxygen. Those who score under 4 require more dramatic lifesaving techniques.

The Apgar test is administered once again at five minutes after birth. If the score is 7 or better at this point, the outlook for the infant is very good. If it's low, it means the baby needs some careful watching, but is still very likely to turn out to be fine.

WHAT IT'S IMPORTANT TO KNOW:
THE STAGES OF CHILDBIRTH

Few pregnancies seem as though they could have been lifted right from the pages of an obstetrical text—with morning sickness that vanishes at the end of the first trimester, first fetal movements felt at precisely 20 weeks, and lightening that occurs exactly two weeks before the onset of labor. Likewise, few childbirth experiences mirror the textbook case—commencing with mild regular contractions that progress at a predictable pace to delivery. Yet just as it's helpful to have a general idea of what a typical woman can expect when she's expecting, it's helpful to know what an average childbirth is like—as long as you are prepared for the likelihood of variations that will make your experience yours alone.

Childbirth is divided (more loosely by nature, more formally by obstetrical science) into three stages. The first stage is labor, with its early, active, and transitional phases ending with the full dilation (opening) of the cervix; the second stage is delivery, culminating in the birth of the baby; and the third is delivery of the placenta, or afterbirth. The whole process averages about 14 hours for first-time mothers, about 8 hours for women who have already had children.

Unless labor is cut short by the need for a cesarean, all women who carry to term go through all three phases of the first stage. Some, however, may not recognize that they are in labor until the second, or even the third, phase because their initial contractions are mild or painless. The third phase of labor is complete once the cervix has dilated to a full 10 centimeters. For a very few women, all of dilatation passes unnoticed; they don't realize they're in labor until they feel the urge to push that signals the second, or delivery, stage.

The timing and intensity of contractions can help pinpoint which phase of labor a woman is in at any particular time. Periodic internal exams, to check on the progress of dilatation, will confirm the progress.

If labor doesn't seem to be progressing along the typical course, many doctors will augment Mother Nature's efforts (with oxytocin, for example), and if that fails, will preempt her entirely with a cesarean section. Others may elect to allow more time before taking such action, as long as both mother and baby are doing well.

Labor Positions

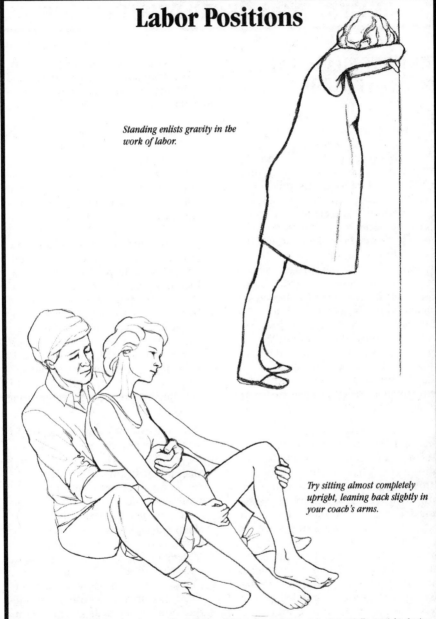

Standing enlists gravity in the work of labor.

Try sitting almost completely upright, leaning back slightly in your coach's arms.

Talk to your practitioner in advance about the possibility of remaining at least partially upright during labor: perhaps standing, walking, or sitting (in a rocking or beanbag chair, or in your husband's arms). Studies show that upright positions can shorten labor by speeding dilatation and descent—though the position that works best and is most comfortable varies from woman to woman. Lying flat on your back can not only slow down labor, but can also compress major blood vessels (especially if you are on a firm surface), possibly interfering with blood flow to the fetus. If you are more comfortable lying down, lie on your side, switching sides and doing pelvic tilts periodically.

THE FIRST STAGE OF CHILDBIRTH: LABOR

THE FIRST PHASE: EARLY OR LATENT LABOR

This is usually the longest and, fortunately, the least intense phase of labor. The dilatation (opening) of the cervix to 3 centimeters and the accompanying effacement (thinning out) that characterize this phase can be reached over a period of days or weeks without noticeable or bothersome contractions, or over a period of two to six hours (and, less commonly, up to 24 hours) of unmistakable labor.

Contractions in this phase usually last 30 to 45 seconds. They are mild to moderately strong, may be regular or irregular (ranging between 5 and 20 minutes apart), and become progressively closer together, but not necessarily in a consistent pattern. Some women don't notice them at all.

You will probably be told to go to the hospital at the end of this phase or the beginning of the next.

What You May Be Feeling or Noticing. The most common signs and symptoms in this phase include backache (either constant or with each contraction), menstrual-like cramps, indigestion, diarrhea, a sensation of warmth in the abdomen, and bloody show (a blood-tinged mucousy discharge). You may experience all of these, or just one or two. The amniotic membranes may have ruptured before the onset of contractions, but it is more likely that they will rupture sometime during labor itself. (If they don't rupture spontaneously, your practitioner may decide to rupture them artificially sometime after you've gone into active labor.)

Emotionally, you may feel excitement, relief, anticipation, uncertainty, anxiety, fear; some women are relaxed and chatty, others tense and apprehensive.

What You Can Do:

❖ Relax. Your practitioner has probably told you not to call until you are in more active labor. Or he or she may have suggested that you call early on if labor begins during the day or if your membranes rupture. Definitely call, however, if your membranes rupture and the amniotic fluid is murky or greenish, if you have any bright red bleeding, or if you feel no fetal activity (it may be hard to notice because you are distracted by contractions, so you might want to try the test on page 202). Although you may not feel like it, it's best if you, not your coach, make the call and talk to your practitioner. A lot can be lost in third-party translations.

❖ If it's the middle of the night, try to sleep (but not on your back; see page 173 for the recommended sleeping position). It's important to rest now, because you probably won't be able to later on in labor. And you needn't fear that you'll sleep through the next phase—the contractions will be too insistent. If sleep eludes you, don't just lie in bed timing contractions—that'll only make labor seem longer. Instead, get up and do things around the house that will distract you. Clean out a closet; put sheets on the baby's bed; finish packing your bag for the hospital (see page 265); make your coach a sandwich to take along; play solitaire; do a jigsaw puzzle.

❖ If it's daytime, go about your usual routine—as long as it doesn't take you far from home. If you have nothing planned, find something to keep you occupied. Try some of the distractions suggested above, take a walk (gravity aids the work of labor), watch TV, make and freeze a casserole or two for easy postpartum dining. Put your husband on alert, but it's not necessary for him to come running home—yet.

❖ Make yourself comfortable. Take a warm bath (only if your membranes haven't ruptured) or a shower (but be careful not to slip); use a heating pad if your back is aching—but *do not* take aspirin or lie on your back.

❖ Eat a light snack if you're hungry (broth, toast with apple butter, or fruit juice). Don't eat heavily, and avoid hard-to-digest foods, such as meats, dairy products, and fats. Not only will digesting a heavy meal compete with the birthing process for body resources, but a full stomach could cause complications if you should need anesthesia later on.

❖ Time contractions for a half-hour span if they seem to be getting closer than 10 minutes apart, and periodically even if they don't. But don't be a clock watcher.

❖ Remember to urinate frequently to avoid bladder distention, which could inhibit the progress of labor.

❖ Use relaxation techniques if they help, but don't start your breathing exercises yet, or you will become bored and exhausted long before you really need them.

What the Coach Can Do:

❖ Practice timing contractions. The interval between contractions is timed from the beginning of one to the beginning of the next. Time them periodically, and keep a record. When they are coming less than 10 minutes apart, time them more frequently.

❖ Be a calming influence. During this early phase of labor, your most important function is to keep the expectant mother relaxed. And the best way to do this is to keep yourself relaxed, both inside and out. Your own anxiety can be transferred to her unwittingly, communicated not just through words but through touch. Doing some relaxation exercises together or giving her a gentle, unhurried massage may help you both. It's too soon, however, to begin using breathing exercises.

❖ Keep your sense of humor, and help her keep hers; time flies, after all, when you're having fun. It'll be easier to laugh now than when contractions are coming fast and hard.

❖ Help distract the expectant mother. Suggest activities that will help keep both your minds off her labor: reading aloud, playing board games or cards, viewing engrossing (and preferably light) television fare, taking short walks.

❖ Offer comfort, reassurance, and support. She'll need them all from now on.

❖ Keep up your own strength so you'll be able to reinforce hers. Eat periodically (not necessarily in front of her), even if she can't. Prepare a sandwich to bring along to the hospital (but nothing with an overpowering or lingering odor that might make you, or your wife, feel queasy—such as salami or tuna).

If You Aren't Making Progress

Progress in labor is measured by the dilatation, or opening, of the cervix and the descent of the fetus through the pelvis. Good progress is believed to require three main components: strong uterine contractions that effectively dilate the cervix; a baby that can fit through the pelvis and is in position for easy exit; and a pelvis that is sufficiently roomy to permit the passage of the baby.

If one or more of these factors is not present, abnormal (or dysfunctional) labor, in which progress is slow or nonexistent, generally occurs. There are several types of abnormal labor:

Prolonged Latent Phase—when little or no dilatation has occurred after 20 hours of labor in a first-time mother, or after 14 hours in one who has delivered previously. Sometimes progress is slow because labor hasn't really begun and the contractions felt are those of false—not true—labor. Sometimes the reason is overmedication before labor was well established. Sometimes, it is theorized, the cause may be psychological: a woman panics when labor begins, triggering the release of chemicals in the nervous system that interfere with uterine contractions.

In general, the practitioner may suggest stimulating a slow first phase of labor with activity (such as walking) or with just the opposite (sleep and rest, possibly aided by the use of relaxation techniques and, if the laboring woman is too agitated to relax naturally, an alcoholic drink or the administration of a sedative). Such treatment will also help rule out false labor (the contractions of false labor will usually subside with activity or a nap).

Once true latent-phase labor has been established, it may be speeded up with an enema or mineral oil, with walking, or with the administration of oxytocin. (Note: it is important to remember to urinate periodically, as a full bladder can interfere with the baby's descent.) If attempts to stimulate labor are unsuccessful, the practitioner may have to consider the possibility that cephalopelvic disproportion (a mismatch between the fetus's head and the mother's pelvis) exists.

Most physicians will perform a cesarean after 24 or 25 hours (sometimes sooner) if sufficient progress has not been made by that time; some will wait longer, as long as both mother and baby are doing well.

Primary Dysfunction of Active Phase—when the second, or active,

THE SECOND PHASE: ACTIVE LABOR

The second, or active, phase of labor is usually shorter than the first, lasting an average of 2 to 3½ hours (though variations on this average are great). The uterus's efforts are more concentrated now, accomplishing more in less time. With contractions becoming stronger, longer, and

more frequent (generally three to four minutes apart and lasting 40 to 60 seconds), the cervix dilates to 7 centimeters. The pattern of contractions still may not be regular. Each contraction probably has a distinct peak (acme or apex) now, which constitutes from 40% to 50% of its total duration. There is less time to rest between contractions.

You will probably be in the hospital by early in this phase.

phase of labor progresses very slowly (less than 1 to 1.2 centimeters of dilatation per hour in women having their first babies, and 1.5 centimeters per hour in those who've had previous deliveries). When any progress, albeit slow, is being made, many practitioners will let the uterus set its own pace—on the theory that the woman will eventually deliver naturally, as two-thirds of those who experience primary dysfunction do. A laboring woman may be able to speed up the work of her uterus by walking, if possible, staying off her back, and keeping her bladder empty. Intravenous fluids will probably be administered during a lengthy labor.

Secondary Arrest of Dilatation—when, during active labor, there is no progress for two hours or more. In about half of these cases, it is estimated, disproportion exists between the fetal head and the pelvis (CPD), necessitating a cesarean delivery. In most other cases, the administration of oxytocin (sometimes along with artificial rupture of the membranes) will reestablish labor, particularly when the cause of the labor slowdown is simply exhaustion. Again, the woman may be able to contribute to the battle against sluggish labor by utilizing gravity when possible (sitting upright, squatting, standing, or walking) and by keeping her bladder empty.

Abnormal Descent of the Fetus—when the baby moves down the birth canal at a rate of less than 1 centimeter per hour in women having their first babies, or 2 centimeters per hour in others. In most such cases delivery will be slow, but otherwise uneventful. Trying to remove with forceps a baby that isn't already at the vaginal outlet, once common practice, is now considered dangerous and unnecessary. Today, stimulation with oxytocin and/or artificial rupture of the membranes is preferred—once CPD and a fetal position that would make vaginal delivery difficult have been ruled out.

Prolonged Second Stage—one that lasts longer than two hours in a first delivery, or slightly less in subsequent deliveries. Many physicians routinely use outlet forceps or perform a cesarean when a second stage goes beyond two hours; others allow the spontaneous vaginal delivery to continue if steady progress is being made and both mother and fetus (whose conditions are being carefully monitored) are doing well. Sometimes the baby's head is gently eased out those last few inches with outlet forceps. Rotation of the head (so that it faces front and will better fit through the pelvis) may also be attempted, either manually or with forceps. Gravity, again, can help; a semi-sitting or semi-squatting position may be most effective for delivery.

What You May Be Feeling or Noticing. The most common signs and symptoms in this phase include increasing discomfort with contractions (you may be unable to talk through them now), increasing backache, leg discomfort, fatigue, increasing bloody show. You may experience all of these, or just one or two. Rupture of the membranes may occur now if it hasn't earlier. (If they don't rupture spontaneously, your practitioner may choose to rupture them artificially sometime during this phase.)

Emotionally, you may feel restless and find it more difficult to relax; or your concentration may become more intense, and you may become completely absorbed in the work at hand. Your confidence may begin to waver, and you may feel as if labor is never going to end; or you may feel excited and encouraged that things are really starting to happen.

What You Can Do:

❖ Start your breathing exercises, if you plan to use them, as soon as contractions become too strong to talk through. (If you have never practiced any of these exercises, some simple breathing suggestions from the nurse may help make you more comfortable.) If the exercises seem to make you uncomfortable or more tense, however, don't feel that you have to use them. Women have given birth without them for centuries.

❖ If your practitioner permits it (some do, particularly if there is no medication being given), drink clear beverages frequently to replace fluids and to keep your mouth moist. If you're uncomfortably hungry, and again if you have your practitioner's okay, have a light snack of a nonfat, non-fibrous food (sorbet, Jell-O, or applesauce, for example). If your practitioner prohibits anything else by mouth, sucking on ice chips can serve to refresh. Some doctors and hospitals, however, discourage even ice chips and use IVs to keep laboring patients hydrated.

❖ Make a concerted effort to relax between contractions. This will become increasingly difficult as they come more frequently, but it will also become increasingly important as your energy reserves are taxed.

❖ Walk around, if possible, or at least change position frequently, seeking those that provide the most comfort. (See page 289 for suggested labor positions.)

❖ Remember to urinate periodically; because of tremendous pelvic pressure, you may not notice the need to empty your bladder.

❖ If you feel you need some pain relief, don't be afraid to discuss it with your attendant. He or she may suggest waiting for 20 minutes or half an hour before actual administration—at which point you may have made so much progress that you won't need it, or you may have found renewed strength and no longer want it.

What the Coach Can Do:

❖ If possible, keep the door of the labor or birthing room closed, the lights low, and the room quiet to promote a restful atmosphere. Soft music, if permitted, may also help. Continue relaxation techniques between contractions. And stay as calm as possible yourself.

❖ Keep track of the contractions. If your wife is on a fetal monitor, ask the practitioner or the nurse to show you how to read it. Later, when contractions are coming one on top of the other, you can alert your wife as each new contraction begins. (The monitor may detect the tensing of the uterus before she can.) You can also encourage her by telling her when each peak is ending. This will give both of you some sense of control over the labor. If there is no monitor, learn to recognize the arrival and departure of contractions with your hand on your wife's abdomen.

❖ Breathe with her through difficult contractions, if that helps her. Don't pressure her to do the breathing exercises if she is uncomfortable with them, they make her tense, or they annoy her.

❖ If she shows any symptoms of hyperventilation (dizziness or lightheadedness, blurred vision, tingling and numbness of fingers and toes), have her exhale into a paper bag (the nurse will be able to supply one if you haven't brought one

On to the Hospital

Getting to the Hospital. Sometime near the end of the early phase or the beginning of the active phase (probably when your contractions are five minutes apart or less, sooner if you live far from the hospital or if this isn't your first baby), your practitioner will tell you to pick up your bag and get going. Getting to the hospital will be easier if you've planned your route in advance, are familiar with parking regulations, and know which entrance will get you to the obstetrical floor most quickly. (If parking is likely to be a problem, taking a cab may be more sensible.) En route, try stretching out on the rear seat with a pillow for your head, your seat belt fastened loosely beneath your belly, and if you have chills, a blanket covering you.

Hospital Admission. Procedures will vary, but you can probably expect something like the following:

❖ If you've preregistered (and it's best if you have), this process will be brief; if you're in active labor, your coach can take care of it.

❖ Once in the labor and delivery suite or birthing unit, you will be taken to a labor or birthing room by your nurse for this shift. Depending on hospital regulations, your husband and other family members may be asked to wait outside while you are being admitted and "prepped." (Note to the coach: This is a good time to make a few priority phone calls, to get a snack, and to arrange for stowing your wife's luggage in her room and for chilling the celebratory champagne. If you aren't called to join your wife within 20 minutes or so, remind someone at the nurses' station that you are waiting. Be prepared for the possibility that you will be asked to put on a sterile gown over your clothes.)

❖ Your nurse will take a brief history, asking, among other things, when the contractions started, how far apart they are, whether your membranes have ruptured, when it was that you last ate.

❖ Your nurse will ask for your signature on routine consent forms.

❖ Your nurse will give you a hospital gown to change into and will request a urine sample. She will check your pulse, blood pressure, respiration, and temperature; look for leaking amniotic fluid, bleeding, or bloody show; listen to the fetal heartbeat with a stethoscope or hook you up to a fetal monitor; and, possibly, evaluate the fetal position and take a fetal blood sample.

❖ Depending on the policies of your doctor and hospital, and possibly, your preferences, your pubic area may be partially shaved, you may be given an enema, and/or an IV may be started.

❖ Your nurse, your practitioner, or a resident doctor will examine you internally to see how dilated and effaced your cervix. If your membranes haven't ruptured spontaneously and you are at least 3 or 4 centimeters dilated (many practitioners prefer to wait until the cervix has dilated to at least 5 centimeters), your membranes may be artificially ruptured—unless you and your practitioner have decided to leave them intact until later in labor. The procedure is painless; all you will feel is a warm gush of fluid.

If you have any questions that haven't been answered before, now is the time for you or your coach to ask them.

along) or into cupped hands. She should then inhale the exhaled air. After repeating this several times, she should feel better. If she doesn't, inform a nurse or your practitioner at once.

❖ Offer constant verbal reassurance (if it doesn't make your wife more edgy); praise, but don't criticize, her efforts (think what you'd like her to say if your roles were reversed). Particularly if progress is slow, remind her to take her labor one contraction at a time, and that each pain brings her closer to seeing the baby.

❖ Massage her abdomen or back, or use counterpressure or any other techniques you've learned, to make her more comfortable. Take your cues from her; let her tell you what kind of stroking or touching or massage helps. If she prefers not to be touched at all (some women find it annoying), then it might be best to comfort her verbally.

❖ Don't pretend the pain doesn't exist, even if she doesn't complain; she needs your empathy. And don't tell her you know how it feels (you don't).

❖ Remind her to relax between contractions.

❖ Remind her to try to urinate at least once an hour.

❖ Don't take it personally if she doesn't respond to—or even seems irritated by—your attempts to comfort her. A woman's moods during labor are mercurial. Stand by to offer support as she needs and wants it. Remember that your role is important, even if you sometimes feel superfluous.

❖ If it is allowed, be sure she has an ample supply of ice chips to suck on or fluids to sip. From time to time ask her if she would like some.

❖ Use a damp washcloth, wrung out in cold water, to help cool her body and face; refresh it often.

❖ If her feet are cold, offer to get out a pair of socks and help her to put them on.

❖ Continue with distractions she finds helpful (card games, conversation between contractions, reading aloud), encouragement, and support.

❖ Suggest a change of position; walk around with her, if that's possible.

❖ Serve as her go-between with medical personnel as much as possible. Intercept questions that you can answer, ask for explanations of procedures, equipment, any medication, so you'll be able to tell her what's happening. For instance, now might be the time to find out if a mirror will be provided so that she can view the delivery. Be her advocate when necessary, but try to fight her battles quietly, perhaps outside the room, so that she won't be disturbed.

❖ If she requests medication, communicate her request to the nurse or doctor, but suggest a waiting period before the administration. During that time, the practitioner will probably want to discuss the need for medication and do an internal exam to check on the progress of labor anyway. It's possible that an encouraging progress report or some time to think it over may give your wife renewed strength to continue unmedicated. Don't be disappointed, however, if she and the doctor decide that medication is needed. Remember, labor isn't a test of pain endurance that your wife will fail if she asks for or accepts medication.

What Hospital Personnel Will Do:

❖ Provide a relaxed, comfortable, supportive environment and answers to your questions and concerns.

❖ Continue monitoring the baby's condition with a stethoscope or electronic fetal monitor, and through observation of the amniotic fluid (greenish-brown staining is a sign of possible fetal distress). Fetal position may be assessed with external palpation.

❖ Continue checking your blood pressure.

❖ Periodically evaluate the timing and strength of contractions and quantity and quality of bloody discharge. (Pads beneath your buttocks will be replaced as needed.) When there is a change in the pattern or intensity of contractions, or the show becomes more bloody, an internal exam will be done to check the progress of your labor.

❖ Possibly, stimulate labor if it is progressing very slowly, by the use of oxytocin or artificial rupture of the membranes if they are still intact, and if this wasn't done earlier.

❖ Administer sedatives and/or analgesics as needed and desired.

THE THIRD PHASE: ADVANCED ACTIVE OR TRANSITIONAL LABOR

Transition is the most exhausting and demanding phase of labor. Suddenly the intensity of the contractions picks up. They become very strong, two to three minutes apart, and 60 to 90 seconds long—with very intense peaks that last for most of the contraction. Some women, particularly women who have given birth before, experience multiple peaks. You may feel as though the contractions never completely disappear, and that you can't completely relax between them. The final 3 centimeters of dilatation, to a full 10 centimeters, will probably take place in a very short time: on average, 15 minutes to an hour.

What You May Be Feeling or Noticing. In transition, you are likely to feel strong pressure in the lower back and/or perineum. Rectal pressure, with or without an urge to push or move your bowels, may cause you to grunt involuntarily. You may feel either very warm and sweaty or chilled and shaky, or alternate between the two. Your bloody vaginal show will increase as more capillaries in the cervix rupture; your legs may be crampy and cold and may tremble uncontrollably. You may experience nausea and/or vomiting, and drowsiness may overcome you between contractions as oxygen is diverted from your brain to the site of the delivery. Not surprisingly, at this point you may feel exhausted.

Emotionally, you may feel vulnerable and overwhelmed; you're reaching the end of your rope. In addition to frustration over not being able to push yet, you may feel discouraged, irritable, disoriented, restless, and have difficulty concentrating and relaxing (it may seem impossible to do either).

What You Can Do:

❖ Hang in there. By the end of this phase, your cervix will be fully dilated, and it will be time to begin pushing your baby out.

❖ Instead of thinking about the work ahead, try to think about how far you've come.

❖ If you feel the urge to push, pant or blow instead, unless you've been instructed otherwise. Pushing against a cervix that isn't completely dilated can cause the cervix to swell, which can delay delivery.

❖ If you don't want anybody to touch you unnecessarily, if your coach's once comforting hands now irritate you, don't hesitate to let him know.

❖ If you find them useful, use breathing techniques you have learned

---

Pain Risk Factors

Your perception of pain may be increased by:	It may be decreased by:
Being alone.	Having the company and support of those you love, and/or of experienced medical personnel.
Fatigue.	Being well rested (try not to overdo things during the ninth month); trying to rest and relax between contractions.
Hunger and thirst.	Having light snacks during early labor; sucking ice chips throughout, drinking fluid if permitted.
Thinking about and expecting pain.	Turning your mind to other thoughts and distractions (though not during pushing); thinking of contractions in terms of how much they accomplish, rather than how much they hurt; and remembering that no matter how intense the discomfort, it will be of relatively brief duration.
Anxiety and stress; tensing up during contractions.	Using relaxation techniques between contractions; concentrating on your breathing or pushing efforts during them.
Fear of the unknown.	Learning as much as you can about childbirth in advance; taking childbirth one contraction at a time; and not worrying about what's to come.
Self-pity.	Thinking about how lucky you are and about the wonderful reward ahead.
Feeling out of control and helpless.	Having good childbirth preparation; knowing enough to feel some measure of control and confidence.

that are appropriate for this stage of labor (or ask the nurse for guidance).

❖ Try to relax between contractions (as much as is humanly possible) with slow, rhythmic chest breathing.

What the Coach Can Do:

❖ Be specific and direct in your instructions, without wasting words. She may find small talk annoying. If she doesn't want your help anymore at some point, don't take it personally. Give her the space she needs for as long as she needs it, but stay nearby in case you can be of help.

❖ Offer lots of encouragement and praise, unless she prefers you to keep quiet. At this moment, eye contact or touch may communicate more expressively than words.

❖ Touch her only if she finds it comforting. Abdominal massage may be offensive now, though counterpressure applied to the small of her back may provide some measure of relief for back discomfort.

❖ Breathe with her through every contraction if it seems to help her through them.

❖ Remind her to take it one contraction at a time. Again, she may need you to warn her when each begins and to tell her as it declines.

❖ Help her relax between contractions, touching her abdomen lightly to show her when a contraction is over. Remind her to use slow, rhythmic breathing.

❖ If her contractions seem to be getting closer and/or she feels the urge to push—and she hasn't been examined recently—inform the nurse or practitioner. She may be fully dilated.

❖ Offer her ice chips frequently, if allowed, and mop her brow with a cool damp cloth often.

What Hospital Personnel May Do:

❖ Continue providing comfort and support.

❖ Continue monitoring your condition and that of the fetus.

❖ Continue noting duration and intensity of contractions, and the progress you are making.

❖ Prepare for delivery, ultimately moving you to a delivery room if you are not delivering in a birthing or labor room.

THE SECOND STAGE OF CHILDBIRTH: PUSHING AND DELIVERY

Up to this point, your active participation in the birth of your child has been negligible. Though you've undeniably taken the brunt of the abuse in the proceedings, your cervix and uterus (and baby) have done most of the work. But now that dilatation is complete, your help is needed to push the baby the remainder of the way through the birth canal and out. This generally takes between half an hour and an hour, but can be accomplished in 10 short minutes or in two, three, or even more very long hours.

The contractions of the second stage are usually more regular than the contractions of transition. They are still about 60 to 90 seconds long, but sometimes farther apart (usually about two to five minutes) and possibly less painful—though sometimes they are more intense. There now should be a well-defined rest period between them, although you may still have trouble recognizing the onset of each contraction.

What You May Be Feeling or Noticing. Common in the second stage is an overwhelming urge to push—although not every woman feels it. You may experience a burst of renewed energy (a second wind) or fatigue; tremendous rectal pressure; very visible contractions, with the uterus rising noticeably with each; an increase in bloody show; a tingling, stretching, burning, or stinging sensation at the vagina as the head crowns; and a slippery wet feeling as the baby emerges.

Emotionally, you may feel relieved that you can now start pushing (though some women feel embarrassed or inhibited); you may also feel exhilarated and excited or, if the pushing stretches on for much more than an hour, frustrated or overwhelmed. In prolonged second stages, the woman's preoccupation is often less with seeing the baby than with getting the ordeal over with; this is a natural, and temporary, reaction, which in no way reflects on her capacity for motherly love.

What You Can Do:
❖ Get into a pushing position (which one will depend upon hospital policy, your practitioner's predilection, the bed or chair you are in, and most important, what is most comfortable and effective for you). A semi-sitting or semi-squatting position is probably the best because it enlists the aid of gravity in the birthing process and may afford you more pushing power.

❖ Give it all you've got. The more efficiently you push, and the more energy you pack into the effort, the more quickly your baby will make the trip through the birth canal. But keep your efforts controlled, coordinating your rhythm closely with the instructions of the practitioner or nurse. Frantic, disorganized pushing wastes energy and accomplishes little.

❖ Don't let inhibition or embarrassment break the pushing rhythm. Since you're bearing down on the whole perineal area, anything that's in your rectum may be pushed out too; trying to avoid this while you're pushing can impede your progress. A little involuntary evacuation (or even a little passage of urine) is experienced by nearly everyone in delivery. No one else in the room will think twice about it, and neither should you. Sterile pads will be used to whisk away any excretion immediately.

❖ Do what comes naturally. Push when you feel the urge, unless otherwise instructed. Take a few deep breaths while the contraction is building; take another and hold it. As the contraction peaks, push with all your might until you can no longer comfortably hold your breath. You may feel as many as five urges to bear down with each contraction. Follow each urge, rather than trying to hold your breath and push through an entire contraction; breath-holding for long periods of time can exhaust you and may deprive the fetus of oxygen. It can also increase the risk of breaking blood vessels in your eyes and face. Taking several deep breaths as the contraction wanes will help restore your respiratory balance. If nothing seems to be coming naturally—and pushing doesn't for every woman—your practitioner

A Baby Is Born

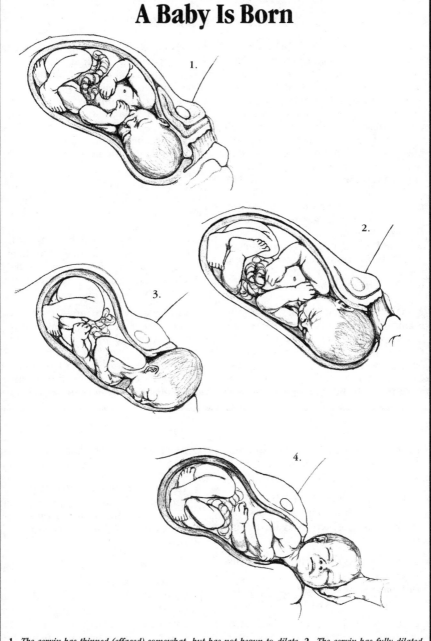

1. *The cervix has thinned (effaced) somewhat, but has not begun to dilate.* 2. *The cervix has fully dilated and the baby's head has begun to press into the birth canal (vagina).* 3. *To allow the narrowest diameter of the baby's head to fit through the mother's pelvis, the baby usually turns sometime during labor. Here the slightly molded head has crowned.* 4. *The head, the baby's broadest part, is out. The rest of the delivery should proceed quickly and smoothly.*

A First Look at Baby

Those who expect their babies to arrive as round and smooth and pink as a Botticelli cherub may be in for a shock. Nine months of soaking in an amniotic bath and a dozen or so hours of compression in a contracting uterus and cramped birth canal take their toll on a newborn's appearance. Those babies who arrived via cesarean section will have a temporary edge as far as appearance goes.

Fortunately, most of the less-lovely newborn characteristics that follow are temporary. One morning, a couple of months after you've brought your wrinkled, slightly scrawny, puffy-eyed bundle home from the hospital, you'll wake to find that the Botticelli cherub has taken its place in the crib.

An Oddly Shaped Head. At birth the infant's head is, proportionately, the largest part of the body, with a circumference as large as the chest. As the baby grows, the rest of the body will catch up. Often the head has molded to fit through the mother's pelvis, giving it an odd, possibly pointed "cone" shape; pressing against an inadequately dilated cervix can further distort the head by raising a lump (called caput succedaneum). The caput will disappear in a day or two, the molding within two weeks—at which point your baby's head will begin to take on that Botticelli roundness.

Newborn Hair. The hair that covers the head at birth may have little resemblance to the hair the baby will have later. Some newborns are virtually bald, some have thick manes, but most have a light cap of soft hair. All will eventually lose their newborn hair (though this may not be apparent), which will gradually be replaced by new growth.

Vernix Caseosa Coating. The cheesy substance that coats the fetus in the uterus is believed to protect the skin from the long exposure to the amniotic fluid. Premature babies have quite a bit of this coating at birth; postmature babies have almost none, except

---

or nurse will help direct your efforts, and redirect them if you lose your concentration.

❖ Relax your entire body, including your thighs and perineum, as you push. Tenseness works against your pushing efforts.

❖ Stop pushing when you're instructed to (as you may be, to keep the baby's head from being born too rapidly). Pant or blow instead.

❖ Rest between contractions, with the help of your coach and the attendants. If you are really exhausted, especially when the second stage drags on, your practitioner may suggest that you don't push for several contractions so you can rebuild your strength.

❖ Don't become frustrated if you see the baby's head crown, then disappear again. Birthing is a two-steps-forward, one-step-backward proposition.

❖ Remember to keep an eye on the mirror (if one is available). Seeing your baby's head crown (and reaching down and touching it, if your practitioner approves) may give you the inspiration to push when the pushing gets tough. Besides, unless your coach is videotaping, there won't be any replays to watch.

in the folds of their skin and under their fingernails.

Swelling of the Genitals. This is common in both male and female newborns, and is particularly pronounced in boy babies delivered via cesarean. The breasts of newborns, male and female, may also be swollen (occasionally even engorged, secreting a white or pink substance nicknamed "witch's milk") due to stimulation by maternal hormones. The hormones may also stimulate a milky-white, even blood-tinged, vaginal secretion in girls. These effects are not abnormal, and disappear in a week to ten days.

Lanugo. Fine downy hair, called lanugo, may cover the shoulders, back, forehead, and temples of full-term babies. This will usually be shed by the end of the first week. Such hair can be more abundant, and will last longer, in a premature baby.

Puffy Eyes. Swelling around the newborn's eyes is often caused by the eye drops that are used to protect the baby from infection, and disappears within a few days. Caucasian babies' eyes are almost always a slate blue, no matter what color they will be later on. In darker-skinned babies, the eyes are usually brown at birth.

Birthmarks and Skin Lesions. A reddish blotch at the base of the skull, on the eyelid, or on the forehead, called a salmon patch, is very common, especially in Caucasian newborns. Mongolian spots—bluish-gray pigmentation of the deep skin layer that can appear on the back, buttocks, and sometimes the arms and thighs—are more common in Asians, southern Europeans, and blacks. These markings will eventually disappear, usually by the time a child is four years old. Hemangiomas, elevated strawberry-colored birthmarks, vary from tiny to about quarter-size. They will eventually fade to a mottled pearly gray, then disappear entirely. Coffee-with-cream-colored (cafe-au-lait) spots can appear anywhere on the body; they are usually inconspicuous, and don't fade. A variety of rashes, tiny "pimples," and whiteheads may also mar the newborn complexion, but all are temporary.

What the Coach Can Do:

❖ Continue giving comfort and support, but don't feel hurt if your wife doesn't seem to notice you're there. Her energies are necessarily focused elsewhere.

❖ Guide her pushing and breathing, using the cues that you have both become familiar with during childbirth preparation; or relay instructions from the nurse or practitioner.

❖ Don't feel intimidated by the finesse and expertise of the professional medical team around you. Your presence is important, too. And in fact, your whispered "I love you" may be more valuable to her at this stage than anything they can offer.

❖ Help her to relax between the contractions—with soothing words, a cool cloth applied to forehead, neck, and shoulders, and, if feasible, back massage or counterpressure to help ease backache.

❖ If it's allowed, continue to supply ice chips to moisten her parched mouth as needed.

❖ Support her back while she's pushing, if necessary; hold her hand, wipe her brow—or do whatever seems to help her. If she slips out of position, help her back up.

❖ Periodically point out her progress. As the baby begins to crown, remind her to keep an eye on the mirror so she can have visual confirmation of what she is accomplishing; when she's not looking, or if there's no mirror, give her inch-by-inch descriptions. Take her hand and touch the head together for renewed inspiration (with the practitioner's okay).

❖ If you're offered the opportunity to "catch" your baby as it emerges or, later, to cut the cord, don't panic. Both are easy—and you'll get step-by-step directions, support, and backup from the attendants.

What Hospital Personnel May Do:
❖ Move you to the room in which you will deliver, if you aren't already there. If you're in a birthing bed, they'll simply remove the foot of the bed to prepare for delivery.

❖ Give support and direction to you as the delivery progresses.

❖ Continue to check the condition of the fetus periodically, usually by attaching the fetal monitor briefly.

❖ About the time the head crowns, prepare for the delivery—spreading sterile drapes and arranging instruments, donning surgical garments and gloves, sponging the perineal area with antiseptic.

❖ Perform an episiotomy just before the head is delivered, if necessary. First a local anesthetic will probably be injected into the perineum. This will be done at the height of a contraction, when the pressure of the baby's head naturally numbs the area; the incision will also be made at the height of a contraction and, if the perineum is anesthetized, will probably be painless.

❖ Elect to use outlet forceps to ease the baby's head out if the second stage lasts more than two hours (some doctors will wait longer if mother and baby are doing well), if the baby shows signs of difficulty tolerating the stresses of labor, if your medical condition prohibits further pushing, or if progress is being impeded because of a slightly irregular fetal presentation or a slight disproportion between fetus and pelvis. (See Forceps Delivery, page 286.) Usually a regional anesthetic will be administered if an epidural or other block hasn't already been given, because forceps delivery can be painful. If forceps aren't feasible or don't work, a cesarean may be the safest delivery route for baby and you.

❖ Once the head emerges, quickly suction the baby's nose and mouth to remove excess mucus, then assist the shoulders and torso out.

❖ Clamp and cut the umbilical cord, possibly with the newborn lying across your abdomen. Your husband may be asked if he would like to do the snipping. Some practitioners prefer to wait until the placenta is delivered or the cord has stopped pulsating before cutting the cord.

❖ Provide initial protective care for the newborn: evaluate his or her condition, and rate it on the Apgar scale at one minute and five minutes after birth (see page 287); give a brisk, stimulating, and drying rubdown; identify the baby by taking his or her footprints and your fingerprint for hospital records, and by attaching an identifying band to your wrist and/or ankle and that of your baby; administer nonirritating eyedrops, to prevent infection; weigh the baby, and wrap him or her to prevent heat loss. (In some hospitals some of these procedures may be omitted; in others many will be attended to later, in the nursery.)

❖ Show your now cleaned-up baby to you and your husband. Unless there is a problem, you and your husband should be able to hold your baby for some significant period. You may, if you wish to, try

breastfeeding (don't worry if you and/or your baby don't catch on immediately—see Getting Started Breastfeeding, page 388).

❖ When you are finished getting acquainted, they will probably whisk baby off to the nursery (at least temporarily) and transfer you to your room.

THE THIRD STAGE OF CHILDBIRTH: DELIVERY OF THE PLACENTA, OR AFTERBIRTH

The worst is over, the best has already come. All that remains is the tying up of loose ends, so to speak. During this final stage of childbirth (which generally lasts anywhere from five minutes to half an hour or more) the placenta, which has been your baby's life support inside the womb, will be delivered. You will continue to have mild contractions of approximately one minute's duration, though you may not feel them. The squeezing of the uterus separates the placenta from the uterine wall and moves it down into the lower segment of the uterus or into the vagina so you can then push it out. Once the placenta is delivered, any necessary stitching up of episiotomy or tears will be taken care of.

What You May Be Feeling or Noticing. Now that the work of labor and delivery is done, you may feel fatigue or, conversely, a burst of renewed energy. You are likely to be very thirsty and, especially if labor has been long, hungry. Some women experience chills in this stage; all experience a bloody vaginal discharge (called lochia) comparable to a heavy menstrual period.

For many women, the immediate emotional reaction is a sense of relief.

There may also be exhilaration and talkativeness; elation, tempered by a new sense of responsibility; impatience at having to push out the placenta or submit to the repair of the episiotomy or tear, though you may be too excited or tired to care. Some women feel a strong closeness to their husbands and an immediate bond with their new baby; others feel somewhat detached (who is this stranger sniffing at my breast?), even resentful (how he's made me suffer!), particularly after a difficult delivery. (See pages 267 and 382 for more on bonding and new-mother love.)

What You Can Do:

❖ Help expel the placenta, by pushing when directed.

❖ Be patient during repair of any episiotomy or tears.

❖ Nurse or hold the baby, once the cord is cut. In some hospitals, and under some circumstances, the baby may be kept in a heated bassinette for a while or be held by the father.

❖ Take pride in your accomplishment, relax, and enjoy! And don't forget to thank your coach.

What the Coach Can Do:

❖ Give your wife some well-earned words of praise—and congratulate yourself for a job well done.

❖ Begin bonding with your baby by holding and hugging him or her now.

❖ Don't forget to do some husband-wife bonding, too.

❖ Ask the nurse for some juice for your wife; she may be very thirsty. After she's been rehydrated, and if both of you are in the mood, break out the bubbly.

❖ Take pictures if you've brought your camera, or tape the baby's first cries if you've brought your tape recorder along.

What Hospital Personnel May Do:

❖ Help extract the placenta. The exact procedure will vary depending upon the practitioner and the situation. Some will pull the cord gently with one hand while pressing and kneading the uterus with the other; others will exert downward pressure on the top of the uterus, asking you to push at the appropriate time. Many physicians will use oxytocin, by injection or IV, after delivery of the placenta to encourage uterine contractions, which will speed expulsion of the placenta and minimize bleeding.

❖ Examine the placenta to be sure it is intact. If it isn't, the practitioner will inspect the uterus manually for placental fragments and remove any that remain.

❖ Cut the cord, if it wasn't cut earlier.

❖ Stitch an episiotomy or tear, if any. A local anesthetic (if none was previously given, or if it has worn off) will probably be injected to numb the area. You will feel a pinch.

❖ Check your vagina to remove clots or sponges used during episiotomy repair.

❖ Sponge-bathe the lower part of your body, help you into a clean gown, and help you put on a perineal pad (sanitary napkin) held in place by a belt.

❖ Wheel you into the recovery room, or to your own room. If you're in a birthing bed, they'll put the foot of the bed back on.

❖ Deliver the baby to the nursery for a bath and some additional protective measures. (If you have rooming-in, the baby will be returned as soon as possible.)

BREECH DELIVERY

As far as the mother and coach are concerned, labor and vaginal delivery of a breech baby don't differ much from that of a vertex (head-down) baby; tips for coping and comforting are virtually identical. The activities of the hospital staff will be different, however, and will vary further depending on the type of breech position and the delivery procedure that the practitioner elects to follow.

Up until the second stage, a vaginal breech labor progesses about the same as a vertex labor. But it is always considered a trial labor, allowed to proceed only as long as it progresses normally. Because of the ever-present possibility that a cesarean may become necessary, you will probably be transferred to a delivery/operating room at the end of the first stage. Depending upon your baby's exact breech position, your doctor will determine the safest and most effective way to proceed. (What is most advisable in such a case also depends on the practitioner's experience. Asking a doctor to perform a procedure for breech extraction that you've read or heard about, but with which he or she is not comfortable, is not in your or your baby's best interest.)

A common procedure is to allow the baby to deliver naturally until the legs and lower half of the torso are out. Then a local anesthetic is administered and the shoulders and head are delivered, with or without the aid of forceps.

A vaginal delivery is not likely to be attempted if the baby is in the complete breech (see page 238) or footling breech (with one leg dangling down) position, if the baby's head is extended (facing upward), if the fetus is estimated to be very large or the mother's pelvis inadequate, if the delivery is premature, or if there are signs of fetal distress.

A large episiotomy is often necessary with a breech, but occasionally it can be avoided. The delivery position for a vaginal breech birth will vary, again depending on the situation and on your practitioner's experience. Some find they have more control if the woman is flat on her back, legs up in stirrups.

Once the baby is delivered, the proceedings continue as with a head-first birth.

CESAREAN SECTION: SURGICAL DELIVERY

You won't be able to participate actively at a cesarean delivery the way you would at a vaginal one. In fact, your most important contribution to the comfort and success of your baby's cesarean birth can be made before you arrive at the hospital—possibly before you even know that you're having a cesarean. That contribution is preparation. Being prepared both intellectually and emotionally for a cesarean, in case it should become necessary, will minimize any disappointment you may feel and help make your surgical delivery experience a positive one.

Thanks to regional anesthesia and the liberalization of hospital regulations, most women (and often their husbands) are able to be participants at their cesarean deliveries. Because they aren't preoccupied with pushing or discomfort, they are often able to relax and enjoy the birth—something women delivering vaginally rarely can do. This is what you can expect in a typical cesarean birth:

❖ Your pubic and/or abdominal hair may be shaved, and a catheter (a narrow tube) will be inserted into your bladder to keep it empty and out of the surgeon's way.

❖ In the operating room, sterile drapes will be arranged around your exposed abdomen, which will be washed down with an antiseptic solution. If you are to be awake for the delivery, a screen will be put up at about shoulder level so that you won't have to see the incision being made.

❖ An IV infusion will be started to provide speedy access if additional medication is needed.

❖ Anesthesia will be administered: either an epidural or a spinal block (both of which numb the lower part of your body but don't knock you out) or a general anesthetic (which does put you to sleep—sometimes necessary in an emergency when the baby must be delivered immediately).

❖ If you've had a regional anesthetic and your coach is going to attend the delivery, he will be suited up in sterile garb. He will sit near your head, so that he can give you emotional support and hold your hand; he will have the option of viewing the actual surgery. (Whether or not you know in advance that you are going to have a cesarean, it's a good idea to discuss with your doctor ahead of time the conditions under which your spouse will or won't be allowed to be with you during surgery.) Usually, if general anesthesia is used, the husband will be asked to wait outside the operating room.

❖ If yours is an emergency cesarean, things may move very quickly. Don't be alarmed by the seeming storm of activity around you. Be prepared for the possibility that hospital policy, and concern for the safety of you and your baby, may dictate that your husband leave during the delivery, which will take only about five or ten minutes.

❖ Once the physician is certain that the anesthetic has taken effect, an incision (a cut) is made in the lower abdomen. If you are awake, you may feel a sensation of being "unzipped," but no pain.

❖ A second incision is then made, this time in the lower segment of your uterus. The amniotic sac is opened, and if it hasn't already ruptured, the fluid is suctioned out; you may hear a sort of gurgling or swooshing sound.

❖ The baby is then eased out, either manually or with forceps, usually with an assistant pressing on the upper portion of the uterus. With an epidural (though not likely with a spinal block), you will probably feel some pulling and tugging sensations, as well as some pressure. If you're eager to see your baby's arrival, ask the doctor if the screen can be lowered slightly, which will allow you to see the actual birth, but not the more graphic details.

❖ Your baby's nose and mouth are then suctioned; you'll hear the first cry, and if the cord is long enough, you will be allowed a quick glimpse.

❖ The cord will be quickly clamped and cut, and while the baby is getting the same routine attention that a vaginally delivered infant receives, the doctor removes the placenta.

❖ Now the doctor will quickly do a routine check of your reproductive organs and stitch up the incisions that were made.

❖ An injection of oxytocin may be given intramuscularly or into your IV bottle, to help contract the uterus and thus control bleeding. IV antibiotics may be given to minimize the chances of infection.

❖ Depending upon your condition and the baby's, as well as hospital rules, you may or may not be able to hold the baby right there in the delivery room. If you can't, perhaps your husband can. If the infant has to be whisked away to the ICU nursery, don't fret. This is standard in many hospitals and doesn't necessarily indicate a problem with a baby's condition. And as far as bonding is concerned, later can be just as good as sooner.

Part 3

OF SPECIAL CONCERN

15
If You Get Sick

E very woman expects to succumb to at least a few of the less desirable pregnancy symptoms during her nine-month stint—morning sickness and leg cramps, for instance, or indigestion and exhaustion. But it surprises some to discover that they're also susceptible to symptoms that have nothing at all to do with pregnancy: those associated with such "civilian" sicknesses as colds, flu, gastroenteritis, even measles and mumps. Though most such illnesses do not affect a pregnancy, an occasional one can. Prevention is, of course, the best way to keep that healthy glow of pregnancy going strong. But when it fails, quick and safe treatment, in most cases under the supervision of your doctor, is essential to protect yourself and your baby from complications.

WHAT YOU MAY BE CONCERNED ABOUT

COMING DOWN WITH A COLD OR FLU

"I've got a terrible cold and I'm worried about it affecting my baby."

M ost women come down with a cold or the flu at least once during their nine months, and though you may be very uncomfortable, a mild illness like this will not affect your pregnancy. However, the medications that you're probably accustomed to taking for these maladies, such as cold tablets and antihistamines, could. So don't take these or any other medications, including aspirin (see page 320) or megadoses of vitamin C, without your doctor's approval. He or she should be able to tell you which cold treatments are safe in pregnancy and which will work best in your case. None, of course, will cure a cold, but some may relieve its symptoms. (See page 321 for information on taking medication during pregnancy.)

If you've already taken a few doses of one medication or another, don't panic. It's very unlikely any harm was done. But do check with your practitioner if you're concerned.

Fortunately for you and your baby, some of the best cold and flu remedies are the safest ones, too:

❖ Nip the cold in the bud, before it blossoms into a nasty case of bronchitis or another secondary infection. At the very first sneeze, go to bed or at least plan on getting a little extra rest.

❖ When you're lying down or sleeping, keep your head slightly elevated to facilitate breathing.

❖ Don't starve your cold, fever—or baby. Stay on the Best-Odds Diet whether you have an appetite or not, forcing yourself to eat if need be. Be sure to have some citrus fruit or juice every day, but don't take extra vitamin C supplements (beyond that in your pregnancy formula) without medical advice.

❖ Flood yourself with fluids. Fever, sneezes, and a runny nose will cause your body to lose fluids that you and your baby urgently need. Keep a thermos of hot grapefruit juice or orangeade (½ cup unsweetened frozen juice concentrate to 1 quart of hot water) next to your bed, and drink at least one cupful an hour. Also try the Jewish penicillin: chicken soup. Medical researchers have proven that it not only replaces fluids but also helps make cold sufferers more comfortable.

❖ Keep your nasal passages moist with a humidifier (see Appendix), and by spraying the inside of your nose with an atomizer filled with salt water.

❖ If your throat is sore or scratchy, or if you're coughing, gargle with salt water (1 teaspoon of salt to 8 ounces of water) at the temperature of hot, but not scalding, tea.

❖ Bring down a fever naturally. Take cool showers or baths, or sponge with tepid water; drink cool beverages; and wear light bedclothes. If your fever reaches 102° degrees or more, call your doctor immediately (see page 320).

Unfortunately, colds tend to last longer during pregnancy, possibly because the immune system slows down a bit in order to protect the baby (a foreign body) from immunological rejection. If your cold or flu is severe enough to interfere with eating or sleeping, if you're coughing up greenish or yellowish sputum, or if symptoms last more than a week, call your doctor. He or she may want to prescribe a powerful cold preparation that is safe for use in pregnancy, or if there is a risk of a bacterial infection, a sputum test may be needed and/or an antibiotic prescribed.

Don't put off calling the doctor or refuse to take a prescribed medication you are assured is safe, because you've heard all drugs are harmful in pregnancy. They aren't.

For that important ounce of prevention next time you're exposed to cold germs, see page 323.

GASTROINTESTINAL ILLS

"I've got a stomach bug, and I can't keep anything down. Will this hurt my baby?"

Fortunately gastroenteritis (an inflammation of the stomach and intestines) usually has a limited life span—often no longer than 24 hours, very rarely longer than 72. And as long as fluid balance is maintained through adequate replacement, even complete lack of solid nourishment for a day or two won't harm your baby.

But the fact that the virus isn't affecting your baby's health doesn't mean that you should ignore it. Take these steps to increase your comfort and speed your recovery while you're waiting for your bug to bug off.

❖ Take to your bed, if possible. Bed rest, particularly in a dark, quiet room, seems to reduce symptoms of gastroenteritis.

❖ Replenish lost fluids. Diarrhea and vomiting are extremely dehydrating. And since fluid intake is more important than solid intake for the short term, it's essential to keep the clear liquids coming. Take them in whatever form they're palatable (water, club soda or seltzer, weak decaffeinated tea, orange juice diluted with an equal quantity of water, or if diarrhea isn't also a problem, diluted apple or grape juice), in small sips as often as possible (aim for every 15 minutes). If you can't even keep these down, suck on ice chips or ice cubes. Avoid the traditional cure of sugary soft drinks—this will only prolong your symptoms. Milk may, too.

❖ Modify your diet. Traditional wisdom says that unless you're really hungry, it's probably better to eat nothing for the first 12 hours or so with a stomach virus. More recent research, however, suggests that continuing solids may actually be preferable to semi-starvation. Check with your physician for advice. Whether you continue solids or wait 12 to 24 hours before digging in, keep your diet simple. At first stick to diluted nonacidic fruit juices, clear broths or bouillon, thinned cream of wheat or rice, unbuttered white toast, boiled or steamed converted white rice, boiled or baked potato without the skin, bananas, applesauce, gelatin desserts (make these with unflavored gelatin and fruit juice instead of sugary mixes). Gradually add, as they become appealing to you, cottage cheese, yogurt, chicken, fish, then cooked vegetables and fruit, before returning to your normal diet.

❖ Supplement, when you can. Getting your vitamin insurance is an especially good idea now; so try to take your supplement when it's least likely to come back up. Don't worry, however, if you can't manage to keep it down for a few days or so; no harm will be done.

❖ Consult with your practitioner. Discuss all of your symptoms, particularly any fever, which may need to be treated. Call again as instructed, and/or if symptoms don't let up after 48 hours. Medication may be necessary.

If others who have eaten with you take ill at the same time, this may be food poisoning instead of a virus. Or if you recently traveled to an exotic destination, parasites or other exotic infectious organisms may be responsible for your distress. Check with your doctor if you suspect this type of infection.

Of course, even better than trying to cure an illness is preventing it in the first place. So always observe the prevention tips on page 323.

GERMAN MEASLES (RUBELLA)

"I was exposed to German measles on a trip out of the country. Do I have to have an abortion?"

That's a question only 1 out of 7 pregnant women need ever confront. The other six are, happily, immune to rubella, or German measles, having contracted it at some other time in their lives (usually during childhood) or because they were vaccinated against it (usually in early adolescence or when they were married). You may not know whether or not you are immune, but you can find out with a simple test—a rubella antibody titer—which measures the level of antibodies to the virus in your blood and is performed routinely at the first prenatal visit by most practitioners. If this test was not performed, it should be now.

If it turns out you're not immune,

you still needn't consider drastic measures immediately. Exposure alone cannot harm your baby. For the virus to do its damage, you have to contract the illness. The symptoms, which show up two or three weeks after exposure, are usually mild (malaise, slight fever, and swollen glands, followed by a slight rash a day or two later) and may sometimes pass unnoticed. A blood test during that time, however, can show whether or not you have an active infection. By 22 weeks it's possible to test a fetus to see if it has been infected (earlier, the infection may not show up), but this is rarely needed.

Unfortunately there is no way of absolutely preventing an exposed woman from coming down with rubella. Gamma globulin shots were once given routinely, but they have been found to be inconsistent in preventing infection. Should you come down with rubella, you will need to discuss with your doctor all the possible risks to your fetus before making a decision about terminating your pregnancy. It's important to understand that the risks involved decrease as a pregnancy progresses. If a woman is infected in the first month, the chance of her baby developing serious congenital malformation is high, about 35%. By the third month, the risk is down to 10% to 15%. After that the risk is very slight.

Fortunately, the chance of being exposed to rubella in this country is small. Since immunization has become routine in the U.S., the disease is becoming more and more rare here. Still, if you aren't immune and don't contract the disease this time around, avoid the concern entirely in subsequent pregnancies by having your doctor vaccinate you after this delivery. As a precaution, you will be instructed not to become pregnant for two or three months following vaccination. But should you conceive acci-

dentally during this time—or if you were vaccinated early in this pregnancy, before you knew you had conceived—don't worry. Though there is a theoretical risk of fetal damage, there have been no reported cases of birth defects of the type associated with congenital rubella in babies whose mothers were inadvertently vaccinated early in pregnancy or conceived soon after vaccination.

TOXOPLASMOSIS

"Though I've given all the cat-care chores over to my husband, just the very fact that I live with cats makes me worry about toxoplasmosis. How would I know if I came down with the disease?"

You probably wouldn't. Most people who are infected show no symptoms at all, though some do notice mild malaise, slight fever, and swollen glands two or three weeks after exposure, followed by a rash a day or two later.

The only way to actually determine if an infection occurs is by means of a blood test; this will indicate if the parasite, *Toxoplasma gondii,* has suddenly developed in a woman who previously showed no antibodies. Check with your practitioner to see if you were tested before pregnancy. If you had antibodies then—very likely if you've been living with cats—you're immune and needn't worry about developing an infection now. If you had no antibodies, you are not immune. In that case, the recommended procedure is to repeat the IgG antibody test every month or two until you deliver. Should tests become positive at any point, it's likely an infection has occurred.[1]

---

1. *Do not* try to test yourself; home tests for toxoplasmosis are highly unreliable.

In that unlikely event (in the U.S., only 1 woman in 1,000 is believed to become infected during pregnancy), a thorough discussion of the options with the doctor, a maternal-fetal subspecialist, or possibly with a genetic counselor, should be the next step. The point in a pregnancy at which the infection occurs is a factor to consider. The risk of a fetus becoming infected in the first trimester is relatively small, probably less than 15%, but the risk of serious damage to the fetus is high. In the second trimester, the likelihood of infection is a little higher, but the risk of fetal damage somewhat smaller. In the last trimester the baby is most likely to be infected, but the risk of serious damage is smallest. Only 1 baby in 10,000 is born with severe congenital toxoplasmosis.

Another factor to consider is whether or not the fetus itself has actually become infected. Recent advances have made it possible to test for fetal infection through amniocentesis, as well as through the examination of a fetal blood and/or amniotic fluid sample, though not usually before 20 to 22 weeks. If there is no fetal infection, the fetus is probably not affected. Finally, it's recommended that if a pregnant woman does show an infection and does not wish to terminate her pregnancy no matter what testing suggests, she should be treated with special antibiotics—possibly for several months. Such treatment appears to greatly reduce the risk of a baby being born with severe problems.

If you weren't tested earlier, then according to the latest research there is no point in testing you now unless you develop symptoms. The tests are not accurate enough to show whether a woman who was never tested before has a new infection or simply shows antibodies from an old infection.

The best "treatment" of toxoplasmosis is prevention. See page 65 for tips on how to avoid infection.

CYTOMEGALOVIRUS (CMV)

"I teach at a nursery school, and I've been told that I should take a leave of absence during my pregnancy because I could contract cytomegalovirus, which could be harmful to my baby."

Although somewhere between 25% and 60% of all preschoolers carry the cytomegalovirus and can excrete it in saliva, urine, and feces for months or even years, the chances that you will pick up the infection from your young charges and pass it on to your baby with adverse results are small. First of all, the virus is not extremely contagious. Second, most adults were infected in childhood. If you were, you can't "catch" CMV from the children you care for now. (If your CMV becomes reactivated, the risks to your baby are smaller than if you have a new infection during pregnancy.) Third, though roughly 1 in 100 babies is born with the virus, only a small percentage of these actually show any of the ill effects commonly associated with CMV infection in utero, which include jaundice, high-tone deafness, and eye problems.

Still some physicians, like yours, suggest that unless a woman knows for sure that she has already been infected (most people don't have this information unless they are tested prenatally, since CMV usually comes and goes with no obvious symptoms), it's a good idea to take a leave of absence from any job that puts her in daily contact with large numbers of pre-schoolers, at least for the first 24 weeks of pregnancy, during which the risks to the fetus are the greatest. Others recommend wearing gloves on the job, washing up carefully after changing diapers (which you should do anyway), and resisting kissing the toddlers in your care or eating their leftovers.

Though pregnant women with toddlers of their own may worry about catching CMV in the nursery, the possibility is so remote that the worry is unnecessary. That doesn't mean, of course, that good hygiene in the home should be ignored—it should be practiced whether you're worried about CMV or not.

Should you come down with what seems like flu or mononucleosis (fever, fatigue, swollen lymph glands, sore throat), however, do check with your doctor. Whether these symptoms represent CMV or another illness, they need treatment.

FIFTH DISEASE

"I read that a disease I had never even heard of before—fifth disease—could cause problems in pregnancy."

Fifth disease—technically "erythema infectiosum," caused by the human parvovirus B19—is the fifth of a group of six diseases that cause fever and rash in children. But unlike its sister diseases (such as chicken pox), fifth disease isn't widely known because its symptoms are mild and can go unnoticed. Fever is present in only 15% to 30% of cases. The rash—which for the first few days gives the cheeks the appearance of having been slapped, then spreads in a lacy pattern to trunk, buttocks, and thighs, recurring on and off (usually in response to heat from the sun or a warm bath) for one to three weeks—is often confused with the rash of rubella and other childhood illnesses. Concentrated exposure from caring for a child sick with fifth disease or from teaching at a school where it is epidemic puts an expectant mother at greater risk of developing the infection than with casual contact.

Recently fifth disease has been linked to a slightly increased risk of miscarriage in women who contract it. But since most women of childbearing age are already immune because they were infected as children, infection of pregnant women is not common. If the disease does cause a miscarriage in one pregnancy, however, a repeat miscarriage due to parvovirus is not likely.

Very rarely, fifth disease may lead to an unusual form of fetal anemia, similar to that in Rh disease. For that reason, women who have fifth disease during pregnancy are generally examined periodically with ultrasound to look for the swelling (resulting from fluid retention) in the fetus that is characteristic of this kind of anemia; if it is found, treatment will probably be necessary.

GROUP B STREP

"I read in a magazine that strep B infection in a mother can kill her baby. It's terrifying to think that I might be carrying it around."

Scary headlines sell magazines, but they do a disservice to readers. Though it's true that a baby who contracts a group B streptococcus infection from its mother at birth can become ill and even die, with modern obstetrical practice this doesn't have to happen.

Since there are no symptoms to indicate a woman is carrying the bacteria, most practitioners do a culture for group B strep (using a vaginal swab) in all their pregnant patients at about 26 to 28 weeks. If the results are positive, the woman is treated with antibiotics as soon as her membranes rupture or when she goes into labor. Studies show that this effectively protects the baby from harm. (Treating earlier may not be helpful because the bacteria have time to regroup and establish another beachhead before labor begins.)

So while you shouldn't worry, you should be sure that you've been tested and that if the test is positive, you are treated at the appropriate time.

LYME DISEASE

"I know I live in an area that's high risk for Lyme disease. Is it dangerous to have when you're pregnant."

Lyme disease—which got its name from Lyme, Connecticut, where it was first diagnosed in the U.S.—is most common among those who spend time in woods frequented by deer, mice, or other animals carrying "deer" ticks, but it can also be picked up in forest-free cities via greenery brought from the country or at a farmer's market. Lyme disease can be passed on to the fetus, but whether or not the fetus can suffer permanent harm isn't entirely clear. It is suspected, but not proven, that the disease may be linked to heart defects in the babies of infected mothers.

The best way to protect your baby as well as yourself is by practicing preventive measures. If you are out in woodsy or grassy areas, or if you handle greenery grown in such areas, wear long pants tucked into boots or socks, and long sleeves; use an insect repellent effective for Lyme ticks on your clothing, but *not* on your skin. When you return home, check your skin carefully for ticks (removing them shortly after they attach almost entirely eliminates the possibility of infection) and shower thoroughly.

If you suspect you've been infected, see your doctor immediately. (Early symptoms may include a blotchy bull's-eye rash at the bite site, fatigue,

headache, fever and chills, generalized achiness, swollen glands near the site of the bite; other possible symptoms are redness or swelling of the eyes, erratic behavior, sore throat, nonproductive [dry] cough, hives or other allover rash.) Prompt treatment may prevent your passing the infection on to your baby, and your becoming seriously ill.

MEASLES

"I'm a teacher, and a child in our school has the measles. Should I be immunized?"

No. Measles vaccine is not given during pregnancy because of the theoretical risk to the fetus from the vaccine, though there have been no reports of malformations among newborns whose mothers were inadvertently vaccinated. Besides, the odds are good that you are already immune to measles, since most women of childbearing age were vaccinated against the disease as children. If you are not immune (your doctor can run a test to determine whether you are), the risk that you will contract measles is small since most, if not all, of the children in your class have been vaccinated against it and are themselves unlikely to come down with the disease. Also reassuring is the fact that measles, unlike German measles, or rubella, does not appear to cause birth defects, though it may be linked to an increased risk of miscarriage or premature labor and is sometimes quite a severe illness in pregnant women. Still, if you are exposed directly to someone with measles and are not immune, your doctor may administer gammaglobulin during the incubation period—between exposure and the start of symptoms to decrease the severity of the illness.

If a pregnant woman contracts measles near her due date, there is a risk of infection in the newborn, which could be serious. Again, gammaglobulin may be administered to reduce the severity of such an infection.

URINARY TRACT INFECTION

"I'm afraid I have a urinary tract infection."

Urinary tract infections (UTIs) are so common in pregnancy that 10% of pregnant women can expect to develop at least one—and those who have already had one have a 1 in 3 chance of an encore. Most often it will be cystitis, a simple bladder infection. In some women cystitis is without symptoms, or "silent," and is diagnosed only after a routine urine culture. In others, symptoms can range from mild to quite uncomfortable (an urge to urinate frequently, a burning sensation when the urine—sometimes only a drop or two—is passed, sharp lower abdominal pain).

Regardless of whether there are symptoms or not, once an infection is diagnosed it should be treated promptly by a physician, with an antibiotic approved for use during pregnancy.[2] Finishing the prescription is vital to preventing a recurrence; don't be tempted to discontinue treatment once you're feeling better.

In 20% to 40% of cases, untreated bladder infection during pregnancy progresses to kidney infection (pyelonephritis), which is more of a threat to mother and baby. This occurs most often in the last trimester, and can lead to preterm labor. The symptoms are the same as those of cystitis but are frequently accompanied by fe-

---

2. Do not take a medication previously prescribed for you or for anyone else, even if it was prescribed for a urinary tract infection.

ver (often as high as 103 degrees), chills, blood in the urine, and backache (in the midback or on one or both sides). Should you experience these symptoms, notify your doctor *immediately.* Antibiotics can generally cure a kidney infection, but hospitalization for intravenous administration will probably be necessary.

Many physicians today try to head off kidney infection by screening pregnant women, at their first visit, for susceptibility. If a culture of the urine turns up bacteria (and it does in about 7% to 10% of pregnant women), antibiotics are administered to prevent the development of cystitis or pyelonephritis.

There are some home remedies and preventives that may also help ward off UTI; used in conjunction with medical treatment, they may help speed recovery when infection occurs:

❖ Drink plenty of fluids, especially water. Unsweetened citrus and cranberry juices may also be beneficial. But avoid coffee and tea (even decaffeinated varieties) and alcohol.

❖ Empty your bladder just before and after intercourse.

❖ Every time you urinate, take the time to be sure your bladder is thoroughly emptied. Leaning forward when you urinate may help to ensure that you empty your bladder completely. Also, it sometimes helps to "double void"; after you urinate, wait five minutes, then try to urinate again. And don't put off urinating—those who chronically "hold it in" increase their susceptibility to infection.

❖ Wear cotton-crotch underwear and pantyhose, and avoid wearing tight under or outer pants. Don't wear pantyhose under slacks. And sleep without panties on.

❖ Keep the vaginal and perineal areas meticulously clean. Wash daily and avoid perfumed soaps, sprays, and powders in the area. Always wipe from front to back after using the toilet. And ask your practitioner about the advisability of using an antibacterial cleansing agent.

❖ Eat unsweetened yogurt or frozen yogurt that contains active cultures when taking antibiotics, to help restore the balance of bacteria in your intestines.

❖ Keep your resistance high by eating a nutritious low-sugar diet (see Best-Odd Diet, page 80), getting plenty of rest, not working to the point of fatigue, and not letting your life get too stressful.

HEPATITIS

"One of the toddlers in the day care center where I work was just diagnosed as having hepatitis A. If I get it, could it affect my pregnancy?"

Hepatitis A is very common (nearly 1 in 3 children comes down with it before the age of five), is almost always a mild disease (often with no notable symptoms), and is not known to be passed on to a fetus or newborn. So it should not affect your pregnancy. Still, you are better off not contracting an infection of any kind. Since hepatitis A is passed by the fecal-oral route, be sure to wash your hands after changing diapers or taking your young charges to the bathroom, as well as before eating. You might also ask your physician about the advisability of immunization against hepatitis A.

"Is hepatitis B contagious? My husband came down with a case of it, which is strange because he isn't in a high-risk category."

Not really so strange. While about 6 in 10 hepatitis B victims fall into the so-called high-risk categories,[3] 1 in 3 cases occur in those with no known risk factors. Since this liver infection, which is most common during the childbearing years of 15 to 39, can be passed from mother to fetus, it's of concern to expectant parents. And since it's transmissible from person to person, it's of particular concern to you. To prevent your becoming infected, you and your husband should take special precautions: no sharing of toothbrushes, razors, or other personal items, and abstention from sexual intercourse. Unlike hepatitis A, for which everyone in the home may be given preventive shots to forestall infection, with hepatitis B only the spouse (or sexual partner) is immunized. So ask your doctor about immunization.

If you haven't been tested for hepatitis B and experience any of its symptoms (yellowing of the skin or whites of the eyes, along with vomiting, abdominal pain, and loss of appetite), ask your doctor about being tested. A test may be a good idea even if you have no symptoms, since many cases of hepatitis are so mild that no symptoms, or only stomach-flu-like ones, are noted.[4]

When an expectant mother (or any-

---

3. At highest risk of hepatitis B, which is transmitted through blood and body fluids, are IV drug users, homosexual men, and heterosexuals with more than one partner in a six-month period. Also at risk are health-care workers and immigrants from China, Southeast Asia, and other high-prevalence areas. Vaccination is available and is recommended for these groups.

4. It's now recommended that all pregnant women be tested for hepatitis B. If a woman tests positive, her family will usually be immunized and her newborn treated with vaccine and immune globulin.

one else) has an active hepatitis B infection, bed rest and a nutritious diet are the mainstays of treatment. Alcoholic beverages must be avoided, but that applies to pregnant women in general anyway. The patient's blood is checked periodically to monitor the progress of the disease. In 95% of cases, full recovery can be expected; in the others, the disease may become very severe or chronic.

If the hepatitis B virus is present in the mother at delivery, bathing the newborn as soon as possible to remove all traces of maternal blood and secretions, and administering hepatitis B vaccine and immune globulin within 12 hours of birth, usually prevent the infection taking hold in the baby. Treatment is repeated at 1 and 6 months, and the child is usually tested at 12 to 15 months to be sure that the therapy has been effective.

There are other forms of hepatitis, such as hepatitis C and hepatitis E (also known as non-A non-B hepatitis). At present it isn't clear whether or not these can be transmitted from mother to child during pregnancy or childbirth.

MUMPS

"A co-worker just came down with mumps. I don't know if I ever had the disease. Would it be dangerous to get it now that I'm expecting?"

Mumps in pregnancy is rare because most young adults today either had the disease or were immunized against it as children. If you can, check with your parents or the doctor who cared for you as a child to see if you are in this category. If you're not, you still may not come down with mumps because it is not highly contagious. Nevertheless, because the disease appears to trigger uterine contractions and thus can lead to

miscarriage in early pregnancy or to premature labor later, you should be alert for the first symptoms of the disease (possibly vague pain, fever, and loss of appetite before the salivary, or parotid, glands become swollen; then ear pain and pain on chewing or on taking acidic or sour food or drink). Notify your doctor of such symptoms immediately, because prompt treatment can reduce the chance of problems developing.

CHICKEN POX (VARICELLA)

"My toddler was exposed to chicken pox at her day care center. If she comes down with it, could the baby I'm now carrying be hurt?"

Not likely. Well insulated from the rest of the world, the fetus can't contract chicken pox, or varicella, from a third party—only from its mother. And you would have to catch it first, which may very well be impossible. There is only a small chance that you didn't have the infection as a child (85% to 95% of today's adult population has had it) and are not already immune. Ask your mother, or check your health records to find out whether you have had chicken pox. If you can't find out for sure, ask your practitioner to run a test to see if you are immune.

Though the chances of your becoming infected are slim even if you aren't immune (about 1 to 5 in 10,000), an injection of varicella-zoster immune globulin (VZIG) within 96 hours of exposure may be recommended. It isn't clear whether or not this will protect the baby should you come down with chicken pox anyway, but it should minimize complications for you, which is significant, since this mild childhood disease can be quite severe in adults, sometimes causing varicella pneumonia. (Whether or not it is even more severe in pregnant women is a matter of debate.) If you should be hit with a severe case, treatment with an antiviral drug may be begun to reduce the risk of complications.

There is a risk of damage to the fetus when the mother is infected, but it is a small one. Even if a fetus is exposed when most vulnerable—during the first half of pregnancy—there's only a 2% to 10% chance of its developing the defects typical of congenital varicella syndrome. When the exposure occurs in the second half of pregnancy, fetal damage is extremely rare.

Chicken pox once again becomes a threat close to term, when a maternal infection can lead to a baby being born with neonatal varicella. The risk is reduced if delivery doesn't occur until the mother develops antibodies and passes them to the fetus through the placenta, which may take 1 to 2 weeks. But if a mother develops chicken pox within 4 or 5 days of delivery, there's a 15% to 30% chance her newborn will arrive infected and will develop the characteristic rash within a week or so. Since neonatal varicella can be extremely serious, VZIG is usually given to the baby. The risk of the newborn being infected is small if maternal infection occurs between 5 and 21 days before delivery, and serious consequences from the disease at that point are rare.

Incidentally, shingles, or herpes zoster, which is a reactivation of the chicken pox virus in someone who had the disease earlier, does not appear to be harmful to a developing fetus, probably because the mother and thus the baby already have antibodies to the virus.

Once the now experimental varicella vaccine is approved for general use, women who are not immune will probably be routinely vaccinated prior to conception, effectively eliminating the issue of chicken pox in pregnancy.

FEVER

"I'm running a fever. Should I take aspirin to bring it down?"

During most of your life, fever needn't be feared or fought. In fact, it is one of the body's most powerful allies in the war against infection. During pregnancy, however, an increase of body temperature to over 104 degrees for a day or more can cause birth defects—particularly during weeks three to seven of pregnancy. Damage may occasionally occur when a temperature as low as 102 degrees is sustained for two or more days. So bringing a fever down promptly—rather than letting it run its course—becomes the safest way to go.

How best to bring a fever down will depend on how high it has gone up, and on your practitioner's recommendations. Call your doctor the same day if you're running a fever of between 100 and 102 degrees; call immediately if it's 102 or higher. For a temperature under 102, home remedies, such as a cool bath (see Appendix), may do the trick without medication. For a higher temperature related to a bacterial infection, acetaminophen teamed with an antibiotic (there are several that are considered safe for use during pregnancy) will probably be prescribed. Aspirin should not be routinely taken for fever (see below).

TAKING ASPIRIN AND NONASPIRIN

"Last week I took two aspirins for a pounding headache, and now I read that

aspirin can cause birth defects. I'm a nervous wreck."

Of the millions of Americans who opened their medicine cabinets today and reached for a bottle of aspirin, few thought twice—or even once—about its safety. And for most people, occasional aspirin use is not only helpful but perfectly harmless. But during pregnancy, there is concern that aspirin, like many other ordinarily innocuous over-the-counter remedies, may be hazardous.

If you've unwittingly taken one or two aspirins on one, or even a few, occasions in the first two trimesters, don't worry—there is no evidence they will hurt your baby. It's estimated that 1 in every 2 pregnant women takes at least one dose of aspirin during pregnancy, with seemingly no ill effect. For the rest of your pregnancy, however, it's advisable to treat aspirin as you would any other drug, taking it only when absolutely necessary and only when recommended by a practitioner who knows you're pregnant.

Aspirin use is most risky in the third trimester, when even one dose can interfere with fetal growth and cause other problems. Because it is an antiprostaglandin, and prostaglandins are involved in the mechanism of labor, aspirin can prolong both pregnancy and labor and lead to other complications during delivery. And since it interferes with blood-clotting, aspirin taken during the two weeks before delivery can increase the risk of hemorrhage at delivery and even bleeding problems in the newborn.

On the other hand, the careful, medically supervised use of low doses of aspirin (less than half a regular-strength tablet a day) to treat immunologic conditions (such as lupus), to stop preterm labor, or to prevent preeclampsia or fetal growth retardation, does not seem to cause such problems.

Indiscriminately popping aspirin substitutes in place of aspirin isn't the logical solution in pregnancy. Though the moderate use of acetaminophen (Tylenol, Datril, Anacin III) in pregnancy appears to pose no problem, it too should be taken only when necessary, and *only* with the approval of your practitioner.

Ibuprofen (Advil, Nuprin, Medipren) is a relatively new entry in the pain reliever sweepstakes. Similar to aspirin in some ways, it may trigger a cross reaction in those sensitive to aspirin. Though there have been no reports of problems when ibuprofen is used early in pregnancy, its use in the last trimester can result in problems in the unborn child, a prolonged pregnancy, and/or a prolonged labor. Because of this risk, don't use this medication at all in the last three months of pregnancy, and use it earlier only if recommended by a physician who knows you are pregnant. (But don't worry about the ibuprofen you took before you found out you were pregnant.)

While caution is imperative in considering the use of these medications, avoiding their use entirely is unwarranted. There are times when pain can not be relieved or a fever brought down in any other way. The most sensible course in pregnancy is first to try to use nondrug remedies (see Appendix) for pain or low-grade fever, and then to resort to nonaspirin acetaminophen products—under medical supervision—if those methods fail.

TAKING MEDICATIONS

"How do I know which medicines, if any, are safe to take during pregnancy, and which aren't?"

No drug, prescription or over-the-counter, is 100% safe for 100% of the people 100% of the time. And when you're pregnant, every time you take a drug there are two individuals at risk, one very small and vulnerable. Although a few drugs have been shown to be particularly hazardous to a developing fetus, many drugs have been used safely during pregnancy, and there are situations in which medication is absolutely essential to life and/or health. Whether you will take a particular medication at a particular time during pregnancy is something you and your physician will have to decide by weighing the drug's potential risks against the benefits it offers. In any case, the general rule should be: take medication only on the advice of a physician who knows you are pregnant, and only when it is absolutely necessary.

Which drug you take in a specific situation will depend on the latest information available on drug safety in pregnancy. The many lists of safe, possibly safe, possibly unsafe, and definitely unsafe drugs may provide some assistance, but most are outdated and unreliable by the time they're published. Package inserts and labels are of limited use, since most warn not to use the product during pregnancy without a physician's orders, even when the product is believed safe. Your best sources of information will be:

❖ A well-informed physician (not all are familiar with drug safety in pregnancy); a maternal-fetal medicine subspecialist may be particularly helpful.

❖ The Food and Drug Administration—contact your regional office or write to the Public Health Service, FDA, Parklawn Building, 5600 Fisher's Lane, Rockville, MD 20857.

❖ The March of Dimes—try your local office first, or contact the National Foundation/March of Dimes,

1275 Mamaroneck Avenue, White Plains, NY 10605.

Once you've made certain that a prescribed drug is considered safe for use during pregnancy, don't hesitate to take it because you're still afraid it might somehow harm your baby. It won't—but delaying treatment might.

If you do need some kind of medication during pregnancy, follow these steps for increased benefit and reduced risk:

❖ Discuss with your physician the possibility of taking the medication in the smallest effective doses for the shortest possible time.

❖ Take the medication when it's going to benefit you the most—a cold medication at night, for instance, so it will help you sleep.

❖ Follow package or doctor's directions carefully. Some medications must be taken on an empty stomach; some should be taken with food or milk. If your physician hasn't given you any instructions, ask your pharmacist for particulars.

❖ Explore nondrug remedies, and use them to supplement the drug therapy—eliminating as many offending allergens from your home as you can, for instance, so your physician can reduce the amount of prescribed antihistamine you take.

❖ Make sure the medication gets where it's supposed to by taking a sip of water before you swallow a capsule or tablet, to make it go down more easily, and by drinking a full glass afterward, to ensure that it is washed speedily down to where it will be absorbed. Taking the medication while sitting or standing, rather than lying down or propped up, may also help speed its passage.

HERBAL CURES

"I wouldn't think of taking any drugs during pregnancy. But would it be all right to substitute medicinal herbs?"

M edicinal herbs *are* drugs—often very powerful ones. Some are so powerful that they're used in laboratories to produce prescription medicines. Others have been used for generations in some societies to induce abortions, and some have been linked to miscarriage. Even in a seemingly soothing cup of tea, some herbs are capable of producing such symptoms as diarrhea, vomiting, and heart palpitations. The use of herbal medicines presents an added risk that isn't present when the remedies come from the drugstore. They are not made under quality-controlled conditions, and may be dangerously strong or impotently weak. They may also contain harmful contaminants, including such allergens as insect parts, pollens, and molds, and even such toxic agents as lead or arsenic.

So treat medicinal herbs as you would any drugs during pregnancy. Do not take them except on the advice of your doctor. If you are experiencing any symptoms that need treatment, check with your practitioner instead of trying to self treat.

Also avoid herbal teas. If you've been drinking herbal teas up until now, don't worry. They obviously haven't made you ill or caused problems in your pregnancy. But from now on, avoid them unless prescribed by your doctor. If you're hankering for the taste of a favorite herbal tea, concoct your own potion by adding any of the following to boiling water or decaffeinated tea: orange, apple, pineapple, or other fruit juice; raspberry, strawberry, orange, or other jam or marmalade; slices of lemon, lime, orange, apple, pear, or other fruit; mint leaves, cinnamon, nutmeg, cloves, or other spices. And never make tea from a plant growing in your backyard unless you are absolutely certain what it is and that it is safe to use in pregnancy.

WHAT IT'S IMPORTANT TO KNOW: STAYING WELL

I n pregnancy, because of the potentially harmful effects of both illness and medication on the unborn baby, the proverbial ounce of prevention is worth far more than a pound of cure. The following suggestions will increase your odds of staying well, whether you're pregnant or not.

❖ Ideally, you should have gotten your immunizations up to date before you conceived (see page 425). If that wasn't done, ask about the results of your rubella (German measles) test to see if you are immune or susceptible to the disease. If you're not immune, try to avoid contact with anyone infected. Also ask about flu shots if flu season is approaching. They can be given during pregnancy and greatly reduce the chances of your coming down with influenza.

❖ Keep your resistance up. Eat the best diet possible (see the Best-Odds Diet, page 80); get enough sleep and adequate exercise; and don't run yourself down by running yourself ragged.

❖ Avoid sick people like the plague. Try to stay away from anyone who has a cold, flu, stomach virus, or anything else noticeably contagious. Distance yourself from coughers on the bus, avoid lunching with a colleague who's complaining of a sore throat, and evade the handshake of a friend with a runny nose (germs as well as greetings can be exchanged in a handshake). Also avoid crowded or cramped indoor spaces when you can. Wash your hands thoroughly after exposure to crowds or riding on public transportation—especially before touching your mouth, nose, or eyes.

❖ At home, limit contact with sick children or a sick spouse as much as possible (have other family members, a sitter, or a nonpregnant friend play nursemaid). Avoid finishing up their lunches, drinking from their cups, and kissing them on the face. Wash your hands after any contact with the patients, their linens, or soiled tissues, especially before touching your own eyes, nose, or mouth. See that they wash their hands frequently, too, and that they cover their mouths when they cough or sneeze. Use disinfectant, such as Lysol spray, on telephones and other surfaces they handle. Isolate contaminated toothbrushes, and replace them when the illness is over.

❖ If your own child or a child you regularly spend time with develops a rash of any kind, avoid close contact and call your doctor at once

unless you already know that you are immune to rubella, German measles, chicken pox, fifth disease, and CMV (cytomegalovirus).

❖ To avoid food poisoning, practice safe food preparation and storage habits: keeping hot foods hot and cold foods cold, refrigerating leftovers quickly, and discarding questionable items. Use nonporous surfaces (such as Formica, glass, stainless steel) rather than porous ones (wood or plastic with dirt-collecting gashes) for food preparation, and keep them scrupulously clean. Hands, too, should be washed before food is handled and after touching raw meat, fish, or eggs. Always cook meats, fish, and poultry thoroughly, and if there is a threat of salmonella in your area, do the same with eggs (eggs that are certified "fresh" and kept refrigerated in the market are the safest). Avoid eating in restaurants that seem to ignore basic sanitation rules (perishable foods are kept at room temperature, kitchen workers and waiters handle food directly with their hands, bathrooms are unclean, and so on).

❖ Keep pets in good health, updating their immunizations as necessary. If you have a cat, take the precautions to avoid toxoplasmosis (page 65).

❖ Avoid outdoor areas where Lyme disease is prevalent, or be sure to protect yourself adequately (see page 316).

❖ Don't share toothbrushes or other personal items.

16
Coping With a Chronic Condition

A nyone who's lived with a chronic condition knows that life can get pretty complicated, what with the special diets, the medications, and the medical monitoring. Anyone who's lived with a chronic condition while being pregnant knows that those complications can double, with the special diet needing to be modified, the medications altered, and the medical monitoring stepped up.

In the past there was another complication for women with chronic conditions who became pregnant: ma-

jor risk to themselves and their babies. Today, happily, thanks to many scientific advances, that complication is much less common and most chronic conditions *are* compatible with pregnancy. Still, special precautions are necessary on the part of both the mother and her medical providers. This chapter outlines those precautions for the most common chronic conditions. Where the recommendations in this chapter differ from your doctor's, be sure to follow those of your doctor, since they probably have been tailored to your personal needs.

WHAT YOU MAY BE CONCERNED ABOUT

DIABETES

"I'm a diabetic, and I'm concerned about the effect of my condition on my baby."

U ntil recently, getting pregnant was a risky business for the diabetic woman, and even riskier for her unborn baby. Today, with expert medical care and guidance and scrupulous

self care, the diabetic woman has just about as good a chance of having a successful pregnancy and a healthy baby as any other pregnant woman does. In fact, diabetic women in one study took such excellent care of themselves throughout their pregnancies that they and their babies had even *fewer* problems than their nondiabetic counterparts.

Making your diabetic pregnancy a success will take a good deal of effort on your part, but the reward—a healthy baby—will make it well worthwhile.

Research has proved that the key to successfully managing a diabetic pregnancy is maintaining euglycemia (normal blood glucose levels). The availability in the past few years of home monitoring, split-dose administration of insulin, and even insulin pumps has made this increasingly possible.

Whether you came into pregnancy a diabetic or developed gestational diabetes along the way, all of the following considerations will be important in working toward a safe pregnancy and a healthy baby.[1]

Doctor's Orders. You will probably see your obstetrician (as well as your internist or endocrinologist) more often than do other expectant moms. You will be given many more orders, and will have to be far more scrupulous in following them.

Good Diet. A diet geared to your personal requirements should be carefully planned with your physician, a nutritionist, or a nurse-practitioner with expertise in diabetes. The diet will probably be high in complex carbohydrates, particularly beans (about half your daily calories should be from carbohydrates), moderate in protein (20% of caloric intake), low in cholesterol and fat (30% of caloric intake, no more than 10% saturated), and contain no sugary sweets. Plenty of dietary fiber will be important (40

to 70 grams daily are recommended), since some studies show that fiber may reduce insulin requirements in diabetic pregnancies. Calories may be restricted, particularly if you are overweight.

The extent of your carbohydrate restriction will depend on the way your body reacts to particular foods. Some women can handle fruit and fruit juices; others experience sharp blood sugar increases on consuming them, in which case they have to get more of their carbohydrates from vegetable, grain, and legume sources than from fruits (and may not be able to partake of certain Best-Odds treats). To maintain normal blood sugar levels, you will have to be particularly careful to get enough carbohydrates in the morning. Snacks will also be important, and ideally they should include both a complex carbohydrate (such as whole-grain bread) and a protein (such as meat or cheese). Your caloric requirement, like that of other pregnant women, will increase by about 300 calories a day over what you needed before pregnancy, and your protein requirement by about 30 grams (an average serving of meat or fish). Skipping meals or snacks can dangerously lower blood sugar, so be sure to eat regularly.

Pregnancy is not a time to be lax about your diet, although exhaustion may tempt you to be. It is, rather, an ideal time to get your dietary act together—for you and for your baby. Perfecting dietary control in a diabetic pregnancy is so important that many specialists recommend in-hospital training for diabetic women prior to conception or early in pregnancy. In some cases, in-hospital training may also be recommended for women who develop diabetes as pregnancy progresses (gestational diabetes).

If morning sickness is a problem at any time during pregnancy, try not to let it interfere with nourishing your

---

1. These are components of a typical diabetic pregnancy program. The one laid out for you by your physician or medical team may differ and is the one you should follow. If you are not already pregnant, your physician will start you on a special program to ready you for conception.

Safe Exercise Heart Rate for Diabetic Pregnancies

It is usually recommended that pregnant women with diabetes not exercise beyond 70% of the maximum safe heart rate for their age group, which is determined by subtracting one's age from 220, then multiplying the result by .70. If you are 30, for example, you would figure it this way: 220 − 30 = 190; then .70 × 190 = 133. This means that 133 beats per minute would be your upper safe limit of exercise intensity, the level you should not exceed.

---

baby and keeping your blood sugar stable.[2] Never fast or skip meals; eating regularly is essential. If you have trouble getting down three large meals, take six to eight small ones, regularly spaced and carefully planned. (See page 105 for some general tips on dealing with morning sickness.)

Sensible Weight Gain. It's best to try to reach your ideal weight before conception (something to remember if you plan another pregnancy). But if you start your pregnancy overweight, don't plan on using the gestational period for slimming down. Getting sufficient calories is vital to your baby's well-being. Weight gain should progress according to the guidelines set by your physician, usually 25 to 30 pounds during the nine months.

Exercise. A moderate exercise program will give you more energy, aid in regulating your blood sugar, and help you get in shape for delivery. But it must be planned in conjunction with your medication schedule and diet plan by or with the help of your medical team. If you experience no other medical or pregnancy complications and are physically fit, such moderate exercise as brisk walking, swimming, and light stationary biking (but not jogging) will likely be suggested. Only light exercise (such as leisurely walking) will be allowed if you were out of condition prior to pregnancy or if there are any signs of problems with your diabetes, your pregnancy, or your baby's growth.

Precautions you may be asked to observe when exercising include taking a snack, such as milk, before your workout; not allowing your heart rate (pulse) during exercise to exceed 70% of the maximum safe heart rate for your age (see box); and never exercising in a warm environment (with temperatures in the 80s or higher). If you are on insulin, you will probably be advised to avoid injecting insulin into the parts of the body being exercised (your legs, for example, if you're walking) and not to reduce your insulin intake prior to exercise.

Rest. Especially in the third trimester, adequate rest is very important. Avoid overtaxing your energies, and try to take some time off during the middle of the day for putting your feet up or napping. If you have a job, especially a demanding one, your doctor may recommend that you begin your maternity leave early.

---

2. If nausea and vomiting interfere with eating, check with your physician about adjusting your insulin intake.

Medication Regulation. If diet and exercise alone do not control your blood sugar, you will probably be put on insulin. If you had been taking oral medication for diabetes prior to conception, you will be switched to injected insulin, which is less likely to adversely affect your fetus, for the duration of your pregnancy. If you need insulin for the first time, you may be hospitalized briefly so that your blood sugar can be stabilized under close medical supervision. Since levels of the pregnancy hormones that work against insulin increase as pregnancy progresses, your insulin dose may have to be adjusted upward periodically. The dose may also have to be recalculated as your size and your baby's size change, or if you are ill or under emotional strain.

Blood Sugar Regulation. You may have to test your blood sugar (with a simple finger-prick method) at least four or as often as ten times a day to be sure it is remaining at safe levels. To maintain euglycemia, you will have to eat regularly (no meal skipping), adjust your diet and exercise as needed, and, if necessary, take medication. If you were insulin dependent before pregnancy, you should be aware that you are more subject to hypoglycemic (low blood sugar) episodes than when you were not pregnant. This is especially common in the first trimester.

Reduction of Other Risk Factors. Since risk in pregnancy is cumulative—the more risk factors, the higher the risk—you should endeavor to eliminate or minimize as many as possible. (See Reducing Risk in Any Pregnancy, page 50.)

Careful Monitoring. Don't be alarmed if your physician orders a great many tests for you (in and out of the hospital), especially during the third trimester, or even suggests hospitalization for the final weeks of your pregnancy. This doesn't mean something is wrong, only that he or she wants to be sure that everything stays right. The tests will primarily be directed toward regular evaluation of your condition and that of your baby, in order to determine the optimal time for delivery and whether any other intervention is needed.

You will probably have regular eye exams to check the condition of your retinas and blood tests to evaluate your kidneys (retinal and kidney problems tend to worsen during pregnancy, but usually return to prepregnancy states after delivery). The condition of your baby and the placenta will probably be evaluated through stress and/or non-stress tests (see page 263), biophysical profiles, amniocentesis (to determine lung maturity and readiness for delivery), and sonography (to size up your baby to be sure it's growing as it should be and so that delivery can be accomplished before he or she's too big for vaginal delivery).

You may be asked to monitor fetal movements yourself three times a day (see page 202 for one way to do this). If you don't feel movement during any test period, call your doctor immediately.

Don't panic if your baby is placed in a neonatal intensive care unit immediately after delivery. This is routine procedure in most hospitals for infants of diabetic mothers. Your baby will be observed for respiratory problems (which are unlikely if the lungs were tested and found to be mature enough for delivery) and for hypoglycemia (which, though more common in babies of diabetics, responds quickly and completely to treatment).

Elective Early Delivery. Because babies of many diabetics tend to be too large for full-term vaginal delivery (particularly when euglycemia has not been maintained throughout pregnancy); because their placentas often begin to deteriorate early (robbing the fetus of vital nutrients and oxygen during the last weeks); and because they are subject to acidosis (abnormal acid-base balance in the blood) and other problems, they are often delivered before term, generally at about 38 or 39 weeks. The various tests mentioned above help the physician to decide when to induce labor or perform a cesarean—late enough so that the fetal lungs are sufficiently mature to function outside the womb, not so late that fetal safety has been jeopardized. Women who developed gestational diabetes, as well as women with pre-existing mild diabetes and sometimes even those with very well-controlled moderate disease, can often carry to term safely.

ASTHMA

"I've been an asthmatic since childhood. I'm concerned that the attacks and the drugs I take for them might harm my baby."

While it's true that a severe asthmatic condition does put a pregnancy at higher risk, studies have shown that this risk can be almost completely eliminated. Asthmatics who are under close, expert medical supervision (preferably by their internist and/or allergist in collaboration with their obstetrician) throughout their pregnancies have as good a chance of having normal pregnancies and healthy babies as nonasthmatics. But though asthma, if controlled, has only a minimal effect on pregnancy, pregnancy often has a considerable effect on asthma. With about one-third of pregnant asthmatics, the effect is positive—their asthma improves. In another third, their condition stays about the same. In the remaining third (usually those with the most severe disease) the asthma worsens, generally after the fourth month.

Whether your asthma is mild or severe, you and your baby will benefit if you get the condition under control before conception or at least early in pregnancy. The following steps will help:

❖ If you smoke, quit immediately. See page 55 for how-to tips.

❖ Identify environmental triggers. The most common offenders are pollens, animal danders (you may need to board your pet at a friend's), dusts, and molds. Tobacco smoke, household cleaning products, and perfumes can also provoke a reaction, and it's a good idea to steer clear of them. (See Allergies, page 157, for tips on avoiding allergens.) If you were started on allergy shots before pregnancy, this treatment will probably be continued. If necessary, such therapy may be begun during pregnancy. Attacks can also be brought on by exercise; these can usually be prevented by taking the medication prescribed by your doctor for this purpose prior to exertion.

❖ Try to avoid colds, flu, and other respiratory infections. (See page 323.) Your doctor may give you medication to ward off an asthma attack at the beginning of a mild cold, and will probably want to treat any but the most minor respiratory infections with antibiotics. You may also be immunized against influenza and pneumococcal infections.

❖ If you have an asthma attack, treat it immediately with your prescribed medication, to avoid depriving the fetus of oxygen. If the medication doesn't help, head for the nearest emergency room or call your doctor immediately.

❖ Take only drugs that have been prescribed by your physician *during your pregnancy,* and take them only as prescribed *for pregnancy use.* If your symptoms are mild, you may not require medication. If they are moderate to severe, there are several medications, both inhaled and ingested, that are considered to be "probably safe" for the fetus. The risks of taking these medications, if any, are quite small compared to the benefits of preventing fetal hypoxia (oxygen deprivation). And as an added benefit, some of these medications actually appear to reduce the risk of pre-eclampsia (see page 204) as well.

❖ Reduce other pregnancy risk factors. Since pregnancy risks are cumulative, you should endeavor to eliminate or minimize as many as possible. (See Reducing Risk in Any Pregnancy, page 50.)

The normal breathlessness that afflicts a majority of women in late pregnancy (see page 234) may be alarming to the asthmatic mother-to-be, but it is not dangerous. However, in the last trimester, as breathing becomes more labored because of the enlarged uterus crowding the lungs, pregnant asthmatics may notice a worsening of asthmatic flare-ups. Prompt treatment is especially important during such attacks.

The tendency toward allergies and asthma is inherited, and so it is wise for asthmatics to postpone exposing their babies to potential food allergens by breastfeeding exclusively for at least six months, thereby delaying the onset of allergic sensitization in their children and possibly reducing their long-term risk of allergy.

CHRONIC HYPERTENSION

"I've had hypertension for years. How will my high blood pressure affect my pregnancy?"

Since increasing numbers of women are choosing to conceive in their 30s and 40s and hypertension (high blood pressure) is more common as one gets older, the condition is showing up in more and more pregnant women. So you're not alone. Still, yours is considered a high-risk pregnancy (see page 339), which means that you will be seeing your doctor or doctors more often (preferably beginning with pre-pregnancy counseling), and will have to follow their advice more faithfully. But assuming that your blood pressure remains under control, with good medical and self care, it is very likely that both you and your baby will come through pregnancy well. Recent studies show that even those hypertensive women who have some kidney impairment can usually have successful pregnancies.

All of the following can help increase the odds of a successful pregnancy:

Relaxation. Pay more than just passing attention to the kinds of relaxation exercises mentioned on page 114. Try, too, any others that are recommended by your physician, such as biofeedback. Studies have shown that relaxation can help lower high blood pressure.

Blood Pressure Monitoring. You may be advised to take your own blood pressure daily, using a home blood pressure kit. Take it when you are most relaxed.

Good Diet. The Best-Odds Diet is particularly important to women with high-risk pregnancies. The one variation that may be recommended by your doctor is limitation of foods high in sodium, though this isn't universal. Do follow any such recommendation rigorously.

Adequate Fluid. Though your first instinct on experiencing a slight swelling of your feet and ankles because of fluid retention may be to cut down on your fluid intake, you should really do just the opposite. Drinking more water (up to a gallon a day), rather than less, will help flush out the excess.

Plenty of Rest. Take rest breaks, preferably with your feet up, both morning and afternoon. If you work at a high-stress job, consider giving it up until after the baby arrives. If you have your hands full at home with other children, get help—paid or volunteer.

Prescribed Medication. If you have been taking medication to control your blood pressure, your physician may okay your continuing it, or he or she may prescribe one that is considered to be safer in pregnancy. There are several blood-pressure-regulating drugs that appear to be safe when taken as directed. Low-dose aspirin may be prescribed to prevent preeclampsia.

Attention to Your Body. Be alert to signs of pregnancy complications (see page 117), and contact your physician immediately if you experience any of them.

Close Medical Monitoring. Your physician will probably schedule more frequent visits for you than for other expectant mothers, and may subject you to many more tests.

If your blood pressure is very high and remains high in spite of medication, and/or you have serious side effects, such as retinal hemorrhages, severely impaired kidney function, or an enlarged heart, the risks of an unfavorable outcome to your pregnancy increase. In such a case, you may, in consultation with your physicians, have to weigh risks against benefits before deciding to attempt a pregnancy or continue with one already under way.

MULTIPLE SCLEROSIS (MS)

"I was diagnosed several years ago as having multiple sclerosis. I've only had two episodes of MS, and they were relatively mild. Will the MS affect my pregnancy? Will my pregnancy affect my MS?"

Multiple sclerosis appears to have little if any effect on pregnancy. Nevertheless, early and regular prenatal care, coupled with regular visits to your neurologist, is a must. Iron supplements will probably be prescribed to prevent anemia and if necessary, stool softeners to combat constipation. Because urinary tract infections are more common in pregnancy, and because they could cause MS symptoms to flare, you may be given antibiotics as a preventive measure if you have a history of UTIs. Labor and delivery are not usually affected by MS, either. Epidural anesthesia, if needed, appears to be safe for use during both.

Nor does pregnancy seem to have much effect on MS. In fact, during pregnancy most women with MS find that their condition stabilizes, though in the later months, as weight gain increases, those with preexisting gait problems may find these exacerbated. If steroids are needed, prednisone in low to moderate doses is considered safe to use. Some other medications used for MS are less so; be sure to have your doctor check out the safety for use in pregnancy of any medication before you take it.

Though risk of relapse doesn't seem to increase during pregnancy, it does in the first six months postpartum. This risk, however, doesn't appear to be as serious as once supposed or to affect the overall lifetime relapse rate or the extent of ultimate disability. To reduce the risk of postpartum relapse, take your iron supplements as prescribed, and try to minimize stress, get adequate rest, and avoid infection and raising your temperature unduly (as in exercise or a hot tub). Going back to work early in the postpartum period may increase both exhaustion and stress, so discuss the risks with your doctor before deciding to return.

Breastfeeding will be possible, even if you occasionally need to take steroid medication; in small doses, very little of the drug passes into the breast milk. If you have to take large doses temporarily, you can pump your milk and discard it, giving your baby formula or previously pumped milk until the drug is gone from your milk. If breastfeeding is stressful for you, consider switching to bottle feeding, partially or completely—and don't feel guilty about your decision. Babies do very well on a good formula.

Most MS mothers manage to stay active for 25 years or more after their diseases are diagnosed, and are able to carry out childcare chores without difficulty. However, if MS does interfere with your functioning while your child is young, see page 334 for tips on baby care for disabled parents.[3]

AN EATING DISORDER

'I've been fighting bulimia for the last ten years. I thought I'd be able to stop the bingeing/purging cycle now that I'm pregnant, but I can't seem to. Will it hurt my baby?"

Not if you quit right away. The fact that you've been bulimic (or anorectic) for a number of years puts your baby and your body at a disadvantage right off the bat—your nutritional reserves are probably low. Fortunately, early in pregnancy the need for nourishment is less than it will be later on, so you have the chance to make up for the abuse done to your body before it can damage your baby.

There has been very little research in the area of eating disorders and pregnancy, partly because these disorders cause disrupted menstrual cycles, allowing very few women with such problems to become pregnant in the first place. But the studies that have been done suggest the following:

❖ A woman with an eating disorder who controls her dangerous habit during pregnancy is as likely as anyone else to have a healthy baby—all other things being equal.

❖ It is important that the practitioner who is caring for her pregnancy be informed of the eating disorder.

❖ Counseling from a professional who is experienced in treating eating disorders is advisable for anyone who suffers from such a problem, but it is essential for the woman who is pregnant. Support groups may also be helpful.

❖ The laxatives, diuretics, and other drugs taken by bulimics are harmful to a developing fetus if the mother continues taking them once she learns she's pregnant. They draw off nutrients and fluids from the mother's body before they

3. Many women with MS are concerned about passing the disease on to their children. Though there is a genetic component to the disease, placing these children at increased risk of being affected as adults, the risk is really quite small. Between 90% and 95% of children of MS mothers remain MS free. If you are concerned nevertheless, see a genetic counselor.

can be utilized to nourish her baby (and later to produce milk); and they may lead to fetal abnormality. These medications, like all others, should not be used by any pregnant woman unless prescribed by a physician who is aware of the pregnancy.

It is also clear that it is necessary for you, and anyone else with an eating disorder, to understand the dynamics of weight gain in pregnancy. Keep in mind the following:

❖ The pregnant shape is beautiful, not fat and repugnant. Whereas excess fat may ordinarily be unhealthy and unattractive, pregnancy weight gain is vital to your baby's growth and well-being as well as to your own health.

❖ Gaining a moderate amount of weight each week in the second and third trimesters of pregnancy is not only normal, it's desirable (see page 147). If you stay within the recommended guidelines (which are higher in those who begin pregnancy underweight), you will be able to lose the weight easily after the baby arrives.

❖ If the weight is gained on high-quality foods as recommended in the Best-Odds Diet, the chances of having a healthy baby increase considerably, as do the chances that you'll recover your figure faster postpartum.

❖ Exercise can help avoid excessive weight gain, and can ensure that what weight is gained ends up in the right places—but it should be exercise appropriate for a pregnant woman (see page 189).

❖ All of the weight gain of pregnancy does not drop off in the first few days after delivery. With sensible eating, the average woman returns to close to her prepregnancy weight about six weeks after delivery, though for some women the weight loss process takes longer. If negative feelings about your body image cause you to slip back into bingeing and purging during the postpartum period (which could interfere with your ability to recover from childbirth, to parent effectively, and to produce milk if you choose to breastfeed), it's important that you continue professional counseling with someone experienced in the treatment of eating disorders or get help if you hadn't previously.

If you cannot seem to refrain from bingeing, vomiting, diuretics or laxatives, or practicing semi-starvation, you should discuss with your physician the possibility of hospitalization until you get your disease under control. If this isn't acceptable, you may want to consider whether this is the right time for you to be pregnant.

PHYSICAL DISABILITY

"I'm a paraplegic because of a spinal-cord injury, and I'm confined to a wheelchair. In spite of a lot of dire warnings and our own fears, my husband and I have wanted a baby for a long while. I've finally become pregnant. Now what?"

Like every pregnant woman, you'll need to deal with first things first: selecting a practitioner. And like every pregnant woman who falls into a high-risk category, your practitioner should ideally be an obstetrician or maternal-fetal subspecialist who has experience dealing with women who face the same challenges and potential risks as you do. If such a person isn't available in your area, you need a doctor who is willing to learn "on the job," and who is able to offer the wholehearted support you and your husband will need. Toward the end of your pregnancy you will also have to start looking for a pediatrician or family doctor who will be supportive of you as a physically challenged parent.

Just which special measures will be necessary to make your pregnancy successful will depend on your physical limitations. In any case, restricting your weight gain to within the recommended range (25 to 35 pounds) will help to minimize the stress on your body. Eating the best possible diet will improve your general physical well-being while decreasing the likelihood of pregnancy complications. And keeping up your physical therapy will help ensure that you have maximum strength and mobility when the baby arrives. It should be reassuring to know that, though pregnancy may be more difficult for you than for other pregnant women, it should not be any more stressful for your baby. There is no evidence of an increase in fetal abnormality among babies of spinal-cord injury patients (or of those with other physical disabilities not related to hereditary or systemic disease).

Women with spinal-cord injuries are more susceptible to such pregnancy problems as kidney infections and bladder difficulties, palpitations and sweating, anemia, and muscle spasms. Childbirth, too, may pose special problems, though in most cases a vaginal delivery will be possible. Because uterine contractions will probably be painless, you will have to be instructed to note other signs of impending labor.

Long before your due date, devise a fail-safe plan for getting to the hospital—one that takes into account the fact that you may be home alone when labor strikes (you may want to plan to leave for the hospital early in labor to avoid any problems caused by delays en route); prepare the hospital staff for your special needs; and be sure you will be able to get around the obstetrical unit in your wheelchair.

Parenting is always a challenge. It will be even more so for you and your husband. Planning ahead will help you meet this challenge more successfully. Make any necessary modifications to your home to make child care easier (you might try to contact other physically disabled mothers to see what tricks they've learned); sign on help (paid or otherwise) to at least get you started; enlist your spouse in the preparations for your baby's arrival, and divide up the household chores and baby care tasks for when baby comes home. Be creative. You don't have to do things "by the book"—do them in the way that works best for you. Breastfeeding, if it's possible, will make life simpler—you won't have to fuss with sterilizing, rush off to the kitchen to prepare a bottle when baby starts to cry, or shop for formula. A diaper service (they can deliver cloth or disposable diapers) will also save effort and time. The changing table should be tailored for you to use from your wheelchair, and the crib should have a drop side so you can take baby in and out easily. If you are going to be the one to bathe baby (though this is a job fathers often like and do well), you will have to arrange a baby tub on an accessible table. Since daily tub baths aren't a must, you can sponge baby on the changing table or on your lap on alternate days. A baby carrier may be a convenient way for you to carry your baby around, leaving your hands free to control your chair. Joining a support group of parents with disabilities can be not only a source of comfort and strength but also a gold mine of ideas and advice.[4]

---

4. For additional practical parenting advice, get a copy of *Aids and Adaptations for Parents with Physical or Sensory Disabilities* by T. Conine et. al (Vancouver, Canada: School of Rehabilitation Medicine, University of British Columbia, 1988).

It won't be easy, for you or for your husband, who may have to be a more-than-equal partner in parenting. But knowing that you're not the first to do it—and that the vast majority of those who have done it before you have reported that the satisfactions are more than worth the struggles—should be reassuring.

EPILEPSY

"I'm epileptic, and I just found out I'm pregnant. Will my baby be okay?"

With expert medical care, preferably beginning before conception, for both your epilepsy and your pregnancy, the odds are very much with you and your baby; epileptics have a 90% chance of having a healthy baby. If you haven't yet begun seeing an obstetrician, do so as soon as possible. And inform the physician who cares for your epilepsy of your pregnancy; close supervision of your condition, and possibly frequent adjustment of medication levels, will be necessary.

Epileptic mothers-to-be don't seem to have an increased incidence of such serious pregnancy and childbirth complications as miscarriage, pre-eclampsia, and premature birth, but they are more likely to experience excessive nausea and vomiting (hyperemesis).

It's believed that the slight increase in the incidence of certain birth defects in the children of epileptic mothers is in great measure attributable to the use of certain anticonvulsant medications during pregnancy, though some appear related to the epilepsy itself. Ideally, a woman with epilepsy should discuss with her doctor ahead of time the possibility of being weaned from her medications prior to conception. If she has to continue medication, it may be possible to switch to a less risky drug (phenobarbital, for example, causes fewer birth defects than phenytoin [Dilantin]; sodium valproate, trimethadione, and paramethadione appear even more hazardous). But she should not stop taking a necessary medication for fear of hurting her baby; not taking it—and having frequent seizures—may be more dangerous to the unborn child.

Since the greatest risk of abnormalities developing exists during the first three months, there is little reason to worry about the effects of medication after that. Sometimes ultrasound or alpha-fetoprotein tests can determine early in pregnancy whether the fetus has been affected. If you've been taking valproic acid (Depakene), the doctor may want to look specifically for neural-tube defects, such as spina bifida.

Epileptic women often develop folate-deficiency anemia (which research shows may also be related to neural-tube defects in their babies), and so many doctors will prescribe a folic acid supplement for pregnant epileptics even though it may rarely increase the number of seizures. Vitamin D supplementation may also be recommended for women on certain anticonvulsants. During the last two months of pregnancy, a vitamin K supplement may be prescribed to reduce the increased risk of hemorrhage in the newborn. Alternatively, the baby will be given an injection of the vitamin at birth.

Most epileptic women find that pregnancy does not have a negative effect on their epilepsy. Half experience no change in their disease, and a smaller percentage find that seizures become less frequent and milder. A few find, however, that their seizures become more frequent and severe. This may be because of individual differences, or because medication has been vomited or overly diluted in the excess body fluid of pregnancy. The problem of losing medication by vomiting can often be minimized by taking a time-release anticonvulsant before going to bed, which allows the medication to build up before vomiting begins in the morning. Ask your doctor about the appropriateness of such a drug for you. If the problem is over-dilution of the medication, it may be necessary for your doctor to readjust the dosage.

Once your baby arrives, if you want to breastfeed, it shouldn't be a problem. Most epilepsy medications pass into the breast milk in such low doses that they are unlikely to affect a nursing baby. But do check with your baby's doctor to be sure the specific medications you are taking are okay. And if your breastfed baby becomes unusually sleepy after you've taken a medication, report this to the doctor. A change may be necessary.

PHENYLKETONURIA (PKU)

"I was born with PKU. My doctors let me get off a low-phenylalanine diet when I was in my teens, and I was fine. But when I discussed getting pregnant with my obstetrician, she said I should go back on the diet and stay on it for my entire pregnancy. Should I take her advice even though I feel perfectly fine on a regular diet?"

Not only should you take her advice, you should thank her for it. It has only recently been recognized that pregnant women with phenylketonuria (PKU) who are *not* on a low-phenylalanine diet put their babies at great risk of being born too small, with small head circumferences, malformations, and possible brain damage. Ideally, as your doctor recommended, the special diet should be resumed before conception and blood levels of phenylalanine kept low

through delivery. The phenylalanine-free milk substitute and measured amounts of other foods permitted on this diet should be supplemented with micronutrients (zinc, copper, etc.) that might otherwise be absent from it. And, of course, all foods sweetened with aspartame (Equal or NutraSweet) are absolutely off-limits.

Though this diet isn't appealing, most mothers feel it's clearly worth the sacrifice to protect their developing babies from harm. If in spite of this incentive, you find yourself slipping off the diet, try to get some professional help from a therapist who is familiar with your type of problem. If counseling doesn't help, you should consider whether it is fair to continue the pregnancy with such heavy odds against your baby.

CORONARY ARTERY DISEASE (CAD)

"My doctor warned me not to get pregnant because I have coronary artery disease. But I did accidentally, and I don't want to abort. I want this baby more than anything."

Your situation isn't as unique as it once might have been. CAD, which is seen more often as women grow older, is becoming more common in pregnancy as more women opt to have their babies at a later age.

Whether or not it's safe for you to continue your pregnancy depends on the nature of your disease. If your disease is mild (you have no limitations on physical activity, and ordinary activity doesn't cause undue fatigue, palpitations, breathlessness, or angina) or moderate (you have slight limitations on physical activity, are completely comfortable at rest, but do experience symptoms with ordinary physical activity), chances are good that you can, under very close medical supervision, safely carry a pregnancy to term. If your disease is severe (you have marked limitations on physical activity, even very light activity causes symptoms, though you are comfortable at rest) or very severe (any physical activity causes discomfort, symptoms are noted even at rest), your doctor will probably tell you that carrying this baby will put your life at risk.

You and your husband will have to decide, with the help of your doctor, just how to proceed. When making that decision, keep in mind that if you don't survive the pregnancy, your baby probably won't either. But even if terminating this pregnancy turns out to be necessary in order to save your life, you aren't necessarily doomed to a life of childlessness. It's possible that your heart condition may be correctable (through open-heart surgery, for example), so that you will be able to go through a future pregnancy safely. If surgery isn't an option, perhaps adoption is, assuming you have the strength for childrearing.

If your cardiologist believes you can weather pregnancy safely, you will probably be given some very strict instructions. They will vary depending on your condition, but they may include:

❖ Avoiding physical and emotional stress; in some cases you may be asked to limit your activities for the duration of your pregnancy, possibly even to stay in bed.

❖ Taking your medication faithfully (be sure it's one that is safe for your baby; many appear to be).

❖ Watching your diet carefully so that you don't gain excess weight, which can put additional strain on your heart.

❖ Eating a low-cholesterol, low-saturated-fat, low-overall-fat diet if your condition requires it, but not a no-fat diet; some fat is essential for healthy fetal development. Moderate sodium restriction (about 2,000 milligrams a day) is usually recommended, but greater restriction isn't. An iron supplement is generally prescribed.

❖ Wearing pressure-graded support pantyhose, to help reduce the pooling of blood in your legs.

❖ Quitting smoking, if you smoke.

Toward the end of your pregnancy, you are likely to begin undergoing frequent ultrasound scans and non-stress tests, so that the physician can keep abreast of your baby's condition. The tests will also help assure you that everything's okay.

If you pass through pregnancy without heart or lung complications, you're not likely to encounter problems during labor and delivery. Nor are you more likely to need a cesarean than other mothers. Outlet forceps (under local anesthesia; see page 286) may be used, however, to reduce the stress of labor and speed the final stage of delivery.

SICKLE-CELL ANEMIA

"I have sickle-cell disease, and I just found out that I'm pregnant. Will my baby be okay?"

Not too many years ago, the answer would not have been reassuring. Today, however, thanks to major medical advances, women with sickle-cell disease have a very good chance of coming through childbirth safely and of winding up with a healthy baby. Even those women with such sickle-cell complications as heart or kidney disease are often able to have a successful pregnancy.

Pregnancy for the woman with sickle-cell anemia, however, is usually classified as high risk. Because of the added stress on her body, her chances of having a sickle-cell crisis increase; and because of the disease the risks of certain pregnancy complications, such as miscarriage and preterm delivery, also increase. Preeclampsia, or toxemia, is also more common in women with sickle-cell anemia, but whether this is because they have sickle cell or because they're black and more subject to hypertension isn't clear.

The prognosis for both you and your baby will be best if you receive state-of-the-art medical care. You should have prenatal checkups more frequently than other pregnant patients—possibly every two to three weeks up to the 32nd week, and every week thereafter. Ideally your obstetrician should be familiar with sickle-cell disease and should work closely with a knowledgeable maternal-fetal subspecialist, internist, or hematologist. It's likely that prenatal vitamin and iron supplements will be prescribed. And probably at least once (usually in early labor or just prior to delivery), and possibly periodically throughout pregnancy (though this treatment is controversial), you will be given a blood transfusion. You are as likely as other mothers to have a vaginal delivery. Postpartum, you may be given antibiotics to prevent infection.

If both parents carry a gene for sickle-cell anemia, the risk that their baby will inherit a serious form of the disease is increased. Early in your pregnancy (if not prior to conception), your husband should be screened for the sickle-cell trait. If he turns out to be a carrier, you may want to see a genetic counselor, and possibly to undergo prenatal diagnosis (see page 42) to see if the fetus is affected.

SYSTEMIC LUPUS ERYTHEMATOSUS (SLE)

"My lupus has been pretty quiet lately. I just became pregnant. Is this likely to bring a flare-up? Will my baby get lupus?"

There's a lot that's still unknown about systemic lupus erythematosus (SLE), an autoimmune disease that affects primarily women between the ages of 15 and 64, black women more often than white. The studies that have been done seem to indicate that pregnancy doesn't affect the long-term course of lupus. During pregnancy itself, some women find their condition improves, others find it worsens. What happens in one pregnancy doesn't predict what will happen in subsequent ones. In the postpartum period, there does appear to be an increase in flare-ups.

The effect of SLE on the pregnancy, however, isn't absolutely clear. It does seem that the women who do best are those who, like you, conceive during a quiet period in their disease. Though their risk of pregnancy loss is slightly increased, their chances of having a healthy baby are excellent. Those with the poorest prognosis are those women with SLE who have severe kidney impairment (ideally, kidney function should have been stable for at least six months before conception) or who have what is called the lupus anticoagulant in their blood. No matter what the severity of a pregnant woman's lupus, it is extremely unlikely that her baby would be born with lupus.

If needed for arthritic symptoms or by women with the lupus anticoagulant, and if taken at the lowest effective doses, both daily doses of aspirin and the steroid prednisone seem to reduce overall risk. Many steroids are safe to use in pregnancy—some because they don't cross the placenta. Some that do cross the placenta are nevertheless safe, and some may actually benefit the fetus by hastening lung maturity.

Because of your lupus, your pregnancy care will be more complicated than most, with more, and more frequent, tests and possibly more limitations. But with you, your obstetrician or maternal-fetal subspecialist, and the physician who treats your lupus all working together, the odds are very much in favor of a happy outcome that will make it all worthwhile.

WHAT IT'S IMPORTANT TO KNOW:
LIVING WITH THE HIGH-RISK OR PROBLEM PREGNANCY

Pregnancy is a "normal" process to be experienced, not an illness to be treated—so the popular gestational dogma goes these days. But if yours is a high-risk pregnancy, you're all too aware that it's not universally true. For many women pregnancy is a time of fear, anxiety, constant medical care, frequent hospitalization, and a feeling that "no one else knows what it's like." Other expectant couples are living with joy and anticipation, but the couple in a high-risk pregnancy may live with:

Fear. While other parents are excitedly preparing for the birth of their baby at the end of nine months, high-risk parents may just be hoping that the fetus they are nurturing will still be alive tomorrow.

Resentment. A woman who is used to being independent may resent her sudden total dependence, especially if her activities are restricted ("Why me? Why do I have to give up my job? Why do I have to stay in bed?"). The anger may be aimed at the baby, at her spouse, or elsewhere. Her husband, of course, may have his own share of resentments ("Why does she get all the attention? Why do I have to do all the work? Does she really have to stay

in bed—and do I really have to stay home with her every evening?"). There may be unspoken resentments, too, about the high cost of her medical care and the lack of lovemaking, if it is restricted.

Guilt. A woman may agonize over what she may have done to make this a high-risk pregnancy, or to lose previous pregnancies, even though in the vast majority of cases, her actions aren't the cause at all. She may worry that she's just being lazy, staying in bed or leaving her job early. She may fear that she's destroying her relationship with her husband or with her other children. Her husband may be saddled with guilt too; he may feel bad that his wife is doing all the suffering, or he may feel remorse for the resentments he's harboring.

Feelings of Inadequacy. A woman who can't have a "normal" pregnancy may consider herself somehow lacking.

Constant Pressure. The high-risk expectant parent often has to keep her pregnancy and its requirements in mind every moment of every day; she'll need to pause almost constantly to ask herself "Can I do this? Is that allowed?" There may be a special diet, activity restrictions or even total bed rest, frequent examinations and tests.

Marital Stress. Any kind of crisis puts stress on a marriage, but a high-risk pregnancy often adds the stress of limited or prohibited sexual intercourse, which may make it hard for the couple to achieve intimacy. There may be added stress from the high cost of a high-risk pregnancy (much of which may not be reimbursed by insurance) and from the loss of income if the expectant mother can't continue working.

Though the ultimate rewards can make all the efforts more than worthwhile, it can be an undeniably tough nine months for the high-risk couple. The following may help make the going a little easier:

Financial Planning. As other parents save for college, you'll need to save for your baby's safe delivery. Knowing in advance that yours will be a high-risk, and thus an expensive, pregnancy is ideal, but it isn't always possible, at least not the first time. If it is, it makes sense to shop around for the best available insurance plan, and to forgo expensive vacations and other lifestyle frills so you can sock away some of the needed cash before the pregnancy begins. If it isn't, start taking belt-tightening steps as soon as you discover your situation.

Social Planning. If your pregnancy requires bed rest, partial or complete, don't resign yourselves to the hermit's life. Invite your best friends to supper in the bedroom (order pizza in and have your husband whip up some Mock Sangrias). Or ask friends in to play Monopoly, Scrabble, or cards, or to view a film that's just come out on video. If you have to miss an important family event, a friend's wedding, or your company's annual party, have your husband attend and record (in

his head, on tape, on video, or with a camera) the goings-on so he can share them with you later. If your sister is getting married 1,000 miles away and the doctor has vetoed traveling, videotape a message of love to her, or write a special poem to be read at the reception. Ask her to videotape the ceremony so you can share it.

Filling Time. Weeks, or even months, in bed may sound like a life sentence. But it can also be a time to do all the things you haven't had time for in your hectic life. Read those bestsellers everyone's been talking about, or some of the old classics that you never got around to enjoying. Join a video club that offers a good selection and good prices (how many other people ever have the time to take advantage of those "two-films-for-the-price-of-one" offers?). Study a foreign language, listen to a good book if you're tired of reading, or cultivate a new interest via audio tapes. Learn to knit or crochet or embroider—and make something for yourself, your husband, your mom, or your doctor if you're too superstitious to make something for your baby. If you're permitted to sit up, get a laptop computer and organize your financial life. Keep a journal of your thoughts, both the good and the bad, as a way both to pass the time and to work out your resentments. Collect some of the best catalogs, and do your shopping by phone or mail.

Childbirth Preparation. If you can't go to Lamaze classes, ask your husband to go and tape them, or to take notes and report on them verbally. If your bedroom is large and the class is small, ask if the others would mind holding at least one session at your home. Though you may feel that learning about normal childbirth may jinx yours, it will be important for you to be as well informed as possible. Read what you can on the subject in this book and elsewhere; even view a childbirth video or two. And though you may feel that you'd rather not know, learn all you can, too, about what delivery is like for someone with your particular problem—from your doctor as well as from books.

Mutual Support. A high-risk pregnancy, particularly when there are a lot of restrictions, is a real test of a marriage. You'll be going through a period of months where many of the normal pleasures of marriage are missing (sex, going out together, weekend trips, for example) and where even the joy of expecting a baby is marred and muddled. To be sure you end up with a healthy baby and a healthy marriage, each of you will have to think about the other's needs. The expectant mother's will be most obvious. She

will need support in everything, from sticking to a restricted diet to sticking to restricted activities. But the needs of the father, who must be providing a lot of this support, may be neglected as a result. Even from her bedridden or otherwise depressingly restricted position, she has to recognize his feelings and let him know how truly important he is in all that is going on.

Sexual Sublimating. Making love doesn't always have to mean sexual intercourse. Read about how to achieve intimacy in pregnancy even when the doctor says "no sex" (page 168).

Getting Support. As with so many of life's crises, being able to talk to others in the same position as yours can help immeasurably. See below for tips that can help.

MOMS HELPING MOMS

Often a woman who has a high-risk or difficult pregnancy, or who has experienced a pregnancy loss, feels that she is unlike everyone else; she is acutely aware that her pregnancy experience is very different from those of her "normal" friends. If you feel this way, you may find comfort and support in a group of women who have had experiences similar to yours.

Discussions may cover such topics as feeling guilty about not being able to have a normal pregnancy; coping with being confined at home or in the hospital; concern over subsequent pregnancies; grieving over the loss of a baby; finding sources of emotional support; dealing with feelings of alienation. A lot of practical advice is also exchanged at support groups—managing your household when confined to bed; keeping your family going when you have a baby in intensive care; getting the best

care for a particular disorder. And continuing with such a group after you feel better also helps you bring your own experience full circle, and helps with your healing while you support other women in need.

If you think you might benefit from a support group, try to find out if there is one in your area (check with your hospital, doctors, midwives, nurses). If there isn't and you have the energy, consider collecting the names of women in similar situations and starting a group yourself.

If you are bedridden and can't attend a support group, try phone meetings with other expectant mothers in bed, hold a meeting at your home occasionally, and subscribe to "LeftSide Lines," the newsletter for women with complicated pregnancies (Sidelines, 2805 Park Place, Laguna Beach, CA 92651).

17
When Something Goes Wrong

Considering the incredibly intricate processes that are involved in the creation of a baby, from the impeccably precise divisions of a fertilized egg to the dramatic transformation of a shapeless bundle of cells into a tiny human form, it's nothing short of miraculous that all goes right most of the time. And it's not surprising that very occasionally something goes wrong—because of genetics, environmental factors, a combination of the two, or just a quirk of nature. Modern medicine, modern sanitation, and an understanding of the significance of diet and lifestyle have all overwhelmingly improved the odds that a pregnancy (and the labor and delivery that follow) will be completed successfully and safely, but some risk still exists. Fortunately, with today's technology on our side, even when something does go wrong, early diagnosis and intervention can often right it.[1]

An obstetrical complication, whether it happens suddenly or was expected, complicates a woman's life as well as her pregnancy. Tips on coping with pregnancy problems that supplement the following medical explanations are under "Living with the High-Risk or Problem Pregnancy," page 339.

Most women go through pregnancy and childbirth without any complications. This chapter, which describes the most common complications, their symptoms and treatments, is not for them. *It should be read only by those women who have a suspected or diagnosed complication; and even then reading should be confined to the problem at issue. Casual reading could lead to not-so-casual, and unnecessary, worrying.*

---

1. Most complications that can occur during the postpartum period are covered in *What to Expect the First Year.*

CONDITIONS THAT MAY CAUSE CONCERN DURING PREGNANCY

HYPEREMESIS GRAVIDARUM

What Is It? This exaggerated form of morning sickness probably occurs in fewer than 1 in 200 pregnancies. Hyperemesis gravidarum, or excessive vomiting of pregnancy, is more common in first-time mothers, in women who are carrying multiple fetuses, and in women who suffered from the condition during a past pregnancy. Psychological stress may be a factor, but so is the sensitivity of the vomiting center in the brain, which seems to vary from person to person.

Signs and Symptoms. The nausea and vomiting of early pregnancy is more frequent and severe than usual, and it may linger longer—sometimes for the full nine months—rather than letting up at the end of the first trimester. If untreated, the frequent vomiting can lead to malnutrition, dehydration, and possibly harm to the health of mother or baby.

Treatment. Milder cases may be controlled with dietary measures, rest, antacids, and antiemetic (antivomiting) medication,[2] but if vomiting continues and adequate weight is not being gained, hospitalization may be necessary. Further tests may be run to rule out nonpregnancy-related causes of vomiting, such as gastritis, an intestinal blockage, or an ulcer. The patient's room may be darkened and her visitors limited to reduce stimulation; she may receive psychotherapy in an effort to reduce tension. If necessary, intravenous feeding may be given, along with an antiemetic. When fluid balance is restored (usually within 24 to 48 hours), a clear liquid diet is begun. If this is tolerated, the patient graduates to six small meals a day. If she still can't keep food down, intravenous feeding may be continued, though some food by mouth will still be encouraged. Occasionally, when the problem persists for long enough to threaten the proper nutrition of the fetus, special nutrients will be added to the intravenous fluids to allow a complete resting of the gastrointestinal tract for a matter of weeks. This is known as IV hyperalimentation. Only very rarely, when the mother's life is in danger, does termination of the pregnancy need to be considered.

ECTOPIC PREGNANCY

What Is It? A pregnancy that implants outside the uterus, most often in a fallopian tube. Early diagnosis and treatment are very effective. Without them, the pregnancy will continue to grow in the tube and the tube will eventually burst, destroying its ability to carry fertilized eggs on their way to the uterus in future conceptions. An uncared-for ruptured tube could also threaten the mother's life.

Signs and Symptoms. Colicky (spasmodic), crampy pain with tenderness,

---

2. Do not take any antivomiting medication without your doctor's approval. Since some of these drugs interact adversely with other drugs, be sure to let your doctor know about any medication you are presently taking before an antiemetic is prescribed.

starting on one side and often spreading throughout the abdomen; pain may worsen on straining of bowels, coughing, or moving. Often, brown vaginal spotting or light bleeding, intermittent or continuous, which may precede pain by several days or weeks. Sometimes, nausea and vomiting, dizziness or weakness, shoulder pain, and/or rectal pressure. If the tube ruptures, heavy bleeding may begin, signs of shock (rapid, weak pulse, clammy skin, and fainting) are common, and pain becomes very sharp and steady for a short time before diffusing throughout the pelvic region.

Treatment. Getting to the hospital immediately is important. New techniques for early diagnosis and treatment of tubal pregnancy have removed most of the risk for the mother while greatly improving the chances of preserving her fertility.

Diagnosis is usually made through a combination of two procedures: (1) a series of highly sensitive pregnancy tests that track the level of the hor-

---

Bleeding in Early Pregnancy

Bleeding in early pregnancy does not necessarily indicate anything serious, but as a precaution, it should always be reported to your practitioner. Be precise in describing the bleeding: Is it intermittent or persistent? When did it start? Is the color bright or dark red, brownish or pink? Is it heavy enough to soak a sanitary pad in an hour, just occasional spotting, or somewhere in between? Is there any unusual odor? Do any tissue fragments (bits of solid material) seem to have been passed with the blood? (If so, try to save them in a jar or plastic bag.) Be sure to report, too, any accompanying symptoms, such as excessive nausea and vomiting, cramps or pain of any kind, fever, weakness, and so on.

Spotting or staining that is not accompanied by such symptoms is not considered an emergency situation; if it begins in the middle of the night, you can wait until morning to call the doctor. Any other kind of bleeding suggests a prompt call or, if the doctor is unavailable, a trip to the emergency room.

The two most common causes of first-trimester bleeding, neither of which is an indication of trouble, are:

Normal implantation of the pregnancy in the uterine wall. Such bleeding, which sometimes occurs when the fertilized egg attaches itself to the wall of the uterus, is brief and light.

Hormonal changes at the time menstruation would ordinarily have occurred. Bleeding is usually light, though an occasional woman experiences what seems like an actual period.

Less common, and more worrisome, causes of first-trimester bleeding include:

Miscarriage. Usually, heavy bleeding is accompanied by abdominal pain and possibly the passage of embryonic material (see page 346).

Ectopic pregnancy. Brown vaginal spotting or light bleeding, intermittent or persistent, is accompanied by abdominal and/or shoulder pain, which can often be quite severe (page 343).

Trophoblastic disease. A continuous or intermittent brownish discharge is the prime symptom (page 348).

Often, however, the actual cause of bleeding in the first trimester remains unidentified and the pregnancy continues to a happy conclusion.

Bleeding in Mid- or Late Pregnancy

Light or spotty bleeding in the second or third trimester is generally not a cause for concern. It is often the result of trauma to the increasingly sensitive cervix during an internal exam or sexual intercourse, or simply of causes unknown. Occasionally, however, it is a sign that immediate medical attention is needed. Since only your practitioner can determine the cause, he or she should be notified if you experience any bleeding—immediately if bleeding is heavy, the same day even if it is only spotty and there are no accompanying symptoms.

The most common causes of serious bleeding are:

Placenta previa, or low-lying placenta. Bleeding is usually bright red and painless. It most often starts spontaneously, though it can also be triggered by coughing, straining, or sexual intercourse. It can be light or heavy, and it usually stops, only to recur later on in pregnancy. See page 356 for further information.

Abruptio placenta, or premature separation of the placenta. Bleeding may be as light as a light menstrual flow, as heavy as a heavy one, or much heavier, depending on the degree of separation. The discharge may or may not contain clots. The intensity of the accompanying cramping, pain, and abdominal tenderness will also depend on the degree of separation. With a major separation, signs of shock from blood loss may be evident. See page 358.

Late miscarriage. When miscarriage is threatening, the discharge may at first be pink or brown; when bleeding is heavy and accompanied by pain, a miscarriage may be imminent. See page 347.

Premature labor. Labor is considered premature when it begins after the 20th week but before the 37th. A mucousy bloody discharge accompanied by contractions could signal preterm labor. See page 361.

mone hCG in the mother's blood (if the levels of hCG fall or fail to rise as the pregnancy progresses, an abnormal pregnancy, possibly in a fallopian tube, is suspected); and (2) high-resolution ultrasound to visualize the uterus and the fallopian tubes (the absence of a gestational sac in the uterus and, though this isn't always visible, a pregnancy developing in a fallopian tube are indications of ectopic pregnancy). If there is any doubt, confirmation is most often made by viewing the tubes directly, by means of a tiny laparoscope inserted through the navel. High-tech diagnostic tools such as these have made early diagnosis of ectopic pregnancies possible, catching 80% of them before they rupture.

Successful treatment of an ectopic pregnancy is also dependent on high-tech medicine. At one time surgery to remove the abnormal pregnancy was routinely performed through a wide incision in the abdomen, but recently laparoscopy has become more common, because it allows for a much shorter hospital stay and a more rapid recovery. The laparoscopy is accomplished via two tiny incisions, one in the navel for the insertion of the viewing instrument, the laparoscope, and another lower in the abdomen for the surgical instruments. Depending on the circumstances, lasers, electrocautery, or even drugs may be used to remove the pregnancy from the fallopian tube. And, except when there has been irreparable damage to the tube, it is usually possible to save it, improving the chances of a successful pregnancy in the future. Since residual material from a pregnancy left in the tube could damage it, a followup test of hCG levels is performed to be sure that the entire tubal pregnancy was removed.

EARLY MISCARRIAGE, OR SPONTANEOUS ABORTION

What Is It? A miscarriage, also called a spontaneous abortion, is the spontaneous expulsion from the uterus of an embryo or fetus before it is able to live outside the uterus. A miscarriage in

If You've Had a Miscarriage

Though it is hard for parents to accept it at the time, when a miscarriage *does* occur it is usually a blessing. Early miscarriage is generally a natural selection process in which a defective embryo or fetus (defective because of environmental factors, such as radiation or drugs; because of poor implantation in the uterus; because of genetic abnormality, maternal infection, random accident, or other unknown reasons) is discarded, probably because it is incapable of survival or is overwhelmingly defective.

All that said, losing a baby, even this early, is traumatic. But don't let guilt compound your misery—*a miscarriage is not your fault*. Do allow yourself to grieve. Sharing your feelings with your spouse, your practitioner, a friend, will help. In some communities, there are support groups for couples who have experienced pregnancy loss. Ask your practitioner if he or she knows of one in your area, or inquire at your hospital. This may be especially important if you've experienced more than one pregnancy loss. For more suggestions on coping with your loss, see page 366.

Possibly the best therapy is getting pregnant again as soon as it is safe. But before you do, discuss possible causes of the miscarriage with your doctor. Most often, miscarriage is simply a random one-time occurrence caused by chromosomal abnormality, infec-tion, chemical or other teratogenic exposure, or chance, and is not likely to recur. Repeat miscarriages (more than two) are often related to hormonal insufficiency in the mother or to the mother's immune system rejecting a "foreign" intruder, the embryo. In both these situations, treatment when you conceive again, or even before, can often prevent a recurrence. Rarely, repeated miscarriages are due to genetic factors that are detectable by prepregnancy chromosome tests of both husband and wife. Check with your doctor about whether such tests are indicated in your case.

Whatever the cause of your miscarriage, many doctors suggest waiting three to six months before trying to conceive again, though sexual relations can often be resumed after six weeks. (Use reliable contraception, preferably of the barrier type— condom, diaphragm—when you get your doctor's okay.) Take advantage of this waiting period—spend it improving your diet and your health habits. Happily, the odds are excellent that next time around you'll have a normal pregnancy and a healthy baby. Most women who have had one miscarriage do not become habitual aborters. In fact a miscarriage is an assurance of fertility, and the great majority of women who lose a pregnancy this way go on to complete one.

the first trimester is referred to as an early miscarriage. Early miscarriage is very common (many doctors believe that virtually every woman will have at least one sometime in her reproductive years), occurring in as many as 40% of conceptions. Most occur so early that pregnancy is not even suspected yet; so these miscarriages often go unnoticed, passing for an unusually heavy and crampy period. Early miscarriage is usually related to a chromosomal or other genetic abnormality in the embryo; to the mother's body failing to produce an adequate supply of pregnancy hormones; or to her having an immune reaction to the embryo.

Signs and Symptoms. Most often, bleeding with cramps or pain in the center of the lower abdomen. Sometimes, severe pain or persistent pain that lasts 24 hours or more unaccompanied by bleeding; heavy bleeding (like a menstrual period) without pain; persistent light staining (that continues for 3 days or more). Clots or grayish matter may be passed as the miscarriage actually begins.

Treatment. If, on examination, the doctor finds that the cervix is dilated, it will be assumed that a miscarriage has occurred or is in progress. In such a case nothing can be done to prevent the loss. In many cases the embryo or fetus will already have died prior to the onset of miscarriage, triggering the spontaneous abortion.

On the other hand, if the fetus is shown to be alive through either ultrasound or a Doppler device and there is no dilatation, the chances are very good that the threatened miscarriage will not occur. Some physicians will suggest no particular treatment on the theory that a doomed pregnancy will abort, therapy or no, and a healthy pregnancy will hang in there (also with or without therapy). Others—

particularly when a woman has had a history of miscarriage or when it is believed that implantation is imperfect—will impose bed rest and restrictions on activities, including sexual intercourse. Female hormones, once given routinely for early bleeding, are now rarely used because there is doubt about their efficacy and concern over the potential harm to the fetus if the pregnancy continues. In very unusual cases, however, patients with a history of miscarriages who have shown evidence of producing too little of the hormone may benefit from progesterone administration.

Sometimes, when a miscarriage does occur, it isn't complete—only parts of the placenta, sac, and embryo are expelled. If you've had, or believe you've had, a miscarriage, and bleeding and/or pain continues, phone your doctor immediately. A D and C (dilation and curettage) will probably be required to stop the bleeding. It's a simple but important procedure, in which the cervix is dilated and any remaining fetal or placental tissue is scraped or suctioned out. Your physician will probably want to evaluate the material for clues to the cause of the miscarriage.

LATE MISCARRIAGE

What Is It? Any spontaneous expulsion of a fetus between the end of the first trimester and the 20th week is termed a late miscarriage. (After the 20th week, when the fetus may be able to live outside the uterus—even if only with a lot of help from the neonatal nursery staff and equipment—the event is labeled a preterm birth.[3]

---

3. When a baby is born dead after the 20th week, it's usually described as a stillbirth rather than a miscarriage. The definitions of late miscarriage and stillbirth may vary from state to state.

The cause of late miscarriage is usually related to the mother's health, the condition of her cervix or uterus, her exposure to certain drugs or other toxic substances, or to problems of the placenta (see page 177).

Signs and Symptoms. A pink discharge for several days, or a scant brown discharge for several weeks, indicates a threatened miscarriage. Heavier bleeding, especially when accompanied by cramping, probably means a miscarriage is inevitable.

Treatment. For a threatened late miscarriage, bed rest is often prescribed. If the spotting stops, this is taken as an indication that it wasn't related to miscarriage, and a resumption of normal activity is usually permitted. If the cervix has started to dilate, a diagnosis of incompetent cervix may be made and cerclage (stitching closed of the cervix) may prevent miscarriage.

Once the heavy bleeding and cramping that signal a miscarriage begin, the treatment is aimed at protecting the mother's health. Hospitalization may be required to prevent hemorrhaging. If cramping and bleeding continue following a miscarriage, a D and C may be necessary to remove anything that remains of the pregnancy.

If the cause of a late miscarriage can be determined, it may be possible to prevent a repeat of the tragedy. If a previously undiagnosed incompetent cervix was responsible, future miscarriages can be prevented by cerclage early in pregnancy, before the cervix begins to dilate. If hormonal insufficiency was to blame, hormone replacement may allow future pregnancies to progress to term. If chronic disease, such as diabetes or hypertension, is responsible, better control can be established. Acute infection or malnutrition can be prevented or treated. And an abnormally shaped uterus or one that is distorted by the growth of fibroids or other benign tumors can, in some instances, be corrected by surgery.

TROPHOBLASTIC DISEASE (HYDATIDIFORM MOLE)

What Is It? In roughly 1 in 2,000 pregnancies in the United States, more often in women over 45 than in younger mothers, the trophoblast—the layer of cells that line the gestational sac and normally give rise to the chorionic villi—convert into a mass of clear tapioca-like vesicles instead of into a healthy placenta. Without its placental support system, the fertilized ovum deteriorates. Known as trophoblastic disease or hydatidiform mole, the condition is probably caused by a chromosomal abnormality in the fertilized egg.

Signs and Symptoms. The first sign of a molar pregnancy is usually an intermittent, though sometimes continuous, brownish discharge. Frequently the normal morning sickness of pregnancy becomes abnormally severe. As the pregnancy progresses, 1 in 5 women may pass a few of these tiny vesicles through the vagina. By the beginning of the second trimester, the uterus is larger than expected and feels doughy rather than firm; no fetal heartbeat can be detected. Preeclampsia (elevated blood pressure, excessive swelling, and protein in the urine), or in some cases loss of weight and other indications of increased thyroid activity, may also be seen. The definitive diagnosis will depend on an ultrasound exam, which will show the absence of embryonic or fetal tissue and the uterus distended with these small vesicles. The ovaries may also be enlarged because of the accompanying high levels of hCG.

Treatment. The cervix is dilated and the contents of the uterus are carefully evacuated, as in a missed miscarriage or a therapeutic abortion. Follow-up is important, since about 10% to 15% of molar pregnancies don't stop growing immediately. If blood hCG levels fail to return to normal, a repeat D and C is performed. If hCG levels remain elevated after a second procedure, the physician will check for a new pregnancy or for spread of the molar tissue to the vagina or lungs. Very rarely, a molar pregnancy becomes malignant (see choriocarcinoma, page 350), so close medical follow-up after a molar pregnancy is especially important (this condition is potentially curable with early diagnosis and treatment).

It is generally recommended that attempts to conceive again following a molar pregnancy be postponed for one to two years. Careful monitoring of a new pregnancy is vital because of the possibility of another mole developing. Since there is some very tentative evidence that links trophoblastic disease to an inadequate intake of animal protein and vitamin A, strict ad-

---

When a Serious Fetal Defect Is Detected

It's the nightmare of everyone who undergoes any kind of prenatal diagnosis: something actually does turn out to be wrong, so wrong that termination of the pregnancy may have to be considered. The fact that such a nightmare becomes a reality only rarely is no consolation to the couples who receive that dreaded abnormal report.

Before you do consider terminating your pregnancy, you should be sure that the diagnosis is correct and that all your options are clear. Get a second opinion, preferably from a genetic counselor or a specialist in maternal-fetal medicine.

If the pregnancy is to be terminated, you may find that comfort is hard to come by. Well-meaning friends and relatives may not understand what you're going through and may underplay what you view as a tragedy with comments like "It's for the best" or "You can try again." Professional support—from your doctor, a therapist, a social worker, or a genetic counselor—may be necessary to help you deal with this difficult situation. Accepting it won't be easy. You'll probably go through all or most of the other stages of grieving—denial, anger, bargaining, depression—before you reach acceptance.

Often, couples who get bad news saddle themselves with an added, and unnecessary, burden: guilt. It's important to realize that birth defects are most often a matter of chance. You wouldn't knowingly hurt your baby, and if you did so unknowingly, you aren't to blame. See page 366 for additional counsel on dealing with the loss of a baby.

If you decide to terminate but are upset about doing so, it may help you to keep in mind that if this diagnosis were not made prenatally, you would have carried your baby, getting to know and love it, for nine months, only to lose it shortly after birth. Or you would have delivered a baby who lingered for months or years, but with no semblance of life as we know it. Instead, by the time your due date rolls around you may have had the opportunity to become pregnant once again—this time, hopefully, with a healthy baby. That in no way, of course, takes away your right to mourn for the loss of this one.

herence to the Protein and Green Leafy and Yellow Vegetables and Yellow Fruit requirements of the Best-Odds Diet (see page 80) should begin before conceiving again, and should continue throughout any subsequent pregnancy.

PARTIAL MOLAR PREGNANCY

What Is It? In a partial molar pregnancy, as in a complete molar pregnancy (above), there is abnormal development of the trophoblast. With a partial mole, however, identifiable embryonic or fetal tissue is present. If the fetus survives, it is often growth-retarded and likely to have a variety of congenital abnormalities, such as webbed (or connected) fingers and toes (syndactyly) and water on the brain (hydrocephalus). If a normal baby is born, it usually turns out that it was part of a multiple pregnancy, with the mole belonging to a twin that had deteriorated.

Signs and Symptoms. These are similar to those of an incomplete or missed abortion. There is usually irregular vaginal bleeding, usually no fetal heartbeat, and a uterus that is either small or normal for the length of the pregnancy. Only a small percentage of women with partial molar pregnancies have an enlarged uterus, as is common in a complete molar pregnancy. Ultrasound and hCG levels are used to diagnose a partial mole.

Treatment. Follow-up and treatment are similar to that for a complete molar pregnancy, and a new pregnancy is not recommended until hormone levels have been normal for six months. Most women can have healthy babies after having had a partial molar pregnancy, but since the risk of a repeat

exists, early ultrasound examination is important in future pregnancies to rule out that possibility.

CHORIOCARCINOMA

What Is It? Choriocarcinoma is an extremely rare cancer related directly to pregnancy. About half the cases develop when there is a hydatidiform mole (page 348), 30% to 40% following a miscarriage, and 10% to 20% after a normal pregnancy.

Signs and Symptoms. The signs of the disease include intermittent bleeding following a miscarriage, a pregnancy, or the removal of a mole, along with elevated hCG levels and a tumor in the vagina, uterus, or lungs.

Treatment. Chemotherapy. With early diagnosis and treatment, survival is the norm and fertility is unaffected, though it is usually recommended that pregnancy be deferred for two years after treatment is complete.

GESTATIONAL DIABETES

What Is It? A temporary condition, similar to other types of diabetes, in which the body does not produce adequate amounts of insulin to deal with the increased blood sugar of pregnancy. (See page 152.)

Diabetes, both the kind that begins in pregnancy and the kind that started before conception, is generally not dangerous for either the fetus or the mother—*if* it is controlled. But if excessive sugar is allowed to circulate in a mother's blood; and thus to enter the fetal circulation through the placenta, potential problems for both mother and baby are serious.

Signs and Symptoms. The first sign may be sugar in the urine, but there may also be unusual thirst, frequent and very copious urination (as distinguished from the also frequent but usually light voiding of early pregnancy), and fatigue (which may be difficult to differentiate from pregnancy fatigue).

Treatment. Fortunately, virtually all of the potential risks associated with diabetes in pregnancy can be eliminated through the scrupulous control of blood sugar levels achieved by good medical and self care. If doctor's instructions are followed (see page 326 for recommended care), the diabetic mother and her baby will have almost as good a chance to come through pregnancy and childbirth well as any other mother and baby.

CHORIOAMNIONITIS

What Is It? This infection of the amniotic fluid and fetal membranes is diagnosed in only 1 in 100 pregnancies, but it is suspected that the true incidence may be much higher. The infection is believed to be a major cause of premature rupture of the membranes as well as of premature labor.

Signs and Symptoms. In some cases, chorioamnionitis is asymptomatic (has no symptoms), particularly at first. Diagnosis is complicated by the fact that there is no simple test that can confirm the presence of infection. Often, the first sign of chorioamnionitis is rapid heartbeat (tachycardia) in the mother. This may also be caused by dehydration, medication, low blood pressure, or anxiety, but should in any case be reported to the practitioner. Then a fever over 100.4 degrees develops, and in many cases there is uterine tenderness. If the membranes have ruptured, there may also be a foul odor from the amniotic fluid; if they are intact, there may be

an unpleasant-smelling vaginal discharge, originating in the cervix. Lab tests will reveal an increased white blood count (a sign that the body is fighting an infection). The fetus may score low on a biophysical profile (see page 263), indicating some distress.

Treatment. Chorioamnionitis can be caused by a wide range of microorganisms, and the treatment will depend upon the particular organism involved as well as on the condition of the mother and the fetus. Usually other reasons for the symptoms will be ruled out, lab tests to try to determine the type of infectious organism involved will be ordered, and the fetus will be monitored before treatment is begun. If the pregnancy is near term and the membranes have ruptured, and/or if the fetus or mother is in trouble, a prompt delivery is generally the preferred course. If the fetus is extremely immature and unlikely to survive outside the uterus and it is acceptable to delay delivery, large amounts of antibiotics that can cross the placenta are given, while the situation is carefully monitored. Delivery is postponed until the fetus is more mature or the condition of mother or baby begins to deteriorate.

Recent medical advances allowing for more rapid diagnosis and treatment have greatly reduced the risk of chorioamnionitis to both mother and baby; further improvement of diagnostic tools teamed with a better understanding of how to prevent such infections in the first place will reduce these risks even further.

PREECLAMPSIA (PREGNANCY-INDUCED HYPERTENSION)

What Is It? Also called toxemia, preeclampsia is a pregnancy-related form of high blood pressure. No one knows what causes PIH, or why it develops most often in first-time moms-to-be, although some research links it to poor nutrition. Other studies suggest tiny doses of aspirin or large doses of calcium may reduce the risk. Toxic substances have been found in the blood of women who become preeclamptic. In a test tube, these substances damage human endothelial cells (the cells that line the blood vessels). It's theorized that they are produced by the body as an immune, or defensive, reaction to a foreign intruder—the baby—when the mechanism that is supposed to work to suppress such a reaction during pregnancy is absent or fails. Further research into this theory may lead to better ways of dealing with toxemia.

Signs and Symptoms. Initially: swelling of hands and face with sudden excessive weight gain (both related to water retention); high blood pressure (140/90 or more in a woman who has never before had high blood pressure)[4]; and protein in the urine. The condition can progress quickly to the severe stage, characterized by a further increase in blood pressure (usually to 160/110 or higher), increased quantities of protein in the urine, blurred vision, headaches, irritability, scanty urine output, confusion, severe gastric pain, and/or abnormal liver or kidney function and blood platelet test results. Untreated, severe preeclampsia can in turn progress very quickly to the very serious eclampsia, characterized by convulsions, and sometimes coma.

Preeclampsia occurs in 5% to 10%

4. In the HELLP syndrome form of toxemia the blood pressure doesn't go up, but there is usually severe upper mid-abdominal pain and nausea. Blood tests show hemolysis, elevated liver enzymes, and a low platelet count.

of pregnancies and, *if it goes untreated,* can lead to permanent damage to the nervous system, the blood vessels, or the kidneys in the mother and growth retardation (because of a reduced blood supply through the placenta) or oxygen deprivation in the baby. Fortunately, in women who are receiving regular medical care, the disease is almost invariably caught early on and treated successfully, avoiding the rare bad outcome.

Occasionally preeclampsia, or pregnancy-induced hypertension, doesn't appear until labor and delivery, or even until the postpartum period. Such a sudden increase in blood pressure may be merely a reaction to stress or may be true preeclampsia. Therefore women who exhibit such elevations of blood pressure are watched very carefully with frequent checks not just of their blood pressure, but of their urine (for protein), their reflexes, and their blood chemistry.

Treatment. Treatment will vary according to the severity of the disease, the condition of both mother and baby, the length of the pregnancy, and the doctor's judgment.

With mild disease, the woman who is near term and whose cervix is ripe (softened and thinned) is usually induced without delay. The woman who isn't is usually hospitalized for complete bed rest (lying on the left side is best) and close observation, usually without diuretics, blood pressure medication, or drastic sodium restriction. In some very mild cases, bed rest at home may be permitted once blood pressure is normalized. If she is allowed to go home, the mother must be monitored by a visiting nurse and must make frequent visits to the doctor's office. She is informed of the danger signs—severe headache, visual disturbances, or upper or mid-abdominal pain—that may warn her that her condition is worsening, and she is expected to seek emergency medical attention immediately should she experience any of them.

Whether the mother is in the hospital or at home, the baby's condition will be assessed regularly: fetal movements will be checked daily, stress and non-stress tests, ultrasound, amniocentesis, and other procedures will be performed as needed. If at any point the mother's condition worsens or the tests of the fetus indicate the baby would be better off outside the uterus, the mother's condition will be evaluated to determine the best mode of delivery. If the cervix is favorable and the baby is not in acute distress, a vaginal induction of labor is ordinarily decided upon. Otherwise a cesarean will be recommended.

Generally a woman with preeclampsia, even mild preeclampsia, will not be allowed to go past her due date (40 weeks), since post-term the environment in the uterus begins to deteriorate more rapidly than normal. Depending on the circumstances, labor will be induced or the baby will be delivered by cesarean.

The prognosis for a pregnant woman with mild preeclampsia is very good when the medical care is appropriate, and pregnancy outcome is virtually the same as for a woman with normal blood pressure.

With severe disease, or if a mild preeclampsia progresses, the treatment is usually more aggressive. Intravenous magnesium sulfate is begun promptly because it almost always prevents convulsions, one of the most serious complications of the disease. (The side effects of this treatment are uncomfortable, but not usually serious.) If the fetus is close to term, and/or if its lungs are determined to be mature, immediate delivery is usually the recommended route. If the fetus is preterm, but at least 28 weeks old, many doctors will still choose to deliver immediately because they believe

it is best for both mother (in order to normalize her blood pressure and improve her general condition) and baby (who they feel will be better off continuing growth in a neonatal intensive care unit than in the less than hospitable environment in its mother's uterus). Women with such severe disease are best delivered in a tertiary hospital (a major medical center), where optimum maternal support as well as neonatal care for the premature infant are available.

Some doctors, however, prefer a more conservative approach (hospital bed rest, medication, and close monitoring of mother and baby) to give the fetus more time to develop before birth, though it isn't clear if this is really a more beneficial approach. Some will administer steroids to the fetus to try to speed lung maturity before delivery, but there is debate over whether or not this is effective. If the mother's blood pressure can't be controlled or there are signs of maternal or fetal deterioration, conservative methods will be abandoned in favor of immediate delivery.

Between 24 and 28 weeks, virtually all physicians try conservative management of preeclampsia, even when it's severe, in order to give the fetus a little more time in the uterus. Before 24 weeks (when the fetus is rarely able to live outside of the uterus and when severe preeclampsia is fortunately uncommon), delivering the pregnancy is sometimes necessary to reverse the preeclamptic process, even though the baby has no chance of survival.

With appropriate and prompt medical care, the chances of a favorable outcome for the preeclamptic mother and, except in rare instances, for her baby are very good.

In 97% of the women with preeclampsia who do not also have chronic hypertension, blood pressure returns to normal following delivery. The drop takes place for the majority of new mothers within the first 24 hours after childbirth, and for most of the others within the first week. If blood pressure doesn't return to normal by the six-week checkup, the doctor will look for underlying disease.

ECLAMPSIA

What Is It? Eclampsia, which can occur before, during, or after childbirth, is the final stage of toxemia syndrome-preeclampsia/eclampsia. It is very unusual for this stage to be reached when good medical care is given.

Signs and Symptoms. Convulsions and/or coma. These are often preceded by spiking blood pressure, seriously increased levels of protein in the urine, and exaggerated reflex reactions, as well as severe headache, nausea or vomiting, irritability, restlessness and twitching, upper abdominal pain, visual disturbances, drowsiness, fever, or rapid heartbeat.

Treatment. The patient is prevented from injuring herself during the convulsions. Oxygen and drugs to arrest the seizures will be administered; the patient's environment will be kept as free of stimuli, such as light and noise, as possible. Labor will generally be induced or a cesarean-section performed when the patient is stable. With optimum care the survival rate is 98%, and the majority of patients rapidly return to normal after delivery, though careful follow-up is necessary to be certain blood pressure returns to normal.

INTRAUTERINE GROWTH RETARDATION (IUGR)

What Is It? Sometimes when the uterine environment is not ideal—because of maternal illness, maternal lifestyle, placental inadequacy, or other factors —a fetus doesn't grow as rapidly as it should. Without intervention, that baby will be born, whether prematurely or at term, small for gestational age (also called small for date). But if IUGR is diagnosed prenatally, as it often is when a mother is receiving regular medical care, steps are taken that may reverse it.

IUGR is more common in first pregnancies and in fifth and subsequent ones. It's also somewhat more common among women who are under 17 or over 34.

Signs and Symptoms. Carrying small is *not* usually a tip-off to IUGR—as

---

Lowering the Risks for the Baby at Risk

If there is any reason to believe that a baby may be less than perfectly healthy at birth, it is important to be sure that he or she comes into the world under the best of all possible conditions. In most cases, this means being delivered in a tertiary hospital, one that is equipped to handle the most serious of newborn emergencies. (Studies show that this is preferable to moving a sick baby after birth.) If yours is a high-risk pregnancy that puts your baby at serious risk, talk to your doctor about arranging to deliver in a tertiary medical center, and then make the necessary arrangements to get there when the time comes. Specially equipped ambulances or even helicopters may be available to transport you there in a hurry, if necessary.

Repeat Low-Birthweight Babies

A mother who has already had a low-birthweight baby has only a slightly increased risk of having another one—and to her advantage, statistics show that each subsequent baby is actually likely to be a bit heavier than the preceding one. Whether or not her subsequent babies will be small depends to a great extent on the reason her first baby was small and whether or not the same factor, or factors, exists the next time she conceives (see page 354).

Whether or not the cause of her previous baby's IUGR is known, the woman who is planning to become pregnant or who has already become pregnant again should pay extra attention to all the factors that can reduce the risk this time around; see page 50.

carrying large, or having gained a lot of weight, is not necessarily a sign that the baby is big. In most cases there are no outward symptoms that might alert a mother to the problem. The practitioner may, after measuring the abdomen with a tape measure, suspect that the uterus or fetus is small for date. The diagnosis can be confirmed, or ruled out, with an ultrasound examination.

Treatment. In some instances, the factors that might lead to a baby failing to thrive in the uterus are easily identifiable and, once identified, can be modified or eliminated. These include inadequate prenatal care (finding a practitioner early and seeing him or her regularly can reduce risk considerably); poor diet and/or inadequate weight gain (a well-balanced pregnancy diet, such as the Best-Odds Diet on page 80, can help remedy both these problems); cigarette smoking (the sooner a mother quits, the better her baby's chances of coming into the world at a fighting weight); alcohol or other substance abuse (professional help may be needed for some women to deal with these problems before they affect their babies).

Certain maternal factors that contribute to poor fetal growth can't be eliminated, but they can be controlled to minimize any threat to a baby's growth. These factors include chronic illness (diabetes, high blood pressure, lung or kidney disease); illnesses related to pregnancy (anemia, preeclampsia); and acute illnesses not related to pregnancy (urinary tract infections). To learn how these are treated in pregnancy, see the specific conditions.

For intervention to be effective, some other risk factors must be altered before pregnancy begins. These include significantly low maternal weight (putting on some weight and improving nutritional status before conceiving again can help); susceptibility to rubella (immunization eliminates the risk); inadequate spacing between pregnancies (less than six months between the end of one pregnancy and the beginning of the next may shortchange the next baby, although excellent nutrition, lots of rest, and top-notch medical care will go a long way toward improving uterine conditions if such a pregnancy has already begun); a malformed uterus or other problems with reproductive or urinary organs (surgery or other therapy may remedy these); exposures to toxic substances or environments, including occupational hazards (see page 72).

Some factors that make a woman somewhat more likely to have a baby who does not grow well are difficult or impossible to alter. These include being poor, uneducated, and/or unmarried (probably because circumstances make it less likely that a woman will receive optimum nourishment and prenatal care); DES exposure before birth (page 40); living at a high altitude (though risk is only very slightly increased); having had a previous low-birthweight baby, a baby who has a birth defect, or multiple miscarriages; carrying twins, triplets, or more; having first- or second-trimester bleeding, placental problems (such as placenta previa or abruptio placenta), or very severe nausea and vomiting that continues after the third month; having too much or too little amniotic fluid, abnormal hemoglobin, or premature rupture of the membranes; or Rh isoimmunization (see page 33). Having been small at birth yourself also puts you at an increased risk of having a small baby. But in almost every instance, optimum nutrition and the elimination of any other existing risk factors can improve the chances for normal fetal growth.

Since most babies who are delivered early are small (though they may be an appropriate size for their gestational age and don't necessarily suffer from IUGR), altering the factors that lead to premature labor and halting premature labor when it begins or is anticipated (see page 218) can have a major impact on the risk of having a low-birthweight baby.

Recent research has turned up a variety of additional factors that may be involved in producing a too-small baby. These include stress (physical, including fatigue, and possibly psychological); inadequate increase in the mother's blood plasma volume; and progesterone deficiency.

When preventive measures fail and IUGR is diagnosed, a variety of approaches may be tried to deal with the problem, depending on the suspected cause. Among the procedures that may be beneficial are bed rest in the hospital, especially if the home environment is less than ideal; improved nutrition, with an emphasis on protein, calories, and iron, and intravenous feedings if necessary; medications to improve placental blood flow or to correct a diagnosed problem that may be contributing to the IUGR; and finally, prompt delivery of the fetus if the intrauterine environment is very poor and can't be improved.

Even when prevention and treatment are unsuccessful and a baby is born smaller than normal, chances of survival and even excellent health are increasingly good thanks to the miracles of modern medicine. And low-birthweight babies often eventually catch up in both growth and development to their higher-birthweight peers.

PLACENTA PREVIA

What Is It? Placenta previa sounds like a disease of the placenta, but it isn't that at all. It refers to the position of the placenta, not its condition. In placenta previa, the placenta is attached in the lower half of the uterus, covering, partially covering, or touching the edge of the os, or mouth of the uterus. In early pregnancy a low-lying placenta is fairly common; but as pregnancy progresses and the uterus grows, the placenta in most cases moves upward.[5] Even when it doesn't move up, it is unlikely to cause a serious problem unless it actually touches

---

5. Even low-lying placentas diagnosed fairly late in pregnancy may occasionally continue to move upward, allowing for a normal delivery at term.

the cervical os. In the small percentage of cases in which it does touch the os, it can cause problems late in pregnancy and at delivery. The closer to the os the placenta is situated, the greater the possibility of hemorrhage. When the placenta blocks the cervix partially or completely, vaginal delivery is usually impossible.

The risk of having placenta previa is higher in women who have scarring of the uterine wall from previous pregnancies, cesareans, uterine surgery, or D and Cs following miscarriage. The need for greater placental surface area due to an increased need for oxygen or nutrients on behalf of the fetus (because of smoking, living at a high altitude, or carrying more than one fetus) may also increase the risk of placenta previa.

Signs and Symptoms. Painless bleeding as the placenta pulls away from the stretching lower portion of the uterus, occasionally before the 28th week but most often between the 34th and 38th, is the most common sign of placenta previa, though an estimated 7% to 30% of women with low-lying placentas don't bleed at all before delivery. The bleeding is usually bright red, not associated with significant abdominal pain or tenderness, and spontaneous in onset, though it can also be triggered by coughing, straining, or sexual intercourse. It can be light or heavy, and often stops, only to recur later. Because the placenta is blocking their way, fetuses with low-lying placentas do not usually "drop" into the pelvis in preparation for delivery.

In women who have no symptoms, the condition may be discovered during a routine ultrasound exam or may not be found until delivery.

When bleeding is present and placenta previa suspected, diagnosis is usually made by ultrasound.

Treatment. Because most early cases of low-lying placenta correct themselves long before delivery (see page 187) and never cause a problem, the condition doesn't require treatment before the 20th week. After that time, when there are no symptoms, the woman with a diagnosed placenta previa may be put on a modified activity schedule with increased bed rest. When there is bleeding, hospitalization is imperative in order to evaluate the condition of mother and baby, and if necessary to try to stabilize them. If the bleeding stops or is very light, conservative treatment is usually recommended. This consists of hospitalization, including bed rest with bathroom privileges, careful monitoring, supplementation with iron and possibly vitamin C, and transfusions as needed until the fetus is mature enough for delivery. A high-fiber diet with stool softeners may be prescribed to reduce the need to strain at the toilet. Occasionally a mother who has had no bleeding for a week, has easy access to the hospital (within 15 minutes' travel time), can be relied upon to stay in bed, and can find an adult who can be with her 24 hours a day (and if necessary drive her to the hospital in a hurry) may be allowed to go home and follow a similar restricted regimen.

The goal is to try to keep the pregnancy going until at least 36 weeks. At that point, if testing finds the lungs mature, the baby may be delivered by cesarean to reduce the risk of massive hemorrhage. Of course, if before that time the mother and/or her baby is endangered by the bleeding, delivery will be postponed no longer, even if this means the baby will be premature. Thanks to the skill and caring of top-notch neonatal intensive care units, most of these babies will do much better connected to lifesaving equipment in the NICU than connected to a bleeding placenta in the uterus.

Roughly 3 in 4 women with diagnosed placenta previa will be delivered by cesarean section before labor starts. If the condition isn't discovered until labor has begun, bleeding is mild, and the placenta is not blocking the cervix, vaginal delivery may be attempted. In either case, results are usually good; though placenta previa once posed a very serious threat, nearly 99% of mothers today come through it okay, as do almost as many of their babies.

PLACENTA ACCRETA

What Is It? Occasionally the placenta grows into the deeper layers of the uterine wall and becomes firmly attached. Depending on how deeply the placental cells invade, the condition may also be called placenta percreta or placenta increta. This condition is most common in women who have scarring of the uterine wall from previous surgeries or deliveries and especially in those with placenta previa or a prior cesarean.

Signs and Symptoms. During the third stage of childbirth, the placenta will not separate from the uterine wall.

Treatment. In most cases the placenta must be removed surgically to stop the bleeding. When the bleeding cannot be controlled by tying off the exposed blood vessels, removal of the entire uterus may be necessary.

ABRUPTIO PLACENTA

What Is It? This condition, in which the placenta separates, or abrupts, from the uterus prematurely, is responsible for roughly 1 in 4 cases of late-pregnancy bleeding. It is more common in older mothers who have had babies before, and in those who

smoke, have hypertension (chronic or pregnancy-induced), have been taking aspirin late in pregnancy, or have had a previous premature separation of the placenta. A short umbilical cord or trauma due to an accident[6] is occasionally the cause of an abruption.

Signs and Symptoms. When the separation is small, bleeding may be as light as a light menstrual flow or as heavy as a heavy one, and may or may not contain clots. There may also be cramping or a mild ache in the abdomen, and uterine tenderness. Occasionally, particularly when there has been trauma to the abdomen, there may be no bleeding at all.

With a moderate separation, bleeding is heavier, the abdomen is tender and firm, and abdominal pain may be more severe, stemming in part from strong uterine contractions. Both mother and baby may show signs of blood loss.

When more than half the placenta separates from the uterine wall, an emergency situation exists for both mother and baby. The symptoms are similar to those for a moderate separation, but more extreme.

The diagnosis is made using patient history, physical examination, and observation of uterine contractions and the fetal response to them. Ultrasound is helpful, but only about half of abruptions can actually be seen on ultrasound.

Treatment. When the separation is small, bed rest often stops the bleed-

---

6. If you sustain an injury and have any signs of abruption, call your doctor immediately. If you have no such signs, do a test for fetal movement after the accident (page 202). Repeat the test after several hours, and again two or three times during the next two days. Signs of abruption and fetal distress may not show up for 24 to 48 hours.

ing and the mother can usually resume her normal routine, with some restriction on activity, a few days later. Though it's not usual, there is the possibility of a repeat bleeding episode or even of a hemorrhage, so close medical supervision for the rest of the pregnancy is necessary. If signs of trouble recur and the baby is near term, delivery may be carried out.

In most cases, a moderate separation also responds to bed rest. But often transfusions and other emergency treatment may also be needed. Careful monitoring of both mother and baby is necessary, and if either shows signs of distress, delivery without delay may be essential.

When the separation is severe, prompt medical action, including transfusions and immediate delivery, is imperative.

At one time the outlook was bleak for both mothers and their babies when a placenta separated prematurely. Today, with expert and prompt medical care, virtually all the mothers with placental abruption and better than 90% of their babies will survive the crisis.

PREMATURE RUPTURE OF THE MEMBRANES (PROM)

What Is It? PROM refers to the rupture of the chorionic membranes, or "bag of waters," before contractions begin. This can happen just hours before the baby is due, or weeks or even months earlier. Why one woman's membranes spontaneously rupture early and another's don't rupture even during labor, and have to be ruptured artificially, isn't clear. There is speculation, however, that the enzyme collagenase, produced by certain bacteria, plays a role by reducing the strength and elasticity of the membranes surrounding the fetus.

Signs and Symptoms. Leaking or gushing of fluid from the vagina; the flow is heavier when the woman is lying down. The practitioner's check of the vagina reveals fluid that is alkaline (rather than acid, as would be the case with urine) coming from the cervix.

Treatment. Most doctors agree that initially, for anywhere from a few hours to a full day, the expectant mother whose membranes rupture prematurely should be closely observed, and that during that time the baby's condition should be evaluated and the mother monitored for contractions and the possibility of infection. During the initial evaluation, the mother is ordinarily admitted to the hospital for bed rest and careful monitoring of her condition and the baby's. Her temperature and white blood count will be checked periodically so that doctors can take action immediately should infection develop, which can lead to premature delivery. A culture from the cervix may be also taken to check for infection, and in some cases intravenous antibiotics will be given even before the results of the culture are in to prevent any infection from moving into the now open amniotic sac. If contractions begin and the fetus is believed to be immature, medication may be given to try to halt them. As long as both mother and baby are all right, this conservative course may be continued until the baby is deemed mature enough for safe delivery. If at any point mother or baby is thought to be in danger, delivery will be carried out promptly. Rarely the break in the membranes heals and the leakage of amniotic fluid stops on its own. If that happens, the mother may be allowed to go home and resume her normal routine while remaining on the alert for signs of further leakage.

Most doctors will try to delay delivery until 33 or 34 weeks of pregnancy.

At that point some will induce labor; others will continue to try to postpone delivery until 37 weeks. (To help them decide whether or not to induce labor, some will perform amniocentesis or check the amniotic fluid in the vagina to determine the maturity of the baby's lungs.) If PROM occurs at 37 weeks or later most physicians will induce, since at this point the negligible risk to the fetus is far outweighed by the risk of infection that comes with a delay of as little as 24 to 36 hours.

With good care, both mother and baby should be fine, though if the baby is premature a long stay in the NICU and other problems may complicate the picture.

CORD PROLAPSE

What Is It? The umbilical cord is a baby's lifeline in the uterus. Occasionally, when the amniotic membranes rupture, the cord slips, or prolapses, through the cervix or even well into the vaginal canal, carried by the rush of amniotic fluid. It then becomes vulnerable to compression by the baby's presenting part as it presses through the cervix and down the canal during delivery. If the cord does become compressed, the vital supply of oxygen to the fetus can be reduced or even cut off. Prolapse is most common in premature labors (because the presenting part of the fetus is so small it doesn't completely fill the pelvis) or when a part other than the head, especially a foot, presents first (because a foot, for example, takes up less space than a head, allowing the cord to slip down). Prolapse is also more common when the membranes rupture before labor begins, rather than after.

Signs and Symptoms. An umbilical cord can prolapse so far that it may be seen hanging from the vagina, or it may just be felt as "something in there." If it becomes compressed, any distress is likely to be evident on the fetal monitor or other tests of fetal well-being.

Treatment. If you should actually see or feel your baby's umbilical cord in your vagina, or you suspect it might have prolapsed, get on your hands and knees to reduce pressure on the cord. If the cord protrudes, support it gently (don't press or squeeze) with warm wet gauze pads or a clean towel or diaper. Have someone rush you to the hospital, or call 911 or your local medical emergency squad.

At the hospital, a saline solution may be injected into your bladder to cushion the cord; a cord that is outside the vagina may be tucked back in and held in place by a special sterile tampon; and drugs may be given to stop labor while you are readied for an emergency cesarean section.

VENOUS THROMBOSIS

What Is It? A blood clot that develops in a vein. Women are more susceptible to clots during pregnancy, delivery, and particularly in the postpartum period. This happens because nature, worried about too much bleeding at childbirth, tends to increase the blood's clotting ability—occasionally too much—and because the enlarged uterus makes it difficult for blood in the lower body to return to the heart. Clots in superficial veins (thrombophlebitis) occur in about 1 or 2 in every 100 pregnancies. Deep vein thrombosis, which if untreated can result in the clot moving to the lungs and threatening the patient's life, is fortunately much less common. Women who are at a somewhat increased risk of developing clots are those who have had previous clots;

are over 30; have had three or more previous deliveries; have been confined to bed for long periods; are overweight, anemic, or have varicose veins; or have undergone mid-forceps or cesarean delivery.

Signs and Symptoms. In superficial thrombophlebitis there is usually a tender, reddened area that runs in a line over a vein that is near the surface in the thigh or calf. In deep vein thrombosis, the leg may feel heavy or painful, there may be tenderness in the calf or thigh, swelling (ranging from slight to severe), distention of the superficial veins, and calf pain on flexing the foot (turning the toes up toward the chin). Ultrasound or other methods may be used to diagnose the blood clot. Any such symptoms, as well as any other unusual leg symptoms, unexplained fever, or speeded up heartbeat should be reported to the practitioner. If the blood clot (embolus) has moved to the lungs, there may be chest pain, coughing with frothy, blood-stained sputum, speeded up heartbeat and breathing rate, blueness of lips and fingertips, and fever. These symptoms require immediate medical attention.

Treatment. The best treatment is prevention: wear support hose if you are prone to blood clots; avoid sitting for more than an hour or so without walking about and stretching your legs; exercise your legs if you are confined to bed; and don't sleep or exercise while lying flat on your back. Once diagnosed, treatment will depend on the degree and type of clot. A superficial thrombus will be treated with rest, leg elevation, local ointments, moist heat, an elastic compression stocking, and possibly, postpartum, with aspirin. With deep vein thrombosis, an anticoagulant drug (almost always heparin) is given, usually

intravenously for a week or 10 days, then under the skin until labor starts, at which point the drug is discontinued. Several hours after delivery it is resumed once more, and continued for the first few weeks postpartum. With a pulmonary embolus, drugs and surgery may be needed, as well as treatment for any accompanying side effects.

PRETERM OR PREMATURE LABOR

What Is It? Labor that begins after the age of viability (20 weeks in most states) and before the 37th week (when the baby is considered full term). There are a wide range of causes associated with preterm labor (see page 218), but in some cases there is no discernible reason for labor to begin early.

Signs and Symptoms. Menstrual-like cramps, with or without diarrhea, nausea, or indigestion; lower back pain or pressure; an achiness or pressure in the pelvis, thighs, or groin; a watery or pinkish or brownish discharge possibly preceded by the passage of a thick, gelatinous mucus plug; and/or a trickle or flow of amniotic fluid from the vagina.

Treatment. Prompt medical attention to the above symptoms is important since treatment can sometimes halt or postpone the early labor, and each day the baby remains in the uterus until term the better its chances of survival. Some doctors will administer a steroid during the delay to spur fetal lung maturation, although it isn't totally clear whether or not this is effective. Only when the mother and/or child are endangered is no attempt made to postpone early delivery.

Postponement or prevention of the

onset of premature labor can often be achieved through limitations on sexual intercourse and other physical activities, bed rest, and if necessary hospitalization. In about half the cases of women who have early strong contractions but no bleeding and a single live fetus, hospitalized best rest alone, without medication, will check contractions. If the membranes are also intact and the cervix has not effaced or dilated, 3 out of 4 of these women will carry to term. Tocolytic agents (drugs that relax the uterus and have the potential to halt contractions) may be administered to improve these odds, but new research has raised questions about their safety and effectiveness. If infection is thought to have triggered labor, antibiotics may also be given.

CONDITIONS THAT MAY CAUSE CONCERN DURING CHILDBIRTH

UTERINE INVERSION

What Is It? Rarely, the placenta doesn't detach completely after delivery of a baby and when it emerges, it pulls the top, or fundus, of the uterus with it—in effect very much like pulling a sock inside out.

Signs and Symptoms. Symptoms of uterine inversion include excessive bleeding and sometimes signs of shock in the mother. The practitioner, pressing down on the abdomen, will not be able to feel the uterus, and in a complete inversion, part of it will be visible in the vagina. Women at slightly higher risk for an inverted uterus (though the risk is still extremely small) are those who have had many prior births or a prolonged labor (over 24 hours); those who have the placenta implanted across the top (fundus) of the uterus or abnormally attached to it; and those who were given magnesium sulfate during labor. The uterus may also invert if it is overly relaxed or if the fundus isn't held in place while the placenta is coaxed out in the third stage of childbirth.

Treatment. In most cases the uterus can be replaced by hand, though sometimes other techniques are used. Intravenous fluid and blood transfusions may be needed if blood loss has been great. Drugs (such as magnesium sulfate) may be given to relax the uterus even further in order to facilitate the replacement. If fragments of placenta remain in the uterus, they may be removed before or after the uterus is replaced. In very rare cases, the uterus can't be replaced manually and abdominal surgery is necessary.

After replacement, pressure will usually be kept on the abdomen to keep the uterus in place, and oxytocin or other drugs given to firm it so it won't reinvert. Antibiotics may be given to prevent infection.

Since a woman who has had one uterine inversion is at an increased risk for another, your practitioner should be informed if you've had an inversion in the past.

UTERINE RUPTURE

What Is It? Rarely, the uterus ruptures or tears during pregnancy or labor (most often during labor). A scar in the uterine wall is the largest single cause of rupture. The scar may be the result of a prior cesarean section with a classic vertical incision; a repaired uterine rupture; uterine surgery (to correct its shape or remove fibroids); or previous uterine perforation. Extremely violent contractions (spontaneous or induced) can also lead to rupture; but this is rare, particularly in a first pregnancy, without a predisposing scar. Rupture is more common in women who have already had five or more children, have a very distended uterus (because of multiple fetuses or excess amniotic fluid), have had difficult labor previously, or are experiencing difficulties in their present delivery (particularly shoulder dystocia, see below, or midforceps delivery). Abnormalities related to the placenta (such as a placenta that separates prematurely or that is attached deeply in the uterine wall) or to fetal position (such as a fetus lying crosswise in the uterus), as well as severe trauma to the abdomen (as from a knife or a bullet), can increase the risk of uterine rupture.

Signs and Symptoms. Uterine rupture is not a complication that the average pregnant woman need be concerned about. But women who are at increased risk of rupture, because of a scarred uterus or any of the other factors above, should know the possible warning signs, just in case: severe abdominal pain, fainting, hyperventilation (deep, fast breathing), rapid heartbeat, restlessness, and agitation. If you experience such symptoms, which are more severe when the rupture is in the upper half of the uterus, seek immediate emergency medical attention. The first sign of actual rupture is usually a searing pain in the abdomen, accompanied by a feeling that something inside is "ripping." This is generally followed by a brief period of relief, then diffuse abdominal pain and tenderness. Unless the rupture is in the lower segment of the uterus, contractions will generally cease. There may or may not be vaginal bleeding. The fetus will be more easily felt through the abdomen and may show signs of distress.

Treatment. Immediate surgical delivery is necessary, followed by repair of the uterus, is possible. If damage is extensive, a hysterectomy may be required. Sometimes a rupture isn't recognized until hemorrhaging occurs after delivery. Again, the uterus may be repaired or removed.

After a rupture, the mother is closely monitored to be sure complications don't occur, and antibiotics may be given to prevent infection. Depending on the situation, she may be allowed out of bed in as few as six hours or not for several days.

SHOULDER DYSTOCIA

What Is It? Dystocia is labor that doesn't progress; in shoulder dystocia labor doesn't progress because the baby's shoulders become stuck on their way through the birth canal after the head has been delivered.

Signs and Symptoms. Delivery stalls after the head emerges and before the shoulders are out. This can occur unexpectedly in a labor that to that point seemed absolutely normal.

Treatment. A variety of approaches may be used to rescue the baby whose shoulder is impacted in the pelvis, including performing an extra-large episiotomy; trying to rotate the baby and maneuver the back shoulder out first; hyperflexing the mother's knees up on her abdomen; applying moderate pressure to the top of the uterus

First Aid for the Fetus

In late pregnancy, absence of fetal activity could be a sign that something is wrong (for a home test, see page 202). Since diminishing activity (generally judged to mean fewer than ten movements in a two-hour period) is often noted before the fetus actually succumbs, it should be reported imme-diately to your practitioner. If he or she is not available, have someone take you to the emergency room or the labor and delivery area of your local hospital immediately. With prompt action it is sometimes possible to re-suscitate the fetus.

and the pelvis; attempting various other maneuvers to force the shoulders out, including breaking the baby's collarbone. If possible (and rarely is it so), it may be preferable to tuck the baby's head back into the vagina and perform a cesarean section.

FETAL DISTRESS

What Is It? The term is used to describe a situation in which the fetus is believed to be in jeopardy, most often because of decreased oxygen flow. The distress may be caused by a variety of problems, including the mother's position putting pressure on major blood vessels; maternal illness (anemia, hypertension, heart disease), abnormally low blood pressure, or shock; placental insufficiency, degeneration, or premature separation; cord compression; prolonged or excessive uterine activity; or fetal infection, malformation, hemorrhage, or anemia.

Signs and Symptoms. The precise signals sent by the fetus vary with the cause of the distress. The mother may notice a change in fetal movement patterns or an absence of movement. The practitioner can pick up heartbeat changes typical of fetal distress with a Doppler stethoscope or on the fetal monitor.

Treatment. When fetal distress is confirmed (see page 280), immediate delivery is usually indicated. If vaginal delivery is not imminent, then an emergency cesarean is usually performed. In some cases the physician may elect to resuscitate the baby in the uterus before doing a cesarean delivery, to decrease the risk that it will suffer from oxygen deprivation. This is usually done by giving the mother medication to slow contractions, which will increase oxygen to the fetus; to dilate the mother's blood vessels and raise her heart rate, which will also enhance blood flow.

VAGINAL AND CERVICAL LACERATIONS

What Are They? Tears in the vagina and/or cervix, which can range from minor to extensive. These occur only occasionally during labor and delivery.

Signs and Symptoms. Excessive bleeding may be the most obvious symptom, though the lacerations may also be evident to the practitioner after the delivery.

Treatment. Generally, all lacerations that are longer than 2 centimeters or that continue to bleed heavily are sutured (stitched). A local anesthetic may be given first, if one wasn't administered during delivery.

POSTPARTUM HEMORRHAGE

What Is It? Postpartum hemorrhage, or heavy bleeding that is difficult to stem, is a very serious but uncommon complication. When treated promptly, it is rarely the life-threatening situation it once was. Excessive bleeding may occur if the uterus is too relaxed and doesn't contract because of a long, exhausting labor; a traumatic delivery; a uterus that was overdistended because of multiple births, a large baby, or excess amniotic fluid; an oddly shaped placenta, or one that separated prematurely; fibroids that prevent symmetrical contraction of the uterus; or a generally weakened condition of the mother at the time of delivery (due to, for example, anemia, preeclampsia, or extreme fatigue).

Excessive bleeding, or hemorrhage, can occur immediately postpartum because of unrepaired lacerations to the uterus, cervix, vagina, or somewhere else in the pelvis or because the uterus has ruptured or inverted (been turned inside out). It can occur up to a week or two after delivery when fragments of the placenta have been retained in the uterus. Infection can also cause postpartum hemorrhage, right after delivery or weeks later. Postpartum hemorrhage occurs more frequently in women who had placenta previa or abruptio placenta prior to delivery. Rarely, the cause of the hemorrhage is a previously undiagnosed bleeding disorder in the mother that is genetic or is caused by the use of aspirin or other drugs that can interfere with blood clotting.

Signs and Symptoms. Abnormal bleeding after delivery: bleeding that saturates more than one pad an hour for more than a few hours or is bright red any time after the fourth postpartum day, especially if it doesn't slow down when you do; a foul smell to your lochia; large blood clots (lemon-size or larger); pain and/or swelling in the lower abdominal area beyond the first few days after delivery.

Treatment. Depending on the cause of the hemorrhage, the physician may try one or more of the following to stem the bleeding: uterine massage to encourage the uterus to contract; the administration of drugs (such as oxytocin, ergometrine, or prostaglandins) to promote the contraction of the uterus; search for and repair of any lacerations; removal of any retained placental fragments. If bleeding isn't quickly arrested, further measures will be taken: intravenous fluids and, if necessary, transfusion; the administration of blood-clotting agents if failure of the blood to coagulate is the problem, and of antibiotics to prevent infection. Rarely, packing of the uterus with gauze to stem bleeding for 6 to 24 hours or the ligation, or tying off, of the major artery in the uterus will be needed. When all attempts to stop the bleeding fail, the removal of the uterus is necessary.

The odds are very good that treatment of postpartum hemorrhage will be successful, and that the new mother will recover quickly.

POSTPARTUM INFECTION

What Is It? An infection related to childbirth, rare in women who are receiving good medical care and have had an uncomplicated vaginal delivery. The most common postpartum infection is endometritis, infection of the endometrium (lining) of the uterus, which is vulnerable after the detachment of the placenta. Endometritis is more likely to occur after a cesarean section that followed a prolonged labor or early rupture of the membranes. It is also more likely to occur if a fragment of the placenta has been retained in the uterus. Also possible is an infection of a laceration to the cervix, vagina, or vulva.

Signs and Symptoms. These vary according to the site of origin. A slight fever, vague lower abdominal pain, and sometimes a foul-smelling vaginal discharge characterize an infection of the endometrium. With infection of a laceration, there will usually be pain and tenderness in the area; sometimes a foul-smelling, thick discharge; abdominal or side pain; or difficult urination. In certain types of infection, the fever spikes as high as 105 degrees and there are chills, headache, malaise. On occasion, there are no obvious symptoms but fever. Any fever postpartum should be reported to your doctor.

Treatment. Treatment with antibiotics is very effective, but it should begin quickly. A culture may be taken to determine the causative organism so that the right antibiotic can be prescribed.

COPING WITH PREGNANCY LOSS

Demise in the Uterus. When you don't hear from your baby for several hours or more, it's natural to fear the worst. And the worst is, of course, that your unborn baby has died. Fortunately, that's rarely the case. But when it does happen, it can be devastating.

You are likely to be in a fog of disbelief and grief after being told that your baby's heartbeat can't be located and that it has died in the uterus. It may be difficult or even impossible for you to carry on with your normal life while carrying around a fetus that is no longer living, and studies show that a woman is much more likely to suffer severe depression after the delivery of a stillborn if the delivery is delayed more than three days after the death is diagnosed. For this reason, your mental state will be taken into account while doctors decide what to do next. If labor is imminent, or has already started, your stillborn baby will probably be delivered normally. If labor isn't clearly about to start, the decision whether or not to induce it immediately, or to allow you to return home until it begins spontaneously, will depend on how far you are from your due date, and on your physical as well as your mental state.

The grieving process you will go through if your fetus has died in utero will probably be very similar to that of parents whose baby has died during or after birth (see below), although sometimes holding the fetus or having a funeral may not be possible or practical.

Death During or After Birth. Sometimes the death occurs during labor or delivery, sometimes just after delivery. Either way, your world comes crashing down. You've waited for this baby for nearly nine months. You've dreamed about it, felt it kick and hiccup, heard its heartbeat. You've picked out a crib, ordered a tiny layette, prepared your friends, family, and life for the new arrival—and now you're going home empty-handed.

There's probably no greater pain

than that inflicted by the loss of a child. And though nothing can banish the hurt you're feeling, there are steps you can take now to make the future more bearable, and to lessen the inevitable depression that follows such a tragedy.

❖ See your baby, hold your baby, name your baby. Grieving is a vital step in accepting and recovering from your loss, but you can't grieve for a nameless child you've never seen. Even if your child is malformed, experts advise that it is better to see him or her than not to, because what is imagined is usually worse than the reality. Holding and naming your baby will make the death more real to you, and ultimately easier to deal with. So will arranging for a funeral and burial, which will also give you another opportunity to say goodbye. And the grave will provide a permanent site where you can visit your baby in future years.

❖ Discuss autopsy findings and other details with the doctor to harden the reality of what happened and to aid you in the grieving process. You may have been given a lot of details in the delivery room, but medications, your hormonal status, and the shock you felt probably prevented you from fully understanding them.

❖ If possible, ask not to be sedated in the hours after you hear the news. Though it will ease your pain momentarily, sedation will tend to blur your recollections and the reality of what happened. This makes it harder to get on with your grieving, as well as depriving you and your spouse of the chance to support each other.

❖ Save a photo (many hospitals take them) or other mementos, so that you'll have some tangible reminders to cherish when you think about your lost baby in the future. As morbid as this may sound, experts say it helps. Try to focus on positive attributes—big eyes and long lashes, beautiful hands and delicate fingers, a headful of hair.

❖ Ask friends or relatives not to remove all vestiges of the preparations you made for baby at home. Tell them you will do it yourself. As well-meaning as their gestures might be, coming home to a house that looks as though a baby was never expected will only add to any tendency to deny what has happened.

❖ Cry—for as long and as often as you feel you need to. Crying is part of the mourning process. If you don't cry now, it will remain unfinished business that you may find you have to attend to later.

❖ Expect a difficult time. For a while you may feel depressed, empty; experience intense sadness; have trouble sleeping; fight with your husband and neglect your other children; even imagine you hear your baby crying in the middle of the night. You will probably feel the need to be a child yourself, to be loved, coddled, and cared for. All this is normal.

❖ Recognize that fathers grieve too, but that their grief may in some cases be or appear to be shorter-lived and/or less intense, partly because, unlike mothers, they haven't carried their baby inside them for so many months. And they often have different ways of dealing with their distress. They may, for example, try to bottle it up, to be strong for their wives. But then the pain often comes out in other ways: bad temper, irresponsibility, loss of interest in life—or they may use alcohol in an attempt to feel better.

Unfortunately, a grieving father may not be much help to his wife, nor she to him, and both may need to seek support elsewhere.

❖ **Don't face the world alone.** If you're putting off getting back into circulation because you dread the friendly faces asking, "Oh, what did you have?" take a friend who can field the questions for you on the first several trips to the supermarket, bank, and so on. Be sure that those at work, at church or synagogue, at other organizations in which you're active, are informed before you return so you don't have to do any difficult explaining.

❖ **Expect that some friends and family may not know how to respond,** and may withdraw for a while. Others, in trying to help, may make thoughtless statements like "I know just how you feel," or "Oh, you can have another baby," or "It's a good thing the baby died before you became attached to it." They don't understand that no one who hasn't lost a baby can know how it feels, that another baby can never take the place of the one you lost, or that parents can become attached to a baby long before birth, sometimes even before conception. If you are hearing such comments frequently, ask a close friend or

When Multiple Fetuses Aren't Thriving

Twins, triplets, and quadruplets, not surprisingly, are more prone to poor fetal growth than singletons, especially in the third trimester. That's why multiple gestations are followed very closely with series of ultrasound checks from the 20th week on. If one or more fetuses are growing poorly, intensive surveillance, usually in the hospital, is needed. The babies will be delivered promptly either when it is determined that the lungs of the larger (or largest) fetus are mature or when it becomes risky for the smaller fetus to continue to remain in the uterus. Fortunately, such circumstances arise very infrequently.*

Nature often attends to such situations on her own. It's believed that

each year thousands more multiple births are conceived than are born. Early in these pregnancies, because the mother's body is unable to support so many fetuses, generally all but one die, often leaving no visible evidence that they ever existed. Sometimes, however, the multiple fetuses continue to struggle on together, all of them suffering, none of them doing well enough to survive. Then, since Mother Nature hasn't taken the initiative, it may be necessary for medical science to take over and salvage one or two rather then letting them all perish.

Usually there is no way a mother can tell that one or more of the fetuses she is carrying is not doing well. But her physician, using ultrasound and other sophisticated diagnostic techniques, can generally assess the condition of the unborn children.

When it's determined that multiple fetuses aren't doing well, and it is too early to deliver them safely, the medical solution is usually to recommend removing one or more of the fetuses (usually those doing least well) from

---

*If you are carrying more than one fetus, be sure to follow the Best-Odds Diet faithfully, with the additions for multiple pregnancies recommended on page 145. This will improve the odds that all your fetuses will thrive.

relative to explain your feelings and to indicate that you would rather that people just say they are sorry about your loss.

❖ Expect your pain to lessen over time. At first there will be only bad days, then a few good days among them; eventually there will be more good days than bad. But be prepared for the possibility that the pain will never go away entirely. The grieving process, with nightmares and intrusive recollections, is often not fully completed for as long as two years, but the worst is usually over in three to six months after the loss. If after six to nine months your grief remains the center of your universe, if you lose interest in everything else and can't seem to function, seek help. Seek help, too, if from the beginning you haven't been able to grieve at all.

❖ Seek support. Like many other parents, you may derive strength from joining a self-help group for parents who have lost infants. But beware of letting such a group become a way of sustaining your rage or grief. If after a year you're still having problems coming to terms with your loss (sooner, if you're having trouble functioning), you should seek individual therapy.

the uterus so that the remaining fetus or fetuses have a better chance of surviving. This procedure may also be recommended if one of the fetuses is seriously malformed (lacking part or all of the brain, for example).

Some physicians reserve such pregnancy reduction for situations where there are four or more fetuses; others will reduce triplets as well, when it seems appropriate. Some researchers suggest that since up until the end of the first trimester nature may still spontaneously reduce the number of fetuses, the best time to consider a reduction is at the end of this time.

If pregnancy reduction is suggested, the expectant parents are faced with the difficult task of deciding whether or not to let the doctors go ahead with this procedure. Before they make their decision, they should get a second opinion to be sure that the evaluation of the tests on their fetuses is accurate. Then they should discuss the risk that all the fetuses may be lost as a result of the procedure with their physician. This risk is lower, of course, when the surgeon has had a great deal of experience and success with the procedure.

Finally, if religion plays an important part in a couple's life, getting some advice from spiritual as well as medical advisors is a good idea. It will probably also be necessary to talk to a specialist in medical ethics (check with your local hospital), a genetic counselor, a maternal-fetal subspecialist, or another counselor familiar with this issue. In these discussions, they will probably find that most ethicists (even some Catholic theologians) believe that trying to save one baby is preferable to letting them all die. (On the other hand, many would question performing a reduction simply for the sake of convenience—because the family doesn't have room for four cribs, for example.) Reading "When a Serious Fetal Defect Is Detected" (page 349) and "Coping with Pregnancy Loss" (page 366) may be helpful.

Once a couple has made their decision, they should accept that it was the best one they could make. If it doesn't go as they'd hoped, they shouldn't blame themselves.

❖ Limit the use of tranquilizers and sedatives. Although they may seem helpful at first, they can interfere with the grieving process—and can also make you dependent on them.

❖ Turn to religion if you find it comforting. Some bereaved parents feel too angry with God to do this, but for many faith is a great solace.

❖ Don't expect that having another baby will resolve any unresolved grief. Do become pregnant again, if that's what you both want—first observing whatever waiting period the doctor recommends. But don't try to conceive in order to feel better, assuage guilt or anger, or gain peace of mind. It won't work, and it could put an unfair burden on

Loss of One Twin

The parent who loses one twin (or more babies, in the case of triplets or quads) has to face celebrating a birth and mourning a death at the same time. If you are in this position, you may feel too depressed to either mourn your lost child or enjoy your living one—both vitally important processes. Typically, the feeling is "I should be thrilled I have one baby, but I'm so upset, I can't take care of him." Understanding why you feel the way you do may help you to feel better:

❖ You've lost the excitement and prestige of being the parent of twins, a fantasy you may have been playing out for months since your multiple pregnancy was diagnosed. Even if you didn't know in advance about the twins, you may feel cheated. Don't feel guilty if you do; your disappointment is normal. Let yourself mourn this loss as well as the loss of your baby.

❖ You feel it will be difficult and embarrassing to explain that you only have one baby to friends and family who have been eagerly awaiting the twins with you. To ease this burden, enlist a friend or relative to spread the word. When you first go out of the house with the baby, take someone with you who can help explain the situation to people you may run into, if you don't feel up to it.

❖ You may feel inadequate as a woman or as a mother because you lost one of your babies, particularly if they were conceived through the use of fertility agents or IVF or GIFT (gamete intrafallopian transfer). Of course, what happened had nothing to do with your value as a woman or mother.

❖ You feel you are somehow being punished—because you really couldn't have taken care of two children, or because you wanted a boy more than a girl (or vice versa), or because you really didn't want twins. Though such guilt is common in parents who experience a pregnancy loss, it is completely unwarranted.

❖ You are concerned that as your surviving infant grows—at birthdays, the first step, the first "ma-ma" and "da-da"—you will be reminded of the lost child and of what could have been. And it's true that you will be. It will help if you and your spouse share your feelings with each other on these occasions, and not try to suppress them.

❖ You worry that your child, as he or she grows older, will be tormented by the loss. Though some surviving twins do seem to feel that someone is missing or appear lonelier than other children, your child should any new arrival. Any decision about your future fertility—either to have another baby or to undergo sterilization—should be postponed until the period of deepest sorrow has passed.

❖ Recognize that guilt can compound grief and make adjusting to a loss more difficult. If you feel that the loss of your baby was your punishment for having been ambivalent about your pregnancy, or for lacking the nurturing or other qualities necessary for motherhood, seek professional support to help you understand that such feelings are in no way responsible for your loss. Seek help, too, if you feel insecure about your womanhood and now

not suffer because of the loss unless you make an issue of it. Providing lots of love and attention will help ensure a secure, happy youngster.

❖ In trying to help, friends and family may overdo the fanfare when welcoming your living child and maintain a polite silence on the topic of your dead one. Or they may tell you to forget the lost child and appreciate your living one. These insensitive attitudes can anger and upset you. Let people know that you need to grieve for the lost baby as well as rejoice in the live one.

❖ You haven't been allowed, or haven't allowed yourself, to grieve. But grieve you must, or you will never come to terms with your loss. Take the steps for grieving parents described on page 366, so that you can more easily accept your baby's death as a reality.

❖ You believe that to enjoy your surviving baby is somehow disloyal to your dead one. Shake this feeling, though it's a natural one. Loving the sibling that your lost baby spent all those months cuddled up with in your uterus is a way of honoring that child, certainly something he or she would have wanted. On the other hand, idealizing the dead baby and making the living one compete with this idealized image could be quite damaging. If you are uncomfortable about having a christening or a circumcision or other baby-welcoming event for the surviving baby, consider holding a memorial ceremony or farewell for the dead baby first or at the same time.

❖ You're experiencing postpartum depression. It's normal, whether you've lost a child or not, for hormones in chaos to make everything harder to deal with and feelings more conflicted. See page 398 for tips on dealing with postpartum depression.

❖ You're afraid that the loss you've experienced and your consequent depression will damage your relationship with your husband. This is very unlikely if you share feelings, both positive and negative, with each other. One study showed that fully 90% of parents who have gone through this experience have found that their marriage was strengthened by helping each other pull through the mourning period.

❖ You feel guilty that your ambivalence is making it difficult for you to care for your baby. Remind yourself that you have no reason to feel guilty about having feelings that are completely normal.

Give yourself some time. Chances are that you'll soon feel better and, if you let yourself, will be able to begin to truly enjoy your new baby.

Why?

The philosophical question "Why?" may never be answered.* But it is usually helpful to the grieving parents to attach some reality to the tragedy by learning about the physical causes of the death of a fetus or newborn. Often the baby looks perfectly normal, and the only way to uncover the cause of death is to carefully examine the history of the pregnancy and do a complete examination of the fetus or baby. If the fetus died in utero or was stillborn, histological examination of the placenta by a pathologist is also important. At first it may not seem that knowing the cause of death will make acceptance of the loss easier, but in the long run it will. Knowing what happened doesn't really tell you why it happened to you and your baby, but it puts a closure on the event, and it will help you prepare for a future pregnancy.

Of course sometimes it's impossible to determine what went wrong, and in that case the grieving couple have to accept the event in light of their own personal philosophy. They may look upon it as God's will, or as a random occurrence over which humans have no control. In any case, the loss of a baby should never be viewed as punishment.

---

*For help in thinking about this question, see *Why Bad Things Happen to Good People* by Harold S. Kushner.

believe your doubts have been confirmed (you couldn't produce a live baby), or if you feel you have failed your family and friends. If you feel guilty even thinking about getting your life back to normal because you sense it would be disloyal to your dead baby, it may help to ask your baby, in spirit, for forgiveness or for permission to enjoy life again.

Part 4

LAST BUT NOT LEAST:

Postpartum, Fathers, and the Next Baby

18
Postpartum: The First Week

WHAT YOU MAY BE FEELING

During the first week postpartum, depending on the type of delivery you had (easy or difficult, vaginal or cesarean) and other individual factors, you may experience all, or only some, of the following:

PHYSICALLY:

❖ Bloody vaginal discharge (lochia), turning pinkish toward week's end

❖ Abdominal cramps (afterpains) as uterus contracts

❖ Exhaustion

❖ Perineal discomfort, pain, numbness, if you had a vaginal delivery, especially if you had stitches (pain is worse with sneezing and coughing)

❖ Incisional pain and, later, numbness in the area, if you had a cesarean (especially a first one)

❖ Discomfort sitting and walking if you had a repair of an episiotomy or tear or a cesarean

❖ Difficulty urinating for a day or two; difficulty and discomfort with bowel movements for the first few days; constipation

❖ General soreness, especially if pushing was difficult

❖ Bloodshot eyes; black-and-blue marks around eyes, cheeks, elsewhere, from vigorous pushing

❖ Sweating, possibly profuse, after the first couple of days

❖ Breast discomfort and engorgement about the third or fourth day postpartum

❖ Sore or cracked nipples, if you are breastfeeding

EMOTIONALLY:

❖ Elation, depression, or swings between the two

❖ Feelings of inadequacy and trepidation about mothering, especially if you're breastfeeding

❖ Frustration, if you're still in the hospital and would like to leave

❖ Little interest in sex or, less commonly, increased desire (intercourse won't be okayed until at least four weeks postpartum)

WHAT YOU MAY BE CONCERNED ABOUT

BLEEDING

"I'd been told to expect a bloody discharge after delivery, but when I got out of bed for the first time and saw the blood running down my legs, I was really frightened."

Don't be alarmed. This discharge of leftover blood, mucus, and tissue from your uterus, known as lochia, is normally as heavy as (sometimes even heavier than) a menstrual period for the first three postpartum days. And though it'll probably seem more copious than it really is, it may total up to two cups before it begins to taper off. A sudden gush on getting out of bed in the first few days is common, and no cause for concern. And since blood and an occasional blood clot are the predominant ingredients of lochia during the immediate postpartum period, your discharge will be quite red for two or three days, gradually turning to a watery pink, then to brown, and finally to a yellowish white over the next week or two. Sanitary napkins, not tampons, should be used to absorb the flow, which may continue on and off for as long as six weeks.

Breastfeeding and the intramuscular or intravenous administration of oxytocin (routinely ordered by some doctors following delivery) may reduce the flow of lochia by encouraging uterine contractions and helping to shrink the uterus back to normal size more quickly. The contraction of the uterus after delivery is important because it pinches off exposed blood vessels at the site where the placenta separated from the uterus, preventing hemorrhage. If the uterus is too relaxed and doesn't contract, excessive bleeding occurs. If while you are in the hospital, you notice any signs of postpartum hemorrhage listed on page 381 (some of which may also indicate infection), notify a nurse immediately. If any of these signs occur once you are home, call your practitioner immediately; if you can't reach him or her, go to the emergency room (at the hospital in which you delivered, if possible) immediately. To learn how postpartum hemorrhage is treated, see page 365.

YOUR POSTPARTUM CONDITION

"I look and feel as though I've been in a boxing ring rather than in a delivery room. How come?"

You probably worked harder birthing your child than most boxers work in the ring. So it isn't surprising that, thanks to powerful contractions and strenuous pushing during delivery, you look and feel as though you've gone several rounds. Many women do, particularly following a labor that was long and/or difficult. Not uncommon postpartum are:

❖ Black or bloodshot eyes (dark glasses will do a cover-up job in public until the eyes return to normal; and cold compresses for 10 minutes several times a day may hasten that return).

❖ Bruises, ranging from tiny dots on the cheek to larger hematomas, or black and blue marks, on the face or upper chest area.

❖ Soreness at the site of incisions (episiotomy or cesarean) or repairs.

❖ Pelvic soreness as a result of stretching (see page 285).

❖ Difficulty taking a deep breath because of overexertion of the chest muscles during strenuous pushing (hot baths, showers, or a heating pad may reduce discomfort).

❖ Pain and tenderness in the area of the coccyx (tailbone) either because of injury to the muscles of the pelvic floor or because the tailbone is actually fractured (heat and massage may help).

❖ General all-over achiness (again, heat may help).

Though looking and feeling as though you've taken a beating is normal postpartum, you should report any of the above or any other unusual symptoms you notice to the nurse or your practitioner without delay.

AFTERPAINS

"I've been having cramp-like pains in my abdomen, especially when I'm nursing."

These are probably "afterpains," which are believed to be caused by the contractions of the uterus as it makes its normal descent back into the pelvis following birth. The contractions are more likely to be felt by, and be more intense in, women whose uterine musculature is flaccid (lacking in tone) because of previous births or excessive stretching (as with twins).

Afterpains can be more pronounced during nursing, when contraction-stimulating oxytocin is released. Mild analgesics may be prescribed if necessary, but the pain should subside naturally within four to seven days. If analgesics don't relieve the symptoms, or if they persist for more than a week, see your practitioner to rule out other postpartum problems, including infection.

PAIN IN THE PERINEAL AREA

"I didn't have an episiotomy, and I didn't tear. Why am I so sore?"

You can't expect some 7 pounds of baby to pass by the perineum unnoticed. Even if the perineum was left intact during the baby's arrival, the area has still been stretched, bruised, and generally traumatized; and discomfort, ranging from mild to not-so-mild, is the very normal result.

"My episiotomy site is so sore, I'm afraid my stitches are infected. But how can I tell?"

The perineal soreness experienced by all vaginal deliverees is likely to be compounded if the perineum was torn or surgically cut. Like any freshly repaired wound, the site of an episiotomy or laceration will take time to heal—usually seven to ten days. Pain alone during this time, unless it is very severe, is not an indication that an infection has developed.

Infection is possible, but very unlikely if good perineal care has been practiced. While you're in the hospital, a nurse will check the perineum at least once daily to be certain that there is no inflammation or other indication of infection. She will also instruct you in postpartum perineal hygiene, which is important in preventing infection not only of the repair site but of the genital tract as well (puerperal fever). For this reason, the same precautions apply for those who were neither torn nor had an episiotomy. Follow this ten-day plan for the care of the perineum:

❖ Use a fresh sanitary pad at least every four to six hours. Secure it snugly so that it doesn't slide back and forth.

❖ Remove the pad front to back to avoid dragging germs from the rectum toward the vagina.

❖ Pour or squirt warm water (or an antiseptic solution, if one was recommended by your practitioner) over the perineum after urinating or defecating. Pat dry with gauze pads, or with the paper wipes that come with some hospital-provided sanitary pads, always from front to back.

❖ Keep your hands off the area until healing is complete.

Though discomfort is likely to be greater if you've had a repair (with itchiness around the stitches possibly accompanying soreness), suggestions for relief are usually welcomed by all recently delivered mothers:

❖ Warm sitz baths, hot compresses, or heat lamp exposure.

❖ Chilled witch hazel on a sterile gauze pad, or a surgical glove filled with crushed ice, applied to the site.

❖ Local anesthetics in the form of sprays, creams, or pads; mild pain relievers may be prescribed by your physician.

❖ Lying on your side; avoiding long periods of standing or sitting, to decrease strain on the area. Sitting on a pillow or inflated tube may help, as may tightening your buttocks before sitting.

---

1. Use a heat lamp only under supervision in the hospital; to use at home, ask for instructions from your practitioner on how to avoid burns.

❖ Doing Kegel exercises (see page 190) as frequently as possible after delivery, and right through the postpartum period, to stimulate circulation to the area, which will promote healing and improve muscle tone. (Don't be alarmed if you can't feel yourself doing them; the area will be numb right after delivery. Feeling will return to the perineum gradually over the next few weeks.)

DIFFICULTY WITH URINATION

"It's been several hours since I gave birth, and I haven't been able to urinate yet."

Difficulty in passing urine during the first 24 postpartum hours is common. Some women feel no urge at all; others feel the urge but are unable to fulfill it. Still others do urinate, but with accompanying pain and burning. There are a host of reasons why bladder function often becomes such an effort after delivery:

❖ The holding capacity of the bladder increases because it suddenly has more room to expand—thus the need for urination may be less frequent.

❖ The bladder may have been traumatized or bruised during delivery, due to pressure created by the fetus, and become temporarily paralyzed. Even when it's full, it may not send the necessary signals of urgency.

❖ Drugs or anesthesia may decrease the sensitivity of the bladder or the alertness of the mother to its signals.

❖ Pain in the perineal area may cause reflex spasms in the urethra, making urination difficult. Edema (swelling) of the perineum may also interfere with urination.

❖ Any number of psychological factors may inhibit urination—fear of pain on voiding, lack of privacy, embarrassment or discomfort over using a bedpan or needing assistance at the toilet.

❖ The sensitivity of the site of an episiotomy or laceration repair can cause burning and/or pain with urination. (Burning may be alleviated somewhat by standing astride the toilet while urinating so that the flow comes straight down, without touching sore spots.)

As difficult as urination may be after delivery, it's essential that the bladder be emptied within six to eight hours—to avoid urinary tract infection, loss of muscle tone in the bladder from overdistension, and bleeding due to the bladder hindering the proper descent of the uterus. Therefore, the nurse will ask you frequently after delivery if you've urinated. She may request that you void for the first time postpartum into a container, so that she can measure your output, and may palpate your bladder to make sure it's not distended.

If you haven't urinated within eight hours or so, your physician may order a catheter (a tube inserted into your urethra) to empty the bladder of urine. You may be able to avoid this with the following:

❖ Take a walk. Getting up from bed and going for a stroll as soon after delivery as you're allowed will help get your bladder (and your bowels) moving.

❖ If you're uncomfortable with an audience, have the nurse wait outside the bathroom while you urinate. She can come back in when you've finished, to give you a demonstration of perineal hygiene.

❖ If you're too weak to walk to the bathroom and must use a bedpan, ask for privacy; be sure the nurse has warmed the pan (if it's metal) and given you warm water to pour over the perineal area (which may stimulate the urge); and sit on the pan instead of lying on it.

❖ Warm the area in a sitz bath or chill it with ice packs, whichever seems to induce urgency for you.

❖ Turn the water on while you try. Running the water in the sink really does help encourage your own faucet to flow.

After 24 hours, the problem of too little becomes one of too much. Postpartum women begin urinating frequently and copiously as the excess body fluids of pregnancy are excreted. If urinating is still difficult, or if output is scant during the next few days, it's possible you have a urinary tract infection. The symptoms of simple cystitis (bladder infection) include pain and/or burning with urination that continues even after the sensitivity of the episiotomy or laceration repair has lessened; frequency and urgency with little urine passed; and, sometimes, a low-grade fever. Symptoms of a kidney infection are more severe, and may include a fever of 101 to 104 degrees and back pain on one or both sides—usually in addition to the symptoms of cystitis. Your physician will want to begin antibiotic treatment specific to the infection-causing organism, if infection is confirmed. You can help speed recovery by drinking plenty of extra fluids. (Also see page 317.)

HAVING A BOWEL MOVEMENT

"I delivered almost a week ago and I haven't had a bowel movement yet. Al-

though I've felt the urge, I've been too afraid that straining would open my episiotomy."

The passage of the first bowel movement after childbirth is a milestone in the postpartum period. Every day that precedes it may be fraught with increasing emotional and physical discomfort.

Several physiological factors may interfere with the return of normal bowel function after delivery. For one thing, the abdominal muscles that assist in elimination have been stretched during childbirth, making them flaccid and possibly ineffective. For another, the bowel itself may have been traumatized by delivery, leaving it sluggish. And, of course, it may have been emptied before or during delivery, and probably remained empty because no solid food was taken for the duration of labor.

But perhaps the most potent inhibitors of postpartum bowel activity are psychological: the unfounded fear of splitting open the stitches; the natural embarrassment over the lack of privacy in the hospital; and the pressure to perform, which often makes performance all the more elusive.

Although reregulating your system is rarely effortless, it isn't necessary to suffer helplessly. There are steps you can take to resolve the problem:

Don't Worry. Nothing keeps you from moving your bowels more effectively than worrying about moving your bowels. Don't worry about opening the stitches—you won't. And don't worry if it takes a few days to get things moving; that's okay, too.

Request Roughage. Select whole grains and fresh fruits and vegetables from the hospital menu, if possible. Supplement the hospital diet, which many patients find constipating, with bowel-stimulating food brought in

from outside. Apples, raisins and other dried fruit, nuts, bran muffins, and small boxes of bran cereal will help. Chocolate—so often a gift to hospital patients—will only worsen constipation.

Keep the Liquids Coming. Not only must you compensate for fluids lost during labor and delivery, you must take in additional liquids—especially water and fruit juices—to help soften stool if you're constipated.

Get Off Your Bottom. You won't be running marathons the day after delivery, but you should be able to take short strolls through the corridors. An inactive body encourages inactive bowels. Kegel exercises, which can be practiced in your bed almost immediately after delivery, will help tone up not only the perineum but also the rectum.

Don't Strain. Straining won't break your stitches open, but it can lead to hemorrhoids. If you do have hemorrhoids, you may find relief with sitz baths, topical anesthetics, suppositories, or hot or cold compresses.

The first few bowel movements may pass with great discomfort. But as stools soften and you become more regular, the discomfort will ease and eventually end.

EXCESSIVE PERSPIRATION

"I've been waking up at night soaked with perspiration. Is this normal?"

What your doctor may call diaphoresis (but is more commonly referred to as perspiration or sweating) is one of the ways the body rids itself of pregnancy-accumulated fluids during the week following delivery. Often perspiration continues to be a problem for several weeks, because of the postpartum hormonal adjustments. Don't worry about it; but do make sure essential fluids are replaced—particularly if you're breastfeeding—by taking extra liquids. An absorbent towel over your pillow may help make you more comfortable if you do most of your perspiring during the night.

As a precaution, it's a good idea to take your temperature, and to report it to your doctor if it's over 100 degrees.

ADEQUACY OF YOUR MILK SUPPLY

"It's been two days since I delivered, and nothing comes out of my breasts when I squeeze them, not even colostrum. I'm worried that my baby is starving."

Not only is your baby not starving, he or she isn't even hungry yet. Babies aren't born with an appetite, or with immediate nutritional needs. And by the time your baby begins to hunger for a breast full of milk (on the third or fourth postpartum day), you will undoubtedly be able to oblige.

Which isn't to say that your breasts are empty now. Colostrum (which provides your baby with enough nourishment for now and with important antibodies his or her own body can't yet produce, while helping to empty the digestive system of excess mucus and the bowels of meconium) is definitely present in the tiny amounts necessary. (A teaspoon or so per feeding is all your baby needs at this point.) But until the third or fourth postpartum day, when your breasts begin to swell and feel full (indicating the milk has come in), it's not that easy to express manually. Even a day-old baby, with no previous experience, is better equipped to extract this premilk than you are.

ENGORGED BREASTS

"My milk finally came in, leaving my breasts swollen to three times their normal size—and so hard, engorged, and painful that I can't bear to put on a bra. Is this what I have to look forward to until I wean my baby?"

If painfully tender, granite-hard breasts the size of an exotic dancer's were indeed what mothers had to look forward to for the duration of the breastfeeding experience, most babies would be weaned before they entered their second week of life. The engorgement, caused by the milk's arrival, can make nursing agonizing for the mother and, if the nipples are flattened by the swelling, frustrating for the baby. The condition can be aggravated when the initial feeding doesn't begin until 24 to 36 hours after birth, as is common in some hospitals.

Happily, the engorgement and its distressing effects gradually diminish once a well-coordinated milk supply-and-demand system is established—within a matter of days. Nipple soreness, too—which usually peaks at about the 20th feeding—generally diminishes rapidly as the nipples toughen up from frequent nursing. Some women, particularly those with fair skin, may also experience nipple cracking and bleeding. This, with proper care (see page 393), is also only temporary.

Until nursing becomes as gratifying and fulfilling as you had hoped it would be—and, believe it or not, painless—there are some steps you can take to reduce the discomfort and speed the establishment of a good milk supply (see Getting Started Breastfeeding, page 388).

When to Call Your Practitioner

During the first six postpartum weeks, there remains the possibility of a post-childbirth complication. It could be signaled by one or more of the following, all of which require *immediate* consultation with your practitioner:

❖ Bleeding that saturates more than one pad an hour for more than a few hours. Have someone take you to the emergency room, or call 911 or your local emergency medical squad, if you can't reach your doctor immediately. En route or while waiting for emergency help to arrive, lie down and keep an ice pack (or a securely tied plastic bag filled with ice cubes and a couple of paper towels to absorb the melting ice) on your lower abdomen (directly over your uterus, if you can locate it, or at the focus of the pain), if possible.

❖ Bright red bleeding any time after the fourth postpartum day. But don't worry about an occasional bloody tinge to your discharge, a brief episode of painless bleeding at about three weeks postpartum, or an increased flow that slows down when you do.

❖ Lochia that has a foul odor. It should smell like a normal menstrual flow.

❖ Large (lemon-size or larger) blood clots in the lochia. Occasional small clots in the first few days, however, are normal.

❖ An absence of lochia during the first two weeks postpartum.

❖ Pain or discomfort, with or without swelling, in the lower abdominal area beyond the first few days after delivery.

❖ After the first 24 hours, a temperature of over 100 degrees for more than a day. But a brief temperature elevation up to 100.4 degrees right after delivery (due to dehydration) or a low-grade fever at the time your milk comes in is of no concern.

❖ Sharp chest pain, which could indicate a blood clot in the lungs. Call 911 or your local emergency medical squad if you can't reach your doctor immediately.

❖ Localized pain, tenderness, and warmth in your calf or thigh, with or without redness, swelling, and pain when you flex your foot—which could be signs of a blood clot in a leg vein (page 360). Rest, with your leg elevated, while you try to reach your doctor.

❖ A lump or hardened area in a breast once engorgement has subsided, which could indicate a clogged milk duct. Begin home treatment (see page 393) while waiting to reach the doctor.

❖ Localized pain, swelling, redness, heat, and tenderness in a breast once engorgement has subsided, which could be signs of mastitis or breast infection. Begin home treatment (page 394) while waiting to reach the doctor.

❖ Localized swelling and/or redness, heat, and oozing at the site of a cesarean incision.

❖ Difficult urination; pain or burning when urinating; a frequent urge to urinate that yields little result; scanty and/or dark urine. Drink plenty of water while trying to reach the doctor.

❖ Depression that affects your ability to cope, or that doesn't subside after a few days; feelings of anger toward your baby, particularly if those feelings are accompanied by violent urges.

ENGORGEMENT IF YOU'RE NOT BREASTFEEDING

"I'm not nursing. I understand that drying up the milk can be painful."

W hether you nurse or not, your breasts will become engorged (overfilled) with milk on the third or fourth postpartum day. This can be uncomfortable, even painful. However, it is blessedly temporary.

Some physicians used to rely on hormones or other drugs to suppress lactation. But because the drugs have serious side effects and are not reliable (they sometimes fail to relieve engorgement, and if they do, it frequently returns when the medication is discontinued), the FDA's Fertility and Maternal Health Advisory Committee has recommended against their use. Since postpartum breast engorgement is a natural process, it is best to let nature resolve it, which it always does eventually.

The breasts are designed to produce milk only as needed. If the milk isn't used, production ceases. Though sporadic leaking may continue for several days, or even weeks, severe engorgement shouldn't last more than 12 to 24 hours. During this time, ice packs or hot showers and mild pain relievers (such as acetaminophen) may be prescribed. Wearing a tight, well-fitting, supportive bra is important until the breasts return to normal.

BONDING

"My new son was premature and I won't get to hold him for at least two weeks. Will it be too late for good bonding?"

B onding, the process of attachment between a mother and her newborn child, has in recent years become a *cause célèbre* in childbirth circles. The term originated in the 1970s, when some studies began to show that the separation of an infant from its mother immediately after birth posed a threat both to their lifelong relationship and to the infant's future relationships with others. Some very positive changes in post-childbirth procedure have come about because of this work. Today, many hospitals permit new mothers to hold their babies moments after birth, and to cuddle and nurse them for anywhere from ten minutes to an hour or more, instead of whisking the newborns off to the nursery the moment the cord is cut.

But as sometimes happens with the popularization of a good idea, the concept of bonding soon became misunderstood and abused (one of the doctors who published the first book on the subject later said: "I wish we'd never written the statement"), with some unfortunate results. Mothers who have surgical deliveries and are unable to see their babies at birth worry that their parent-child relationship will be forever tarnished. The same worry haunts parents whose babies must be in neonatal intensive care for several days or weeks, giving them little bonding opportunity. So frantic have some parents become about the necessity for instant bonding that they are demanding it even at risk to their infants.

Of course, initial bonding in the delivery room is nice. This early meeting of mother and baby gives them a chance to make contact, skin to skin, eye to eye. It's the first step in the development of a lasting parent-child bond. But only the *first* step. And it doesn't have to take place at the moment of birth. It can take place later in a hospital bed, or through the port-holes of an incubator, or even weeks later at home. When your parents were born, they probably saw little of their mothers and even less of their fathers until they went home—usually ten days after birth—and the vast majority of this "deprived" generation grew up with strong, loving family ties. Mothers who had the chance to bond at birth with one child and not with another usually report no difference in their feelings toward the children. And adoptive parents, who often don't meet their babies until hospital discharge (or even much later) manage to foster strong bonds. Some experts believe, in fact, that bonding doesn't really take place until somewhere in the second half of the baby's first year. Certainly it is a complex process that isn't accomplished in minutes.

It's never too late to tie the bonds that bind. So, instead of wasting energy regretting the time you've lost, prepare to make the most of the lifetime of mothering you have ahead.

"I've been told that bonding brings mother and child closer together, but every time I hold my baby, she seems like a stranger to me."

Love at first sight is a concept that flourishes in romantic books and movies but rarely materializes in real life. The kind of love that lasts a lifetime usually requires time, nurturing, and plenty of patience to develop and deepen. And that's as true for the love between a newborn and its parents as it is between a man and a woman.

Physical closeness between mother and child immediately after birth does not guarantee instant emotional closeness. Feelings of affection don't flow as quickly and surely as lochia; those first few postpartum seconds aren't automatically bathed in the glow of maternal love. In fact, the first sensation a woman experiences after birth is far more likely to be relief than love—relief that the baby is normal and, especially if her labor was difficult, that the ordeal is over. It's not at all unusual to see that squalling and unsociable infant as a stranger—with very little connection to the cozy, idealized little fetus you carried for nine months—and to feel little more than neutral toward him or her. One study found that it took an average of over two weeks (and often as long as nine weeks) for mothers to begin having positive feelings toward their newborns.

Just how a woman reacts to her newborn at their first meeting may depend on a variety of factors: the length and intensity of her labor; whether she received tranquilizers and/or anesthetics during labor; her previous experience (or lack of it) with infants; her feelings about having a child; her relationship with her husband; extraneous worries that may preoccupy her; her general health; and, probably most important of all, her personality. *Your* reaction is normal for *you*.

And as long as you feel an increasing sense of comfort and attachment as the days go by, you can relax. Some of the best relationships get off to the slowest starts. Give yourself and your baby a chance to get to know and appreciate each other, and let the love grow naturally and unhurriedly.

If you don't feel a growing closeness after a few weeks, or if you feel anger or antipathy toward your baby, discuss these feelings with your pediatrician. It's important to work them out early on, to prevent lasting damage to your relationship.

ROOMING-IN

"In childbirth class, having the baby room-in with me sounded like heaven. Since I gave birth, it's been more like hell. I can't get the baby to stop crying— yet what kind of mother would I be if I asked the nurse to take her?"

Y ou would be a very human mother. You've just completed the more-than-Herculean task (Hercules couldn't have done it) of giving birth and are about to embark on an even greater challenge: child rearing. Needing a few days' rest in between is nothing to feel guilty about.

Of course, some women handle rooming-in with ease. They may have had easy deliveries that left them feeling exhilarated instead of exhausted. Or they may have had experience caring for newborns, their own or other people's. For these women, an inconsolable infant at 3 A.M. may not be a joy, but it's not a nightmare, either. For a woman who's been without sleep for 48 hours, however, whose body has been left limp from an enervating labor, and who's never been closer to a baby than a diaper ad, such predawn bouts can leave her wondering tearfully: "Why did I ever decide to become a mother?"

Playing the martyr can raise motherly resentments against the baby, feelings the baby will be likely to sense. If, instead, the baby is sent back to the nursery between feedings at night, mother and child, both well rested, may have a better chance to get acquainted when morning comes.

Full-time rooming-in is a wonderful new option in family-centered maternity care—but it's not for everyone. You are *not* a failure or a bad mother if you don't enjoy, or feel too tired for, rooming-in. Don't be pushed into it if you don't think you want it; and once you've committed yourself, don't feel you can't change your mind. Partial rooming-in (during the day but not at night) may be a good solution for you. Or you might prefer to get a good night's sleep the first night and start rooming-in on the second.

Be flexible. Be more concerned with the quality of the time you spend with your baby in the hospital than the quantity. Round-the-clock rooming-in will begin soon enough at home. And by then, if you are sensible now, you should be emotionally and physically ready to deal with it.

GOING HOME

"My labor was almost effortless, and I feel great. Why should I have to stay in the hospital if I have nothing to recover from?"

C hances are *you* don't have to stay in the hospital. Though ten-day hospital stays were once considered a necessary precaution after giving birth, it's now recognized that a woman who's had an uncomplicated delivery really doesn't need any hospitalization. Your baby, on the other hand, generally does. A minimum of two, but an average of three, days of observation is fairly standard in most hospitals, although that standard may be adjusted at the discretion of your pediatrician—and occasionally a pediatrician will allow for discharge within 24 hours after birth. The major reason for a delay in discharge is to watch for jaundice (a yellowing of the skin), which develops in more than 50% of newborns within the first 24 to 36 hours after birth. Though jaundice is rarely a major complication, many pediatricians prefer to keep the newborn in the hospital an extra day or two, or until it clears up. Others allow for early discharge in mild cases, assuming the infant is otherwise in good health, and providing that the doctor will be able to see him or her within a few days.

Of course, no one can hold you or your baby hostage in the hospital against your will. You have the right to sign yourself and your baby out of the hospital AMA (against medical advice) at any time—if you take full legal, written responsibility for the possible consequences. But unless you have a degree in medicine, it would be extremely unwise to play doctor. If either your pediatrician or obstetrician recommends a prolonged stay, ask for an explanation—but do follow their professional advice. And try to make the best of your extended sojourn, getting as much rest as you can while you still have the chance.

Even if your doctors authorize your early release, you'd be wise to think twice if you don't have full-time help (either hired or volunteer) waiting for you. It's important to rest postpartum—in the hospital or at home.

"I had a rough labor and a major episiotomy, and I feel awful. But my doctor told me I have to go home this afternoon, even though I only gave birth early this morning."

P hysicians are put in a difficult position these days. Under pressure from hospitals and insurance providers, many are forced to discharge patients from the hospital sooner than their medical judgment dictates, sometimes as early as eight hours after delivery. If you really feel unwell and unready to go home, say so. Insist that you (or your husband or other family member) see the hospital's patient advocate or administrator and explain that you do not feel up to going home. You may be able to persuade them that discharging you would be unwise. Or they may allow you to stay AMA (against medical advice), in which case you, and not your insurance carrier, will probably have to foot the bill.

If you are sent home early in spite of your efforts, ask that the fact that you were discharged against your own wishes be noted on your chart. When you get home, be certain that you

have someone with you round the clock (a family member, a friend, or a hired baby nurse), get plenty of bed rest (pretend you're still in the hospital), and pay close attention to your body's signals (keeping in mind the signs and symptoms of postpartum problems; see page 381).

RECOVERY FROM A CESAREAN SECTION

"How different will my recuperation be from that of a woman with a vaginal delivery?"

R ecovery from a cesarean section is similar to recovery from any major abdominal surgery—with a delightful difference: Instead of losing an old gallbladder or appendix, you gain a brand-new baby.

Of course there's another difference, slightly less delightful. In addition to recovering from surgery, you'll also be recovering from childbirth. Except for a neatly intact perineum, you'll experience all the same postpartum discomforts you would have had if you'd delivered vaginally—afterpains, lochia, breast engorgement, fatigue, hormonal changes, hair loss, excessive perspiration, and the baby blues. (See this chapter and the next for tips on how to deal with all of these.)

As for your surgical recovery, you can expect the following in the recovery room:

Anesthesia Aftereffects. Until your anesthesia wears off, you will be observed carefully in the recovery room. You may be very shaky and sensitive to temperature change. If you've had a general anesthetic, your memory of this time may be fuzzy or totally absent. Since everyone responds differently to drugs—and each drug is different—whether you are clear-headed and alert in a few hours or not for a day or two will depend upon you and upon the medications you were given. If you feel disoriented, or have hallucinations or bad dreams, your coach or an understanding nurse can help you get back to reality when you waken.

It will take longer for spinal or epidural anesthesia to wear off—which they usually do from the toes up. You will be encouraged to wiggle your toes and move your feet as soon as you can. If you've had a spinal block, you will have to stay flat on your back for about 8 to 12 hours. You may be allowed to have both your husband and your baby visit with you in the recovery room.

Pain Around Your Incision. Once the anesthesia wears off, your wound, like any wound, is going to hurt—though just how much depends on many factors, including your personal pain threshold and how many cesareans you've had. (The first is usually the most uncomfortable.) You will probably be given pain relief medication as needed, which may make you feel woozy or drugged. It will also allow you to get some needed sleep. You needn't be concerned if you're nursing; the medication won't pass into your colostrum, and by the time your milk comes in, you probably won't need any medication.

Possibly, Nausea, With or Without Vomiting. This isn't always a problem, but if it is, you may be given an antiemetic preparation to prevent vomiting. (If you vomit easily, you might want to talk to your doctor about giving you such a medication before nausea appears.)

Breathing and Coughing Exercises. These help rid your system of any leftover general anesthetic, and help to expand your lungs and keep them clear to prevent pneumonia. Such necessary lung calisthenics may be very uncomfortable if you do them correctly. You may be able to minimize this discomfort by "splinting" your incision with a pillow.

Regular Evaluations of Your Condition. A nurse will check your vital signs (temperature, blood pressure, pulse, respiration), your urinary output and vaginal flow, the dressing on your incision, and the firmness and level of your uterus (as it shrinks in size and makes its way back into the pelvis). She will also check your IV and urinary catheter.

Once you have been moved to your hospital room, you can expect:

Continuing Evaluation of Your Condition. Your vital signs, your urinary output and vaginal flow, your dressing, and your uterus, as well as your IV and catheter (as long as they remain in place) will be checked regularly.

Removal of the Catheter After 24 Hours. Urination may be difficult, so try the tips on page 377. If they don't work, the catheter may be reinserted until you can urinate by yourself.

Afterpains. These start about 12 to 24 hours after delivery. See page 376 for more about these occasional uncomfortable contractions.

Removal of the IV. About 24 hours after surgery, or when your bowels begin to show signs of activity (by producing gas), your IV will be discontinued and you will be allowed some fluids by mouth. Over the next few days, you will probably be able to progress to soft foods, and then to a normal diet. Even if you feel as though you are starving, don't try to circumvent doctor's orders by having someone sneak in a Big Mac. Take it easy getting back to your normal diet. If you are breastfeeding, be sure to get plenty of fluids.

Referred Shoulder Pain. Irritation of the diaphragm following surgery can cause a few hours of sharp shoulder pain. An analgesic may help.

Possible Constipation. It may be a few days until you have a bowel movement, and that's all right. A stool softener or mild laxative may be prescribed to help move things along. Try some of the tips given on page 378, but exclude the roughage for the first few days. If you haven't had a movement by the fourth or fifth day, you may be given a laxative, an enema, or a suppository.

Encouragement to Exercise. Before you are out of bed, you will be encouraged to wiggle your toes, flex your calves, bend your feet up at the ankles, push against the end of the bed with your feet, and turn from side to side. You can also try these: (1) Lie flat on your back, bend one knee, and then extend the other leg while tightening your abdomen slightly. Slide the bent leg slowly back down; repeat with the other leg. (2) Lie on your back, knees pulled up, feet flat on the bed, and raise your head for about 30 seconds. (3) On your back, knees bent, tighten your abdomen, and reach with one arm across your body to the other side of the bed, at about waist level. Reverse. These exercises are intended to improve circulation, especially in your legs, and prevent the development of blood clots. (But be prepared for some of these to be quite painful, at least for the first 24 hours or so.)

To Get Up Between 8 and 24 Hours after Surgery. With the help of the nurse, you'll sit up first, supported by the raised head of the bed. Then, using your hands for support, you will slide your legs over the side of the bed and dangle them for a few minutes. Then, slowly, you'll be helped to step down on the floor, your hands still on the bed. If you feel dizzy (which is normal), sit right back down. Steady yourself for a few more minutes before taking a couple of steps. Those steps may be extremely painful. Stand as straight as you can, though the temptation to hunch over to ease the discomfort may be great. (This difficulty in getting around is temporary; in fact, you may soon find yourself more mobile than the vaginal deliveree next door—and you will certainly have the edge in sitting.)

To Wear Elastic Stockings. These improve circulation and are also intended to prevent blood clots in the legs.

Abdominal Discomfort. As your digestive tract (temporarily put out of business by surgery) begins to function again, trapped gas can cause considerable pain, especially when it presses against your incision line. The discomfort may be worse when you laugh, cough, or sneeze. Tell the nurse or doctor about your problem and they will suggest some possible remedies. Narcotics are not usually recommended because they can prolong the problem, which ordinarily lasts just a day or two. You may get a small enema or a suppository to help release the gas. Or you may be advised to walk up and down the corridor. Lying on your left side or on your back, your knees drawn up, taking deep breaths while holding your incision, may help. If the pain remains severe, a tube may be inserted in your rectum to allow the gas to escape.

Time with Your Baby. You can't lift the baby yet, but you can cuddle and feed him or her. (If you're nursing, place the baby on a pillow over your incision.) Depending on how you feel, and on hospital regulations, you may be able to have modified rooming-in. Some hospitals even allow full rooming-in.

Sponge Baths. Until the stitches are removed (or absorbed), you probably won't be allowed a real bath or shower.

Removal of Stitches. If your stitches or

clips aren't self-absorbing, they will be removed about four or five days after delivery. And although the procedure isn't very painful, you may find it uncomfortable. When the dressing is off, look at the incision with the nurse or doctor; ask how soon you can expect the area to heal, which changes will be normal, and which might require medical attention.

In most cases, you can expect to go home three to five days postpartum.

WHAT IT'S IMPORTANT TO KNOW:
GETTING STARTED BREASTFEEDING

Ever since Eve put Cain to suckle for the first time, breastfeeding has been coming naturally to mothers and newborns. Right?

Well, not always—at least not immediately. Though nursing does come naturally, it comes naturally a little later for some mothers and babies than for others. Sometimes there are physical factors that foil those first few attempts; at other times it's just a simple lack of experience on the part of both participants. But whatever might be keeping your baby and your breasts apart, it won't be long before they're in perfect synch—as long as you don't give up first. Some of the most mutually satisfying breast-baby relationships begin with several days of fumbling, of bungled efforts, and of tears on both sides.

Knowing just what to expect and how to deal with setbacks can help ease the mutual adjustment:

❖ Start as soon as possible after birth. Right in the delivery room is best, when that's feasible. (See Breastfeeding Basics, page 389.) But sometimes mother's not in any con-

dition to nurse, sometimes baby isn't—neither of which means they won't be able to start successfully later. (Even if you and the baby feel well, this first nursing experience won't necessarily go smoothly. You both have a lot to learn.)

❖ Don't let hospital bureaucracy break your tentative connection because of insensitivity, ignorance, and unnecessary rules. Enlist the support of your doctor in advance to be sure that you will be allowed to nurse in the delivery room if all goes normally. Also, arrange for full or partial rooming-in, or for a demand-feeding schedule (having the nursery bring the baby when he or she is hungry) if the staff will oblige. If the baby is with you all day, this may mean limiting visiting privileges to just your husband, which is probably for the best anyway since it allows the three of you to get to know each other while maintaining the relaxed atmosphere needed for nursing. Or you could have the nursery take the baby during visiting hours.

Breastfeeding Basics

1. Get into a comfortable position.

2. Use your thumb and index finger to pull the nipple erect.

3. Tilt the nipple slightly upward, toward the roof of the baby's mouth.

4. Bring the nipple toward the baby's cheek so that it brushes the corner of his or her mouth. This will stimulate the rooting reflex (or you can use a spare finger to do this), which makes the baby turn its mouth toward the touch.

5. Repeat steps 3 and 4 several times; the baby should eventually take the nipple in his or her mouth. (Let the baby take the initiative; don't stuff the nipple into an unwilling mouth.)

6. Be sure the areola and the nipple, not just the nipple, are in the baby's mouth. Sucking on just the nipple won't compress the milk glands and can cause soreness and cracking.

Also be sure that it is the nipple that the baby is busily milking. Some infants are so eager to suck that they will latch on to any part of the breast (even if no milk is forthcoming), and this gumming of sensitive tissue can cause a painful bruise.

7. Use your finger to press the breast away from the baby's nose to prevent interference with breathing.

8. You can assure yourself that your baby is suckling if there is a strong steady rhythmic motion visible in his or her cheek.

9. If your baby has finished suckling but is still holding on to the breast, pulling it out abruptly can cause injury to the nipple. Instead, break the suction first by depressing the breast or by putting your finger into the corner of the baby's mouth to admit some air.

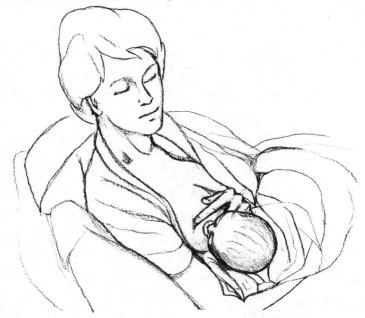

Whatever is comfortable for you and the baby is a good position; prop with pillows as necessary. And be sure not to block the baby's tiny nose with your breast.

❖ Don't let sleeping babies lie if it means that they'll sleep through a feeding. If you have rooming-in, you're not likely to have a problem with this. You'll be able to demand-feed the baby when he or she is hungry and let the baby sleep when he or she's sleepy. If you're dependent on the nursery staff to bring the baby—on their schedule, not junior's—you may find that feeding time is over before the baby wakes. Don't let this happen. If the baby isn't awake on arrival at your room, wake him or her. This sounds crueler than it actually is. Gently set the baby on the bed in a sitting position, one hand holding up the chin, the other supporting the back. Next, bend the baby forward at the waist. The moment he or she stirs, quickly adopt the nursing position. If your baby is swaddled, loosen the blanket so he or she can be close to you.

❖ Be patient if your baby is still recovering from delivery. If you received anesthesia or had a prolonged, difficult labor, you can expect your baby to be drowsy and sluggish at the breast for a few days. This is no reflection on you, your nursing ability, or your baby. There's no danger the baby will starve in the meantime, since newborns have little need for nourishment during the first days of life. What they do need, though, is nurturing. Cuddling at the breast is just as important as suckling.

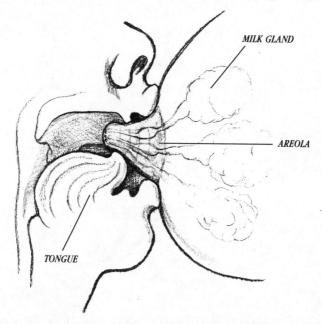

Baby and Breast—A Perfect Feeding Team

MILK GLAND

AREOLA

TONGUE

Be sure that the nursing baby has the areola and not just the nipple in his or her mouth. This way the milk can be efficiently and, eventually, painlessly extracted.

❖ Make sure your baby's appetite and sucking instinct aren't sabotaged between feedings. It's routine in some hospital nurseries to quiet a crying baby between mother's feedings with a bottle of sugar water. This can have a twofold detrimental effect. First, it satisfies the baby's still-delicate appetite for hours. Later, when brought to you for feeding, if your baby doesn't want to nurse, and your breasts aren't stimulated to produce milk, a vicious cycle will have begun. Second, because the rubber nipple requires less effort, the baby's sucking reflex becomes lazy. Faced with the greater challenge of tackling the breast, he or she may just give up. *Don't let anyone talk you into the sugar water.* Give strict orders—through your pediatrician —that supplementary feedings are not to be given to your baby in the nursery unless medically necessary.[2]

❖ Don't try to feed a screaming baby. It's hard enough for an inexperienced suckler to find the nipple when calm. When your baby is overexcited, it may be impossible. Rock and soothe him or her before you start nursing.

❖ If you're having trouble establishing breastfeeding, ask for assistance from hospital personnel or from your practitioner. If you are lucky, a lactation specialist will join you at your first baby feeding to provide hands-on instruction, helpful hints, and perhaps literature. If this is not

a policy in your hospital (or you are somehow bypassed), you can find empathy and advice by calling your local La Leche League chapter.

❖ No matter how frustrating nursing becomes, try to stay calm. Start out as relaxed as you can. Clear out the visitors 15 minutes before feeding time, and don't think about your hospital bill or anything else that might upset you. Then try to remain cool throughout the nursing period, no matter how badly it's going. Tension not only hampers your ability to give milk, it can cause anxiety in your baby. An infant is extremely sensitive to its mother's moods, and reacts accordingly.

WHEN THE MILK COMES IN

Just when you and your baby seem to be getting the hang of it, your milk comes in. Up until now, your baby has been getting tiny amounts of colostrum (premilk), and your breasts have been quite comfortable. Then, within a few hours, your breasts become swollen, hard, and painful. Nursing is difficult for the baby and agonizing for you.[3] Fortunately, this period of engorgement is brief. While it lasts, there are a variety of ways of relieving it and the accompanying discomfort:

❖ Nurse more often, for shorter periods—a four-hour schedule can lead to engorgement, and 20-minute nursing periods to sore nipples; both make nursing difficult in the long run for mother and baby. Start

---

2. You may also want to discuss with your pediatrician the pros and cons of a pacifier being given to your baby in the nursery. On the one hand, it could get him or her hooked on a rubber nipple; on the other, it may be comforting when there's no one to cuddle with in the middle of the night.

3. A few lucky new mothers don't experience engorgement when their milk comes in, possibly because their babies were vigorous nursers from birth; there is also less engorgement with subsequent babies.

off with 5 minutes on each breast, gradually building up to 15 minutes on each by the third or fourth day.

❖ Don't be tempted to skip or skimp on a feeding because of pain. The less your baby sucks, the more en-

gorged you will become. Don't favor one breast because it is less sore or because the nipple isn't cracked; the only way to toughen up nipples is to use them. Use both breasts at every feeding, even if only for a few minutes—but nurse from the

---

Best-Odds Nursing Diet

The levels of protein, fat, and carbohydrates in your breast milk aren't usually affected by the levels of these nutrients in your diet; however, levels of some vitamins are (A and B_{12}, for example). But though the quality of your milk isn't always directly related to the quality of your diet, the quantity of milk usually is. Women whose diets are deficient in protein and/or calories, for example, may produce milk of good composition but in smaller amounts. To make good breast milk, and plenty of it, continue taking your pregnancy (or pregnancy/lactation) vitamin-mineral supplement, and adhere closely to the Best-Odds Diet on page 80, with modifications:

❖ Increase your caloric intake to about 500 calories per day over your prepregnancy requirements. This is flexible, and as during pregnancy, you can let your scale be your guide. If you have a lot of fat stores from pregnancy (or before), you can take fewer calories, as the fat will be burned to produce milk (and you will lose weight). If you are underweight, you will probably need more than 500 additional calories daily (the recommended daily allowance assumes some use of fat stores, which you don't have). No matter what your weight, you may find that you need still more calories as the baby grows and demands more milk. Again, you will be able to determine this by checking your

scale. If your weight starts dipping below the ideal, increase your daily intake.

❖ Increase your calcium requirement to five servings per day.

❖ Reduce your protein intake to three servings per day.

❖ Drink at least eight glasses of fluids (milk, water, broths or soups, and juices); take more during hot weather and if you've been perspiring a lot. (Though it's all right to drink moderate amounts of tea or coffee, and an occasional alcoholic beverage, don't count them in your fluid allowance since they have a dehydrating effect.) Excess is not best, however; flooding yourself with fluid (more than 12 glasses per day) can paradoxically *slow* milk production. Thirst and urinary output can help you gauge your needs.

❖ Splurge occasionally. You've served your nine-month sentence of abstinence; you're entitled to your just desserts, at least once in a while. The key is moderation. Small amounts of sugar won't interfere with milk production, but a steady diet of sweets can, by dulling your appetite for necessary nutrients. Ditto for other nutritionally superfluous foods, such as potato chips, french fries, white bread; eat them only *after* you've fulfilled your nutritional obligations.

less sore one first, since the baby will suck more vigorously when hungry. If both nipples are equally sore (or not sore at all), start off the feeding with the breast you used last.

❖ Use a breast pump on each breast before nursing to lessen the engorgement so that your baby can get a better hold on the nipple, and to get milk flow started. After nursing, empty the second breast if the baby hasn't already done so.

❖ Use ice packs to reduce engorgement. Or a hot shower or hot soaks, if you find them more soothing.

❖ Support is important in a nursing bra, but pressure against your sore and engorged breasts can be painful. Whenever leaking isn't a problem—and especially after nursing —leave the flaps of your nursing bra open.

SORE NIPPLES

T ender nipples sometimes compound the difficulties of early nursing. Most toughen up quickly. But in some women, particularly those who are fair-skinned, the nipples become sore and cracked. To relieve the discomfort:

❖ Expose sore or cracked nipples to the air as much as possible. Protect them from clothing and other irritations and surround them with a cushion of air by wearing breast shells (not shields).

❖ Let nature—and not the cosmetic companies—take care of your nipples. Nipples are naturally protected and lubricated by sweat glands and skin oils. A commercial preparation should be used only when nipple cracking is severe, and

then should be as pure as possible. Do not use lanolin, which may be contaminated, or petroleum-based ointments (such as Vaseline). Instead, apply vitamin E squeezed from opened capsules directly onto the nipples. Wash nipples only with water—never with soap, alcohol, tincture of benzoin, or premoistened towelettes—whether your nipples are sore or not: Your baby is already protected from your germs, and the milk itself is clean.

❖ Vary your nursing position so a different part of the nipple will be compressed at each feeding.

❖ Relax for 15 minutes or so before feeding. Relaxation will enhance the let-down of milk, whereas tension will only hinder it.

OCCASIONAL COMPLICATIONS

O nce nursing is established, it generally continues uneventfully until weaning. But once in a while, complications occur, among them:

Clogged Milk Ducts. Sometimes a milk duct clogs, causing milk to back up. Since this condition (characterized by a small, red, and tender lump on the breast) can lead to infection, it's important to try to remedy it quickly. The best way to do this is to offer the affected breast first at each feeding, and to let your baby empty it as completely as possible. If he or she doesn't do the job, any remaining milk should be expressed by hand or with a breast pump. Keep pressure off the duct by making sure your bra is not too tight, and by varying your nursing positions to put pressure on different ducts. Also, check to see if dried milk is blocking the nipple after nursing. If so, clean it off with sterile cotton dipped in boiled and cooled water. Do not use this time to wean the baby; discontinuing nursing now will only compound your problem.

Breast Infection. A more serious complication of breastfeeding is mastitis, or breast infection, which can occur in one or both breasts, most often between the 10th and 28th postpartum day, in an estimated 7% to 10% of mothers—usually first-timers. The factors that can combine to cause mastitis are failure to empty breasts completely of milk at each nursing, germs gaining entrance into the milk ducts through a crack or fissure in the nipple (usually from the baby's mouth), and lowered resistance in the mother due to stress, fatigue, and inadequate nutrition.

The most common symptoms of mastitis are severe soreness, hardness, redness, heat, and swelling of the breast, with generalized chills and a fever of about 101 to 102 degrees. If you develop some of these symptoms, contact your doctor. Prompt medical treatment is necessary, and may include bed rest, antibiotics, pain relievers, increased fluid intake, and ice or moist heat applications. During treatment you should continue to nurse. Since the baby's germs probably caused the infection in the first place, they won't harm him or her. And emptying the breast will help to prevent clogged milk ducts. Nurse first on the infected breast, and empty it with a pump if the baby doesn't. If the pain is so excruciating that you can't nurse, try pumping your breasts while lying in a tub of warm water with your breasts floating comfortably. Don't use an electric pump.

Delay in treating mastitis could lead to the development of a breast abscess, the symptoms of which include excruciating, throbbing pain; localized swelling, tenderness, and heat in the area of the abscess; and temperature swings between 100 and 103 degrees. Treatment includes antibiotics and, generally, surgical drainage under anesthesia. Breastfeeding with the affected breast must be halted, and a breast pump should be used regularly to empty it until healing is complete and breastfeeding can be resumed. In the meantime, nursing can continue on the unaffected breast.

Don't let breast and nursing problems with your first baby discourage you from nursing future babies. Engorgement and nipple soreness are far less common with subsequent births.

BREASTFEEDING AFTER A CESAREAN

How soon you can breastfeed your newborn after a surgical delivery will depend on how you feel and how your baby is doing. If you are both in good shape, you can probably introduce baby to breast in the delivery room after the surgery is completed, or in the recovery room shortly afterward. If you're groggy from general anesthesia or your baby needs imme-

---

Medication and Breastfeeding

Be sure to tell any physician who prescribes medication for you that you are nursing your baby. Many medications are safe to use when nursing; some others are not. It is usually best to take medication just after you finish a feeding, so that levels in your milk will be lowest when you nurse again.

diate care in the nursery, you may have to wait. If after 12 hours you still haven't been able to get together with your baby, you should probably inquire about using a pump to express milk (at this point it is actually premilk, or colostrum) to get lactation started.

You may find breastfeeding after a cesarean uncomfortable at first—most mothers do. It will be less so if you try to avoid putting pressure on the incision: place a pillow on your lap under the baby; lie on your side; or use the football hold, again supported by a pillow, to nurse. Both the afterpains you experience as you nurse (see page 376) and the soreness at the site of the incision are normal and will lessen in the days ahead.

BREASTFEEDING TWINS

Breastfeeding, like just about every aspect of caring for newborn twins, seems as though it will be impossible until you get into the rhythm of it. Once you have a routine, it is not only possible but very rewarding. To successfully nurse twins, you should:

❖ Fulfill all the dietary recommendations for lactating mothers (see the Best-Odds Nursing Diet), with these additions: 400 to 500 calories above your prepregnancy needs for *each* baby you are nursing (you may need to increase your caloric intake as the babies grow bigger and hun-

grier, or decrease it if you supplement nursing with formula and/or solids, or if you have considerable fat reserves you would like to burn); an additional serving of protein (for a total of four) and an additional serving of calcium (six total) or a calcium supplement.

❖ Drink 8 to 12 cups of fluid a day—but not more, because too much may suppress milk production.

❖ Get as much help as you can with housework, meal preparation, and infant care, in order to conserve your energy.

❖ Explore the various feeding options: nurse one baby, bottle-feed the other; alternate feedings of bottle and breast with each baby; or nurse each separately (which can take ten hours or more a day), or both together. Combining individual and group feedings, and giving each infant at least one private feeding a day, is a good compromise that encourages mother-baby closeness. Father might give a bottle to the other baby at these feedings. Such relief bottles, given by the father or another helper, can be either formula or expressed milk.

❖ Recognize that the twins have different personalities, needs, and nursing patterns, and don't try to treat them identically. Keep records to be sure both are fed at each feeding.

19
Postpartum: The First Six Weeks

WHAT YOU MAY BE FEELING

During the first six weeks postpartum, depending on the type of delivery you had (easy or difficult, vaginal or cesarean), how much help you have at home, and other individual factors, you may experience all, or only some, of the following:

PHYSICALLY:

❖ Continued vaginal discharge (lochia), turning brownish, then yellowish-white

❖ Fatigue

❖ Some pain, discomfort, and numbness in the perineum, if you had a vaginal delivery (especially if you had stitches)

❖ Diminishing incisional pain, continuing numbness, if you had a cesarean delivery (especially if it was your first)

❖ Continued constipation (although this should be easing up)

❖ Gradual flattening of your abdomen as your uterus recedes into the pelvis (but only exercise will bring you fully back to prepregnancy shape)

❖ Gradual loss of weight

❖ Breast discomfort and nipple soreness until breastfeeding is well established

❖ Achiness in arms and neck (from carrying the baby)

❖ Hair loss

EMOTIONALLY:

❖ Elation, depression, or swings between the two

❖ A sense of being overwhelmed, a growing feeling of confidence, or swings between the two

❖ Decreased or increased sexual desire

WHAT YOU CAN EXPECT AT YOUR POSTPARTUM CHECKUP

Your practitioner will probably schedule you for a checkup four to six weeks postpartum.[1] During that visit, you can expect the following to be checked, though the exact content of the visit will vary depending upon what your particular needs are and your practitioner's style of practice.

❖ Blood pressure

❖ Weight, which will probably be down by 17 to 20 pounds or more

❖ Your uterus, to see if it has returned to prepregnant shape, size, and location

❖ Your cervix, which will be on its way back to its prepregnant state, but will still be somewhat engorged and its surface possibly eroded

❖ Your vagina, which will have contracted and regained much of its muscle tone

❖ The episiotomy or laceration repair site, if any; or, if you had a cesarean delivery, the site of your incision

❖ Your breasts, for any abnormalities

❖ Hemorrhoids or varicose veins, if you have either

❖ Questions or problems you want to discuss—have a list ready

At this visit, the practitioner will also discuss with you the method of birth control that you will be using. If you plan on using a diaphragm and your cervix has recovered sufficiently, you will be fitted for one; if not, you may have to use condoms until you can be fitted. If you're not breastfeeding and plan to take birth control pills, they may be prescribed now.

WHAT YOU MAY BE CONCERNED ABOUT

FEVER

"I've just returned home from the hospital and I'm running a fever of about 101 degrees. Could it be related to childbirth?"

Thanks to Dr. Ignaz Semmelweiss, the chances of a new mother developing childbed (or puerperal) fever today are extremely slight. It was in

1847 that this young Viennese physician discovered that if birth attendants washed their hands before delivering babies, the risk of childbirth-related infection could be greatly reduced (though at the time, his theory was considered so outlandish that he was driven from his post, ostracized, and later died a broken man). And thanks to Sir Alexander Fleming, the British scientist who developed the first infection-fighting antibiotics, the occasional case that does occur is easily cured.

The most severe cases of infection usually begin within 24 hours of delivery. A fever on the third or fourth

---

1. If you had a cesarean, your physician may also check your incision at about three weeks postpartum.

day, when you are already at home, could possibly be a sign of postpartum infection—but it could also be caused by a virus or other minor problem. A low-grade fever (of about 100 degrees) occasionally accompanies engorgement when your milk first comes in. Report any fever that lasts more than four hours during the first three postpartum weeks to the doctor—even if it's accompanied by obvious cold or flu symptoms or vomiting—so that its cause can be diagnosed and any necessary treatment started. See page 365 if postpartum infection is suspected or diagnosed.

DEPRESSION

"I have everything I have always wanted: a wonderful husband, a beautiful new baby—why do I feel so blue?"

Why should roughly one half of all new mothers be so miserable during one of the happiest times of their lives? That's the paradox of postpartum depression, for which experts have yet to provide any definitive explanations or solutions.

Hormones, so often the culprit fingered in the case of a woman's mood swings, may offer some rationale. Levels of estrogen and progesterone drop precipitously after childbirth and may trigger depression, just as hormonal fluctuations prior to menstruation may do. The fact that sensitivity to hormonal fluctuations varies from woman to woman is believed to explain at least partially why, though all women experience the same shift in hormone levels after delivery, only about 50% suffer from postpartum depression.

But there are a host of other factors that probably contribute to the postpartum blues—which are most common around the third day after delivery, but which can strike at any time during the first year, and which afflict second-time mothers more often than first-timers:

The Shift from Center Stage to Backstage. Your baby is now the star of the show. Visitors would rather run to the nursery than sit at your bedside inquiring after your health. This change in status will accompany you home; the pregnant princess is now the postpartum Cinderella.

Hospitalization. When you're eager to get home and begin mothering, you may be frustrated by the lack of control you have over your life and your baby's in the hospital.

Going Home. It's not unusual to feel overwhelmed and overworked by the responsibilities that greet you (particularly if you have other children and no help).

Exhaustion. Fatigue from a strenuous labor and from too little sleep in the hospital is compounded by the rigors of caring for a newborn, and often contributes to the feeling that you aren't equal to the demands of motherhood.

A Sense of Disappointment in the Baby. He or she's so small, so red, so puffy, so unresponsive—not quite the all-smiles Ivory Snow baby you'd pictured. Resultant guilt adds to depression.

A Sense of Disappointment in the Birth and/or in Yourself. If unrealistic expectations of an idealized childbirth experience weren't realized, you may feel (unnecessarily) that you've somehow failed.

A Feeling of Anticlimax. Childbirth—the big event you'd schooled for and looked forward to—is over.

Feelings of Inadequacy. A novice mother may wonder, "Why did I have a baby if I can't take care of it?"

A Sense of Mourning for the Old You. Your carefree, possibly career-oriented, self has died (at least temporarily) with your baby's birth.

Unhappiness over Your Looks. Before you were fat and pregnant; now you're just fat. You can't stand wearing maternity clothes, but nothing else fits.

Probably the only good thing that can be said about postpartum depression is that it doesn't last very long—about 48 hours for most women. And though there's no cure other than the passage of time, there are ways of fading those baby blues:

❖ If the blues arrive at the hospital, try to have your husband bring in a special dinner for the two of you; limit visitors if their chattering grates on your nerves, have more of them if they cheer you up. If it's the hospital that's getting you down, inquire about early discharge. (See Going Home, page 384.)

❖ Fight fatigue by accepting help from others, by being less compulsive about doing things that can wait, by trying to squeeze in a nap or rest period when your baby is sleeping. Use feeding times as rest periods, nursing or bottle-feeding in bed or in a comfortable chair with your feet up.

❖ Follow the Best-Odds Nursing Diet (see page 392) to keep your strength up (minus 500 calories and three calcium servings if you're not breastfeeding). Avoid sugar (especially combined with chocolate), which can act as a depressant.

❖ Occasionally unwind with your husband over a cocktail after the baby's evening feeding, but be careful not to overdo—too much can lead to morning-after depression.

❖ Treat yourself to dinner out, if possible. If not, make believe. Order dinner in (or let your husband cook), dress up, create a restaurant ambiance with candlelight and soft music. And keep your sense of humor handy, in case the baby decides to interrupt your romantic interlude.

❖ Look good so you'll feel good. Walking around in a robe all day with unkempt hair would depress anyone. Shower before your husband leaves in the morning (or you may not have a chance again); comb your hair; put on makeup if you ordinarily wear it. Buy an attractive new outfit (washable, of course) that fits loosely now but can be belted so that it continues to fit as you lose weight.

❖ Get out of the house. Go for a walk with the baby or, if someone volunteers to sit, without the baby. Exercise helps chase away the baby blues and will help you get rid of any postpartum flab that might be adding to your depression. But don't do too much too soon.

❖ If you think your misery might like some company, get together with any new mothers you know, and share your feelings with them. If you don't have any newly delivered friends, make some. Ask your pediatrician for names of new mothers in your neighborhood, or contact women who were in your childbirth class, possibly organizing a weekly after-birth reunion. Or join a postpartum exercise class.

❖ If yours is the kind of misery that would rather be by itself, indulge in some solitude. Though depression usually feeds on itself, some experts believe that this is not true of the postpartum variety. If going out with cheerful people, or having cheerful people visit, makes you feel worse—don't do it. Don't, however, leave your husband out in the cold. Communication in the immediate postpartum period is vital for you both. (Husbands, too, are susceptible to postpartum depression, and yours may need you as much as you need him.)

Severe postpartum depression, which requires professional therapy, is extremely rare—affecting fewer than 1 in 1,000 women. If your depression persists for more than two weeks and is accompanied by sleeplessness, lack of appetite, a feeling of hopelessness and helplessness—even suicidal urges or violent or aggressive feelings toward the baby—seek counseling promptly.

"I feel terrific, and have since the moment I delivered three weeks ago. Is all this good feeling building up to one terrific case of letdown?"

It's an unfortunate fact that feeling good doesn't get the kind of attention that feeling bad does. There's no shortage of articles in magazines and newspapers, or chapters in books, about the 50% of newly delivered women who suffer from postpartum depression; but there's little or nothing written about the other 50% who feel terrific after giving birth.

Baby blues are common, but they're by no means an absolute requirement of the postpartum period. And there's no reason to believe that you're in for an emotional crash just because you've been feeling buoyant. Since the majority of baby blues cases occur within the first postpartum week, it's pretty safe to assume you've escaped them. If you'd like to play it even safer

(or if you'd like to prevent depression occurring when you wean), see the tips for fading those baby blues, above.

The fact that you're not suffering from postpartum depression, however, doesn't mean your family has escaped this problem completely. Studies show that while new fathers are unlikely to be depressed when their wives are, their risk of falling into a postpartum slump increases dramatically when the new mother is feeling great. So be sure that your husband isn't experiencing the baby blues. And if he is, use some of the tips on page 398 to help him over them. If his depression persists, or if it is so severe that it interferes with his work and other activities, then be sure that he seeks professional help.

RETURNING TO PREPREGNANCY WEIGHT AND SHAPE

"I knew I wouldn't be ready for a bikini right after delivery, but I still look six months pregnant a week later."

Though childbearing produces more rapid weight loss than the Scarsdale, Stillman, and Mayo Clinic diets combined (an average of 12 pounds at delivery), most women don't find it quite rapid enough. Particularly after they catch a glimpse of their postpartum silhouettes in the mirror—which can still look distressingly pregnant. But happily, most will be able to pack away their maternity jeans within a month or two.

Of course, how quickly you return to your prepregnant shape and weight will depend on how many pounds and inches you put on during pregnancy. Women who gained 25 pounds or so should be able to shed the weight, without dieting, by the end of the second month. Others will find that delivery won't make thighs and hips thickened by overindulgence during pregnancy magically disappear. But sticking to the Best-Odds Nursing Diet (see page 392) if they are breastfeeding (or to the Diet minus the 500 extra nursing calories and the extra calcium serving[2] if they are not) should start them on the way to slow, steady weight loss. After the first six weeks, non-nursers can go on a good, well-balanced reducing diet, such as Weight Watchers. Nursing mothers with considerable amounts of excess body fat can cut their caloric intake somewhat without cutting into milk production and also lose weight. They will usually take off any remaining excess poundage when they wean their babies.

Getting back into shape is a problem even for those women who didn't gain excess weight. No one comes out of the delivery room looking much slimmer than when they went in. Part of the reason for that protruding postpartum abdomen is the still-enlarged uterus, which will be reduced to pre-pregnancy size by the end of six weeks, reducing your abdominal girth in the process. (You can follow the progress of your uterus by asking the nurse or your practitioner to show you how to palpate it in your abdomen. When you can no longer feel it, it has slipped back into the pelvis.) Another reason for your bloated belly is leftover fluids, 5 pounds or so of which will flush out within a few days after delivery. But the rest of the problem is stretched-out abdominal muscles and skin, which may sag for a

lifetime unless a concerted exercise effort is made. (See Getting Back into Shape, page 408.)

BREAST MILK

"Does everything I eat, drink, or take get into my breast milk? Could any of it harm my baby?"

F eeding your baby outside the womb doesn't demand quite as Spartan an existence as feeding him or her inside did. But as long as you're breastfeeding, a certain amount of restraint in what goes into you will ensure that everything that goes into your baby is safe.

The basic fat-protein-carbohydrate composition of human milk isn't dependent on what a mother eats. If a mother doesn't eat enough calories and protein to produce milk, her body's stores will be tapped and the baby will be fed—until the stores run out. Some vitamin deficiencies in the mother's diet will, however, affect the vitamin content of her breast milk. So will excesses of some vitamins. A wide variety of substances, from medications to seasonings, can also show up in milk, with varying results.

To keep breast milk safe and healthful:

❖ Follow the Best-Odds Nursing Diet (page 392).

❖ Avoid foods to which your baby seems sensitive. Garlic, onion, cabbage, dairy products, and chocolate are common offenders, causing bothersome gas in some, though by no means all, babies. Infants with discriminating palates may also be displeased by the taste a strong seasoning may impart.

❖ Take a vitamin supplement especially formulated for pregnant and/ or lactating mothers. Do not take

---

2. It may be a good idea for women who are not nursing to continue to get adequate calcium to prevent the development of osteoporosis later in life. If necessary, take a calcium supplement to get your intake up to 1,200 mg daily.

any other vitamins without the advice of your physician.

❖ Do not smoke. Many of the toxic substances in tobacco enter the bloodstream, and eventually your milk. (Besides, smoking near the baby can cause respiratory problems for him or her and may even be associated with sudden infant death syndrome, or crib death.)

❖ Do not take any medications or recreational drugs without consulting your physician. Most drugs pass into the breast milk, and even in small doses can be harmful to a tiny infant. (Particularly dangerous are antithyroid, antihypertensive, and anticancer drugs; penicillin[3]; narcotic drugs, including heroin, methadone, and prescription painkillers; marijuana and cocaine; tranquilizers, barbiturates and sedatives; lithium; hormones, such as most birth control pills; radioactive iodine; bromides.) Often, safe substitutes can be found for a medication you must take; or perhaps a particular medication can be discontinued for the duration of nursing. (Do make sure that any doctor who prescribes a medication for you is aware that you are breastfeeding.)

❖ Avoid alcohol entirely, or have a single drink only occasionally. Daily imbibing or binge drinking can make baby drowsy, depress the nervous system, and may slow motor development.

❖ Restrict your intake of caffeine. One cup of caffeinated coffee or tea a day probably won't affect your baby. Six cups could make him or her jittery.

❖ Don't take laxatives to promote regularity (some of them will have a laxative effect on your baby); increase your fiber intake instead.

❖ Take aspirin or aspirin substitutes only with your practitioner's approval, but don't take more than the recommended dose, and don't take the drugs frequently.

❖ Avoid excessive amounts of chemicals in the foods you eat, and opt for the foods that are close to their natural state. Read labels to steer clear of foods composed largely of synthetic chemicals.[4] Avoid saccharin, since it passes into the breast milk and has been shown in animal studies to cause cancer. Aspartame, on the other hand, seems to pass into the breast milk in only small quantities and appears safe to use. But be sure the foods you consume that contain aspartame aren't full of a lot of other chemicals.

❖ Minimize your ingestion of incidental pesticides. A certain amount of pesticide residue in your diet (from produce, for example), and thus in your breast milk, is inevitable—and not proven to be harmful to a nursing infant. But though hysteria about possible breast milk contamination is unwarranted, it's prudent to keep your baby's exposure to pesticides as low as you can without giving up eating. Peel vegetables and fruits or scrub with detergent and water; eat low-fat milk products, lean meats, white-meat poultry with the skin removed, and limited amounts of organ meats. (The pesticides ingested by animals are stored in fat, skin, and possibly organs.)

❖ Avoid eating any fish that might be

---

3. Exposure to penicillin at this early age could lead to a baby developing a sensitivity, or allergy, to the drug.

4. See *What to Eat When You're Expecting* for a list of safe, unsafe, and questionable chemicals used in foods.

contaminated. (The same rules for safe fish and seafood consumption that apply to pregnant women apply to lactating women; see page 130.)

LONG-TERM CESAREAN RECOVERY

"I am just now going home, four days after a cesarean. What can I expect?"

To Need Plenty of Help. Paid help is best for the first week, but if that's not possible, ask your husband, mother, or another relative to lend a hand. It's best not to do any lifting (including the baby) or any housework, at least for the first week. If you must lift the baby, lift from waist level, so you use your arms, not your abdomen. Bend at the knees, not at the waist.

Little or No Pain. But if you do hurt, a mild pain reliever should help. Don't take medication, however, if you are breastfeeding, unless it has been approved by your doctor.

Progressive Improvement. Your scar will be sore and sensitive for a few weeks, but will improve steadily. A light dressing may protect it from irritation and you will probably be more comfortable wearing loose clothing. Occasional sensations of pulling or twitching and other brief pains in the region of the scar are a normal part of healing and will eventually subside. Itchiness may follow. The numbness of the abdomen around the scar will last longer, possibly several months. Lumpiness in the scar tissue will probably diminish (unless you tend to get that kind of scar), and the scar may turn pink or purple before it finally fades.

If pain becomes persistent, if the area around the incision turns an an-gry red, or if a brown, gray, green, or yellow discharge oozes from the wound, call your doctor. The incision may have become infected. (A small amount of clear fluid discharge may be normal, but report it to your physician anyway.)

To Wait at Least Four Weeks Before Resuming Sexual Intercourse. Depending on how your incision is healing and when your cervix returns to normal, your doctor may recommend that you wait anywhere from four to six weeks for actual intercourse (though other kinds of lovemaking are certainly permissible). See page 404 for tips on making postpartum intercourse more successful. You are, incidentally, much more likely to find resumption of intercourse comfortable than are women who delivered vaginally.

To Be Able to Start Exercising Once You Are Free of Pain. Since the muscle tone of your perineum probably hasn't been compromised, you may not need to do Kegel exercises, though they can benefit anyone. Concentrate instead on those that tighten the abdominal muscles. (See Getting Back into Shape, page 408.) Make "slow and steady" your motto; get into a program gradually and continue it daily. Expect it to take several months before you're back to your old self.

RESUMING SEXUAL RELATIONS

"My doctor says I have to wait six weeks before having sex. Friends say that isn't necessary."

It's fairly safe to assume that your doctor is more familiar with your medical condition than your friends are. And his or her restriction is probably based on what's best for you, taking into consideration the kind of labor and delivery you had, whether or not you had an episiotomy or laceration, and the speed of healing and recovery. Some practitioners, of course, apply the six-week rule routinely to all their postpartum patients, regardless of condition. If you think that's the case with your doctor and you're feeling up to making love, ask if he or she will consider bending the rule for you. This will be possible only if your cervix has healed and the lochia has stopped. And, for your own comfort, you probably will also want to wait until intercourse no longer causes discomfort in your perineal area.

Should your plea be denied, however, it's wise to follow your doctor's orders. Waiting the full six weeks can't hurt (at least not physically), while not waiting might.

LACK OF INTEREST IN MAKING LOVE

"Ever since the baby was born I just don't feel very interested in sex."

Sex takes energy, concentration, and time—all of which are in particularly short supply in the lives of new parents. Your libido—and your husband's—must regularly compete with sleepless nights, exhausting days, dirty diapers, and an endlessly demanding baby. Your body is still recuperating from the trauma of childbearing; your hormones are readjusting. Fears (of pain, of doing some damage internally, of not being the same, of becoming pregnant again too soon) may plague you. If you are breastfeeding, this may unconsciously be satisfying your sexual needs. Or making love may stimulate uncomfortable leakage of milk. All in all, it's not surprising—

and perfectly normal—if your sexual appetite, no matter how voracious it once was, is temporarily suppressed. (On the other hand, some women have strong sexual drives now, particularly in the immediate postpartum period, when there is engorgement of the genital region.)

If your problem is lack of interest, there are many ways to make making love good again. Which ones will work for you will depend on you, your husband, and your problems:

Make Time Your Ally. It takes at least six weeks for your body to heal, and sometimes much longer—especially if you had a difficult delivery or a cesarean. Your hormonal balance won't be back to normal until you start menstruating, which, if you are breastfeeding, may not be for many months. Even if the doctor's given you the go-ahead, don't feel obligated to make love if it doesn't feel good, emotionally or physically. And when you do, start slowly, possibly with cuddling and petting but no penetration.

Don't Be Discouraged by Pain. Many women are surprised and disheartened to find that postpartum intercourse can really hurt. If you've had an episiotomy or a laceration, there may be discomfort (ranging from slight to severe) for weeks, even months, after the stitches have healed. You may also have pain with intercourse, although it may be less severe, if you delivered with the perineum intact—and even if you've had a cesarean. Until the pain eases, you can try to minimize it in the ways described in Easing Back into Sex, facing page.

Find Alternative Means of Gratification. If intercourse isn't pleasurable yet, seek sexual satisfaction through mutual masturbation or oral sex. Or if you're both too pooped to pop, find pleasure in just being together. There's

Easing Back into Sex

Lubricate. Lowered hormone levels during the postpartum period (which may not rise in the nursing mother until her baby is either partially or totally weaned) can make the vagina uncomfortably dry. Use a lubricating cream, like K-Y Jelly, until your own natural secretions return.

Medicate, If Necessary. Your practitioner may prescribe an estrogen cream to lessen pain and tenderness.

Inebriate. Don't get drunk, of course (since too much alcohol can interfere with sexual enjoyment and perfor-

mance, and if you're breastfeeding can be harmful to your baby), but do feel free to enjoy a glass of wine with your husband before making love, to help both of you relax physically and emotionally. It will also dull some of your pain, plus lessen your fear of feeling it and his fear of causing it. Or use other relaxation techniques to banish fear.

Vary Positions. Side-to-side or woman-on-top positions allow more control of penetration and put less pressure on the episiotomy site. Experiment to find what works best for you.

---

absolutely nothing wrong (and everything right) about lying in bed together, cuddling, kissing, and swapping baby stories.

Keep Your Expectations Realistic. Don't expect simultaneous orgasms the first time you make love after delivery. Some usually orgasmic women don't have orgasms at all for several weeks, or even longer. With love and patience, sex will eventually be as satisfying as ever—or more so.

Readjust Your Sex Life to Dovetail with Your Life with the Baby. When your companionable two becomes a crowded three, you can no longer make love when and where you want to. Instead you'll have to either grab it when you can (if the baby is napping at 3 o'clock on Saturday afternoon, drop everything) or make a point of planning ahead. Don't feel that unspontaneous sex can't be fun. Instead, think of the advance planning as giving you the opportunity to look forward to making love (the baby will be asleep at 8—can't wait!). Accept interruptions—there will be many—with a

sense of humor, and try to start again where you left off as soon as possible. And should sex turn out to be less frequent than before, strive for quality, not quantity.

Don't Be a Perfectionist. A lot of postpartum exhaustion is natural; learning to become parents is certainly taxing. But some of it is unnecessary, often caused by trying to do too much too soon. Pack away your white gloves and forgo the dusting sometimes. Use frozen vegetables instead of fresh. Cut some dispensable corners, so that you occasionally have sufficient energy left for loving.

Communicate. A really good sexual relationship must be built on trust, understanding, and communication. If, for instance, you're too wrapped up in motherhood one night to feel sexy, don't beg off with a headache. Be honest. A husband who's been included in parenting since conception is most likely to understand. If intercourse is painful, don't be a martyr. Explain to your spouse what hurts, what feels good, what you'd rather put off until another time.

Don't Worry. Despite how you may be feeling now, you will live to love again, with as much passion and pleasure as ever. (And because shared parenthood can often bring couples closer together, you may find the flame not only rekindled, but burning brighter than before.) Worry now can only put an unnecessary damper on your sexual relationship.

BECOMING PREGNANT AGAIN

"I thought that breastfeeding was a form of birth control. Now I hear you can get pregnant while nursing, even before you start menstruating again."

How completely you can rely on nursing as a means of birth control depends on how completely devastated you would be if you became pregnant again now. If you're like most brand-new parents, tummy-to-tummy pregnancies just months apart are not your idea of perfect family planning. And if that is indeed the case, breastfeeding by itself shouldn't be relied on for contraception.

It's true that on the average, women who nurse resume normal menstrual cycles later than those who don't. In nonlactating mothers menstruation usually begins somewhere between four and eight weeks after delivery, whereas in lactating women the average is somewhere between three and four months. As usual, however, averages are deceptive. Nursing women have been known to begin menstruating as early as 6 weeks and as late as 18 months postpartum. The problem is, there's no sure way to predict when you will again begin menstruating, though several variables can influence the timing. For example, frequency of

feeding (more than three times a day seems to suppress ovulation better), duration of nursing (the longer you nurse, the greater the delay in ovulation), and whether or not feedings are being supplemented (your baby's taking bottles, solids, even water, can interfere with the ovulation-suppressing effect of nursing).

Why worry about birth control before that first menstrual period? Because the point at which you ovulate for the first time after delivery is as unpredictable as when you menstruate. Some women have a sterile first period; that is, they don't ovulate during that cycle. Others ovulate before the period, and therefore can go from pregnancy to pregnancy without ever having had a menstrual period. Since you don't know which will come first, the period or the egg, caution in the form of contraception is highly advisable. For information on choosing birth control methods, see *What to Expect the First Year.*

Of course accidents can happen. Medical science has yet to develop a method of contraception (with the possible exception of sterilization) that is 100% effective. So even if you've been using contraception—and especially if you haven't been—pregnancy is still a possibility. Unfortunately, the first symptom of pregnancy you would ordinarily look for (absence of menstruation) will not be apparent if you've been nursing and not menstruating. But because of hormonal changes (there are different sets of hormones in operation during pregnancy and lactation), your milk supply will probably diminish noticeably soon after a new pregnancy is established. You might, in addition, experience any or all of the other symptoms of pregnancy (see page 2). Of course, if you do have any suspicion that you might be pregnant, the best thing to do is to visit your practitioner as soon as possible. Because it is virtually impossible to do a good job of nourishing both a breastfed infant and a developing fetus at the same time, it is highly inadvisable to continue nursing during a new pregnancy.

HAIR LOSS

"My hair seems to be falling out suddenly."

D on't order a hairpiece. This hair fall is normal, and will stop well in advance of baldness. Ordinarily the average head sheds 100 hairs a day, which are being continually replaced. During pregnancy (as when you're taking oral contraceptives), the hormonal changes keep those hairs from falling out. But the reprieve is only temporary. Those hairs are slated to go, and they will—within three to six months of delivery (or after you stop taking the Pill). Some women who are breastfeeding exclusively find that hair fall doesn't begin until they wean their baby or supplement the nursing with formula or solids.

To keep what hair you do have healthy, be sure to stay on the Best-Odds Postpartum diet, to continue your pregnancy vitamin supplement, and to treat your hair with kindness. That means shampooing only when necessary, using a conditioner to reduce the need to untangle, using a wide-toothed comb if you do have to untangle, and avoiding the application of heat (with blow dryers, curling irons, or hot rollers). It may also be a good idea to avoid further damage by postponing permanents, hair colorings, and hair relaxing treatments until your tresses seem back to normal.

Just because you lost a lot of hair following this pregnancy doesn't mean you will if there's a next time. Your body's reaction to each pregnancy, as you are sure to find out, can be very different.

TAKING TUB BATHS

"I seem to be getting a lot of contradictory advice about whether or not tub baths are all right in the postpartum period. Are they?"

A t one time, new mothers weren't permitted to set foot in a tub until at least one month after delivery, because of fear of infection from the bathwater. Today, because it's known that still bathwater does not enter the vagina, infection from bathing is no longer considered a threat. Some physicians, in fact, recommend tub baths in the hospital (when a tub is available) because they believe bathing removes lochia from the perineum—and from between the folds of the labia—more efficiently than showering. In addition, the warm water is comforting to the episiotomy site, relieves soreness and edema in the area, and soothes hemorrhoids.

Still, your doctor may prefer that you hold off on bathing until you are home, or even later. If you're eager to bathe (especially if you have no shower at home), discuss the issue with him or her. You may be able to get a dispensation.

If you do bathe during the first week or two following delivery, be sure the tub is scrubbed meticulously before it's filled. (But be sure you're not the one who does the scrubbing.) And get help getting into and out of the tub during the first few postpartum days, when you're still likely to be shaky.

EXHAUSTION

"It's nearly two months since I had the baby, but I feel more tired than ever. Could I be sick?"

Many a new mother has dragged herself into her doctor's office and complained of overwhelming chronic fatigue—convinced that she's fallen victim to some fatal malady. The nearly invariable diagnosis? A classic case of motherhood.

Rare is the mother who escapes this maternal fatigue syndrome, characterized by tiredness that never seems to ease up and an almost total lack of energy. And it's not surprising. There's no other job as emotionally and physically taxing as that of being a mother. The strain and pressures are not, as in most other jobs, limited to eight hours a day or five days a week. (And mothers don't get lunch hours or coffee breaks, either.) Motherhood for first-timers also adds the stress inherent in any new job: there's always something new to learn, mistakes to be made, problems to solve. If all this isn't enough to produce symptoms, add the energy that goes into breastfeeding, the strength sapped by toting around a rapidly growing infant and accompanying paraphernalia, and night after night of broken sleep.

Check with your doctor to be sure there is no physical cause for your exhaustion. If you get a clean bill of health, be assured that time, experience, and your baby sleeping through the night will gradually help relieve much of your fatigue. And once your body adjusts to the new demands, your energy level should pick up a bit, too. In the meantime, try the tips for relieving postpartum depression (page 398), which is closely tied to fatigue.

WHAT IT'S IMPORTANT TO KNOW:
GETTING BACK INTO SHAPE

It's one thing to look six months pregnant when you *are* six months pregnant, and quite another to look it when you've already delivered. Yet most women can expect to be wheeled out of the delivery room not much trimmer than when they were wheeled in—with a little bundle in their arms and several still around their middles. As for the pencil-thin skirts optimistically packed for the going-home trip, they're likely to stay packed, with maternity jeans the depressing substitute.

How soon after you become a new mother will you stop looking like a mother-to-be? With active exercise, that old prepregnancy figure (or a newly slender one) is only a couple of months away.

"Who needs exercise?" you may wonder. "I've been in perpetual motion since I got home from the hospital. Doesn't that count?"

Unfortunately, not much. Exhausting as it is, that kind of activity won't tighten up the perineal and abdominal muscles that have been left saggy by pregnancy. Only an exercise program will.

You can start a postpartum exercise program as early as 24 hours after delivery. But be careful not to overdo it. The following is geared for healthy women who've had uncomplicated vaginal deliveries. If you've had a surgical or a traumatic one, check with your doctor before beginning.

GROUND RULES

❖ Start each session with the least strenuous exercise, as a warm-up.

❖ Keep your exercise sessions brief and frequent, rather than doing one long session a day (this tones muscles better).

❖ If you have the time and really enjoy exercise, take a class for new mothers or buy a postpartum exercise book and develop an extensive program. If those prospects are unappealing, doing just a few simple routines regularly can also get you back into shape, especially if you gear them directly to problem areas, such as abdomen, thighs, buttocks, and so on.

❖ Do exercises slowly, and don't do a rapid series of repetitions with inadequate recovery time after each.

❖ Rest briefly between exercises (the muscle buildup occurs then, not while you are in motion).

❖ Don't do more than recommended, even if you feel you can.

❖ Quit before you feel tired: If you overdo it, you usually won't feel it until the next day—by which time you may be unable to exercise at all.

❖ Don't let mothering stop you from mothering yourself—your baby will love lying on your chest as you exercise.

❖ Do not do knee-chest exercises, full sit-ups, or double-leg lifts during the six-week postpartum period.

Kegel exercises can be done in any comfortable position. All the others are done in the basic position: lying on your back, knees bent, feet about 12 inches apart, soles flat on the floor; your head and shoulders should be supported by cushions, and your arms resting flat at your sides (see page 190). The early exercises can be done in bed; the others are best done on a harder surface, such as the floor. (An exercise mat is a good investment because the baby can try his or her first tentative crawls on it later.)

Head Lifts

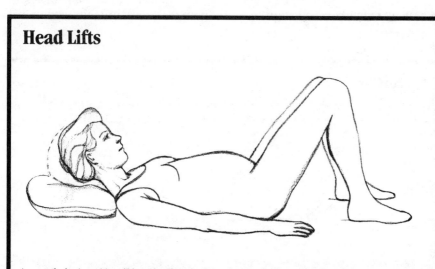

Assume the basic position. Take a deep breath; then raise your head very slightly, exhaling as you do. Lower your head slowly, and inhale. Raise your head a little more each day, gradually working up to lifting your shoulders slightly off the floor. Don't try full sit-ups for at least three or four weeks—and then only if you have always had very good abdominal muscle tone.

PHASE ONE: 24 HOURS AFTER DELIVERY

Kegel Exercises. You can begin these immediately after delivery (see page 190 for directions), though you won't be able to feel yourself doing them at first. This exercise can also be performed in bed or in a sitz bath. Or while you're urinating—contract to stop, then relax to release the flow of urine. Repeat several times. As the muscles regain tone, you will be able to allow just a few drops of urine to pass between repetitions.

Deep Diaphragmatic Breathing. In the basic position, place your hands on your abdomen so you can feel it rise as you inhale slowly through your nose; tighten the abdominal muscles as you exhale slowly through your mouth. Start with just two or three deep breaths at a time, to prevent hyperventilating. (Signs that you've overdone it are dizziness or faintness, tingling, or blurred vision. See page 294 for tips on dealing with hyperventilation.)

PHASE TWO: THREE DAYS AFTER DELIVERY

Three days after you deliver, you can begin doing more serious exercises—but only if you are sure that the pair of vertical muscles of your abdominal wall (called the recti abdominis) have not separated during pregnancy. Fairly common, especially in women who have had several children, this separation (or diastasis) will get worse if you do anything even mildly strenuous before it heals. Ask your nurse or doctor about the condition of these muscles, or examine them yourself this way: As you lie in the basic position, raise your head slightly with your arms extended forward; then feel for a soft lump below your navel. Such a lump indicates a separation.

You may be able to help correct a diastasis, if you have one, with this exercise: Assume the basic position; inhale. Now cross your hands over your abdomen, using your fingers to draw the sides of your abdominal

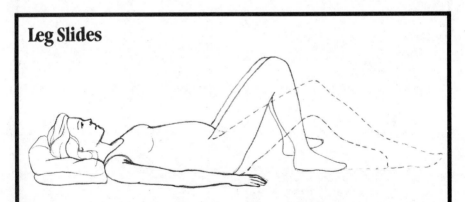

Leg Slides

Assume the basic position. Slowly extend both legs until they are flat on the floor. Slide your right foot, flat on the floor, back toward your buttocks. Keep the small of your back against the floor. Slide your leg back down. Repeat with your left foot. Start with three or four slides per side, and increase gradually until you can do a dozen or more comfortably. After three weeks, move to a modified leg lift (lifting one leg at a time slightly off the floor and lowering it again very slowly), if it is comfortable.

muscles together as you breathe out while raising your head slowly. Inhale as you lower your head slowly. Repeat three or four times, twice a day. When the separation has closed, or if you've never had one, move on to the exercises described here: Head Lifts, Leg Slides, and Pelvic Tilts.

The Pelvic Tilt (see illustration, page 191). Lie on your back in the basic position. Inhale as you press the small of your back against the floor. Then exhale, and relax. Repeat 3 or 4 times to start, increasing gradually to 12, and then 24.

PHASE THREE: AFTER YOUR POSTPARTUM CHECKUP

Now, with your practitioner's permission, you can resume a more active exercise schedule. You can gradually return to, or begin, a program that includes walking, jogging, swimming, aerobics, bicycling, or similar activities. But don't try to do too much too soon. A postpartum exercise class run by a qualified instructor may be the best way to begin.

Exercise postpartum will do more than flatten your tummy and tighten your perineum. The perineal exercises will help you avoid stress incontinence (leaking of urine), a dropping (prolapse) of pelvic organs, and sexual difficulties. Abdominal exercises will reduce the risk of backache, varicose veins, leg cramps, edema, and the formation of blood clots in the veins (thrombi), as well as improve circulation. Regular exercise will also promote healing of your traumatized uterine, abdominal, and pelvic muscles, and hasten their return to normal tone. Planned activity will also help the pregnancy- and delivery-loosened joints return to normal, and will prevent further weakening and strain. Finally, exercise can have a psychological benefit (ask any runner), improving your ability to handle stress and to relax—and minimizing the chance of postpartum blues.

20
Fathers Are Expectant, Too

Mothers- and fathers-to-be today share not only the joys of pregnancy, childbirth, and childrearing, but the worries as well; and the chances are good that there is considerable overlap in what concerns each member of your expectant (or newly delivered) team. Yet fathers are entitled to a few worries of their own—and to some very special reassurance, not only during the pregnancy and the birth, but in the postpartum period as well.

And so this chapter—dedicated to the equal, but often neglected, partner-in-reproduction. But it isn't intended for fathers' eyes only—any more than the rest of the book is intended only for mothers'. An expectant mother can gain some valuable insights into what her husband is feeling, fearing, and hoping by reading this chapter; an expectant father can gain a better understanding of the physical and emotional changes his wife will undergo during pregnancy, childbirth, and the postpartum period while at the same time better preparing himself for his own role in the unfolding drama.

WHAT YOU MAY BE CONCERNED ABOUT

FEELING LEFT OUT

"So much attention has been focused on my wife since she became pregnant that I hardly feel I have anything to do with it."

In generations past, the male involvement in the reproductive process ended once his sperm had fertilized his wife's ovum. Fathers-to-be watched pregnancy from afar, and childbirth not at all.

Great strides have undeniably been made in the past decade for fathers' rights. But social re-education hasn't changed the fact that pregnancy takes place within a woman's body. Or the fact that some fathers are lost in what is still largely a woman's shuffle and end up feeling forgotten, left out—even jealous of their wives.

Sometimes the woman is unwittingly responsible, sometimes the man is. Either way, it's vital that the father's feelings are resolved before resentment grows and is allowed to spoil what should be one of the most wonderful experiences of *both* parents' lives. The best way to accomplish this is for you to get involved in as many aspects of your wife's pregnancy as you can:

See an Obstetrician (or Midwife). Your wife's—as often as she does, if possible. Most practitioners will encourage the husband to attend the monthly appointment. If your schedule won't permit a monthly visit, perhaps you can arrange to attend the landmark appointments (when the heartbeat will first be heard, for instance) and prenatal tests (especially the sonogram, when you can see the baby).

Act Pregnant. You don't have to show up for work in maternity clothes or start drinking a quart of milk a day. But you can do your wife's pregnancy exercise routine with her; give up junk food for nine months; quit smoking, if you're a smoker. And when someone offers you a drink, tell them, "No thanks, we're pregnant."

Get an Education. Even Harvard Ph.D.s have a lot to learn when it comes to pregnancy and childbirth. Read as many books and articles as you can. Attend childbirth classes with your wife; attend classes for fathers, if they are available in your community. Talk to friends and colleagues who've become new fathers recently.

Make Contact with Your Baby. Your wife may have the edge in getting to know the baby prenatally because it's comfortably ensconced in her uterus, but that doesn't mean that you can't start to get to know the new family member, too. Talk, read, sing to your baby frequently; he or she can hear your voice now, and will recognize it after delivery. Enjoy baby's kicks and squirms by resting your hand or your cheek on your wife's naked abdomen each night—it's a nice way to share intimacy with her, too.

Shop for a Layette. And a crib, and a stroller. Help your wife decorate the nursery. In general, become active in picking out, planning, and preparing for the baby's arrival.

Talk It Out. Your wife may be leaving you out unintentionally—she may not even be aware that you'd like to be more involved. It's very likely that she'd be as happy to make you a part of her pregnancy as you would to be a part of it.

FEAR OF SEX

"Even though the doctor has assured us that sex is safe throughout pregnancy, I often have trouble following through for fear of hurting my wife or the baby."

Never is sex more a mind-over-matter situation—for both partners—than during pregnancy. This is true particularly as gestation advances and the mind (and libido) must confront a very sizable matter: the expanding pregnant belly and its precious contents.

Fortunately, you can put your mind to rest over the matter. As vulnerable as mother and baby may seem to an anxious father contemplating intercourse, in a normally progressing low-risk pregnancy, neither one is. (There are a few caveats, particularly in the last two months, detailed in Making Love During Pregnancy, page 164.)

Not only can making love to your wife not do her any harm (assuming the caveats are observed), but because pregnancy is a time for emotional and physical closeness, it can do her a world of good. And as for your baby, though basically oblivious to the whole event, he or she may be pacified by the gentle rocking motion of intercourse and of the contracting uterus during orgasm.

MOODINESS

"Ever since we got the positive pregnancy test, my wife and I seem to be going through opposite mood swings. When she's feeling good, I'm feeling down, and vice versa."

More studies recently have been focusing on the "pregnant" father because it's becoming more and more apparent that even though he doesn't carry the fetus, he can experience many of the prenatal symptoms that are common in pregnant women. Depression, during pregnancy and postpartum, is one of those symptoms. Although in about 1 in 10 cases both parents succumb to depression at the same time, most of the time the depression occurs in just one partner at a time. This may be because signs of depression in a loved one give us the inner strength to rise above our own feelings and to become supportive.

You needn't worry about your pregnancy depression—it's common and likely to be self-limiting—but you should take steps to relieve it. Keep active and try not giving in to your down feelings; talk your feelings over with your wife (if she seems up to listening), with a friend who recently became a father, or even with your own father; avoid alcohol and other drugs, which can aggravate depression and mood swings; and prepare for the baby both mentally and practically (by participating in shopping, painting the nursery, arranging your finances, etc.). You can also try some of the other tips recommended for mothers experiencing prenatal depression (see page 104). If nothing works, and your depression deepens and begins to interfere with your work and other aspects of your life, then seek professional help—from a member of the clergy, from your physician, from a therapist, or from a psychiatrist.

IMPATIENCE WITH YOUR WIFE'S MOOD SWINGS

"I know it's my wife's hormonal changes that are making her so weepy and volatile. But I don't know how much longer I can be patient."

If patience is a virtue, you're going to have to be very virtuous for the rest of your wife's pregnancy. Although the stabilization of hormone levels by the fourth month eases the pronounced premenstrual-like weepiness and moodiness of early pregnancy, the stresses of being pregnant continue. And many women continue to be subject to sudden bursts of emotion and feelings of vulnerability right up to delivery. It doubtless won't be easy, and at times you may find it close to impossible. But there's also little doubt that your efforts will pay off. Touchiness met with understanding will dissipate faster than touchiness met with anger and frustration; shoulders offered to your wife for a 15-minute cry won't have to carry around the weight of her unvented anxiety for days at a time.

Try to keep in mind that pregnancy is *not* a permanent condition, and that the changes in your wife's emotional status are as transient as the changes in her figure.

Be aware, too, that postpartum depression can also afflict dads, and these same tips can help lift you out of the baby blues later.

SYMPATHY SYMPTOMS

"If it's my wife who's pregnant, why am I having morning sickness?"

You may well be among the estimated 11% to 65% (depending on the study) of expectant fathers who suffer from the couvade syndrome during their wives' pregnancies. The symptoms of couvade (which comes from the French for "to hatch") most often appear in the third month and again at delivery, and can mimic virtually all the normal symptoms of pregnancy—including nausea and vomiting, abdominal pain, appetite changes, weight gain, food cravings, constipation, leg cramps, dizziness, fatigue, and mood swings.

Many theories have been suggested to explain couvade—all, some, or none of which may be appropriate to you: sympathy for and identification with the pregnant wife; jealousy over being left out, and a resultant desire for attention; guilt over being responsible for putting the wife in such an uncomfortable situation; stress from living with a woman who's become irritable, moody, and possibly off-limits sexually; and anxiety over the impending addition to the family.

Of course your symptoms could also indicate illness, so it's a good idea to see a doctor. But should an examination show no physical problem, couvade is a likely diagnosis. The underlying cause, if you can identify it, may offer a clue to the cure. For instance, if the cause is jealousy, becoming more involved in your wife's pregnancy may relieve your morning sickness. Or if it's anxiety over handling a newborn for the first time, taking a course in infant care, reading a copy of *What to Expect the First Year*, or spending some time with a friend's baby might prove helpful. Even if you can't put your finger on any one cause for your symptoms, talking out your feelings about pregnancy, childbirth, and parenthood with your wife may alleviate your sympathy pains. So might discussing them with other expectant parents in your childbirth class. Should none of this help, be assured that your reactions are normal, and that all symptoms that don't go away during pregnancy will disappear soon after delivery.

Equally normal, of course, is the father who doesn't have a sick day during his wife's pregnancy. Not suffering from morning sickness or not putting on weight doesn't mean an expectant father doesn't empathize and identify with his wife.

ANXIETY OVER YOUR WIFE'S HEALTH

"I know pregnancy and childbirth are safe today, yet I still can't stop worrying that something will happen to my wife."

There's something undeniably vulnerable about a pregnant woman—and something very natural about your desire, as a loving husband, to want to protect your wife from any possible harm. But you can relax. Your wife is in virtually no danger. Women very, very rarely die as a result of pregnancy or childbirth anymore—and the vast majority of those who do haven't had the benefits of prenatal care or adequate nourishment.

But even though pregnancy doesn't pose a serious physical threat to your wife, you can help make it a safer and more comfortable experience for her: by making sure she gets the best medical care possible and that she eats the best possible diet (see Chapter 4); by letting her get extra rest while you do the laundry, make dinner, or clean the house; and by giving her the kind of emotional support she can't get from anyone else (no matter how far obstetrical science advances, pregnant women will always be *emotionally* vulnerable).

ANXIETY OVER THE BABY'S HEALTH

"I'm so afraid that something will be wrong with the baby, I can't even sleep at night."

Mothers-to-be by no means hold a corner on the worry market. And like almost every expectant mother, virtually every expectant father worries about his unborn baby's health and well-being. Happily, nearly all such worry is needless. The odds that your baby will be born both alive and completely normal are overwhelming—far better than was the case in previous generations.

Happily, too, you don't have to just sit back and hope for the best. You can actually take some steps to help ensure your baby's good health:

❖ Be sure your wife gets good medical care from the very beginning of her pregnancy; be sure she keeps all her prenatal appointments and follows her practitioner's orders.

❖ Encourage her to follow the Best-Odds Diet, which will significantly better the odds of having a healthy baby. If you follow it with her, not only will she be more likely to stay faithful to it, but you'll earn the added benefit of better health yourself.

❖ Make certain that she abstains from alcohol, drugs, and tobacco. Research shows you can best help her do this by abstaining yourself, at least when you are with her. If you think this is a big sacrifice, consider all the sacrifices she's making to have your baby.

❖ Reduce both physical and emotional stress in her life as much as possible. Help around the house, take over some of the chores that have traditionally been hers, encourage her to reduce her work load if her life is too frantic. If your social calendar is usually filled to overflowing, see that it's cut back and that more evenings are spent at home relaxing. If they work for both of you, try doing some relaxation exercises (see page 114) together.

❖ Become familiar with the signs of possible trouble in pregnancy (see page 117), and later in the postpartum period (page 381). If your wife seems to be experiencing any of these, make sure that the appropriate action is taken promptly. If necessary, make the call to her doctor or take her to the emergency room. She may be too embarrassed or too sick to take the needed steps herself.

❖ Share your fears with your wife, and let her share hers with you. This will serve to unburden you both, or at least make your burden of worries easier to carry.

Of course, even the most reassuring statistics and the best preventive measures probably won't be able to banish all your worries; only the birth of a healthy baby will do that. But knowing you're doing all you can toward that important end will make the waiting—and the sleeping—a little easier.

ANXIETY OVER LIFE CHANGES

"Ever since I saw him on a sonogram, I've

*been looking forward to our son's birth.
But I've also been worrying about
whether I'll like being a father."*

Y ou and probably every first-time
father-to-be in history. At least as
much, and possibly even more, than
the expectant mother, the expectant
father worries about impending parenthood and about the effect it will
have on his life. The most common
areas of concern include:

Can I Afford a Larger Family? Especially today, when childrearing costs
are going through the roof (as are the
costs of maintaining or enlarging that
roof), many fathers-to-be lose sleep
over this very legitimate question. But
once the baby comes, they often find
that the alteration of priorities makes
available the money that's needed for
the newborn. Opting for breastfeeding over bottle-feeding if that's possible, accepting all hand-me-downs that
are offered (new clothes start to look
like hand-me-downs after a few
spitting-up episodes, anyway), letting
friends and family know which gifts
you really need rather than allowing
them to fill baby's shelves with silver
spoons and other dust-gatherers, can
all help reduce the cost of caring for
the new arrival. If the new mother is
planning not to go back to her job
right away and this concerns you from
a financial standpoint, recognize that
weighed against the costs of quality
child care, a business wardrobe, and
commuting, the amount of income
lost may really be minimal.

Will I Be a Good Father? Few people
are born good fathers (or mothers, for
that matter). They learn to meet the
challenge in time through on-the-job
training, persistence, and love. But if
you feel you'll be more comfortable
with the tasks at hand if you're formally prepared, by all means take a
parenting class—if one is available in

your area—to learn how to diaper,
bathe, feed, hold, dress, and play with
your baby. If a class isn't available, or
if you have an unquenchable thirst for
such preparation, dive into a pile of
childcare books.

How Will We Divide the Child Care?
This wasn't an issue for fathers a generation or two ago, when child care
was widely considered woman's
work. But most of today's fathers are
aware, to some degree, that parenting
is a two-person job (at least when
there are two parents), although
they're not exactly sure what the division of labor should be. Don't wait
until baby needs his first midnight diaper change or his first bath to decide
this question. Start negotiating now.
Some details may change once you
really start operating as parents (she
committed to the diaper changes but
you turn out to be more proficient at
it), but exploring the options in theory now will make you feel more confident about how baby care is going to
work in practice later.

Will We Have to Give Up Our Social
Lives? You won't have to give up your
social life entirely after baby is born,
but you should expect it to change
somewhat—at least if both of you plan
to be active participants in parenting.
A new baby does, and should, take
center stage, pushing some old lifestyle habits at least temporarily aside.
Parties, movies, and shows may have
to be squeezed in between feedings;
dinners for two in your favorite restaurant may come less frequently,
with more meals being taken in "family" restaurants that tolerate squirming infants. Your taste in friends may
change, too; couples without children
may suddenly have little in common
with you and you may start gravitating
toward other stroller-pushers for empathetic companionship.

Will Our Husband-Wife Relationship Change? Every set of new parents finds that their relationship undergoes some change after childbirth. And anticipating this change during pregnancy is an important first step in dealing with it postpartum. No longer will being alone together be as simple as closing the blinds and taking the phone off the hook; from the moment baby comes home from the hospital, spontaneous intimacy and complete privacy will be precious, often unattainable, commodities. Romance may have to be planned (for the two hours grandma's taken him to the park, for instance) rather than spur of the moment, and interruptions may be the rule (you can't take a baby off the hook). But as long as you both take the trouble to make time for each other—whether that means skipping your favorite television show so that you can share a late dinner after baby's in bed, or giving up Saturday golf with the guys so you can make love during baby's morning nap—your relationship will weather the changes well. Many couples, in fact, find that becoming a threesome ultimately deepens; strengthens, and improves their twosome. (For more tips on nurturing your relationship as you nurture your baby, see *What to Expect the First Year.*)

YOUR WIFE'S LOOKS

"As petty as this might seem, I'm afraid my wife's going to get fat and flabby during pregnancy, and stay that way afterward."

If it were in your wife's obstetrical interest to gain 50 pounds with pregnancy, you (and the countless other expectant husbands who share your "petty" concern) would have no option, of course, but to accept fat and flab as the price of a healthy baby.

But such calories-are-no-object weight gains just aren't medically justifiable —and can, in fact, lead to unnecessary complications during both pregnancy and delivery. A moderate, steady, carefully monitored weight increase of between 25 and 35 pounds, gained on a diet of highly nutritious food, gives your baby the best odds for healthy development and safe delivery—and your wife the speediest return to slenderness after childbirth. (See the Best-Odds Diet, page 80; Weight Gain, page 147).

Sticking to a rigid diet even for two weeks isn't easy. Sticking to one for nine months can be close to impossible, unless the dieter has the support, understanding, and assistance of those close to her. In the case of your wife, that's you. Not only do many husbands fail to provide their wives with that help, they may unwittingly sabotage their efforts. Husbands have probably done more to undermine their wives' diets than Hershey's and Sara Lee put together—either by bringing temptation into the house, ordering it in restaurants, or even offering it directly to their wives ("Come on—one bite won't hurt!").

With the following tips, you'll be able to become your wife's best ally in her campaign to gain weight moderately and eat sensibly during pregnancy—while protecting your own selfish interests (a slim wife):

Lead Your Wife Not into Temptation. If you must indulge in dietary indiscretion, do so out of your home and away from your wife. You can't expect her to live happily on broiled meats, steamed vegetables, and fresh fruit while you gorge on burgers, fries, and Heavenly Hash ice cream beside her.

Practice What You Preach to Her. What's good for the goose and the gosling is good for the gander, too. Your staying close to the Best-Odds

Diet (recognizing that you don't need all that protein or calcium) will not only support your wife, but probably will benefit your health as well.

Don't Be Too Preachy. If she slips, nagging will only help her to fall faster and farther. Remind, don't remonstrate. Prod her conscience, don't try to become it. Signal her quietly when in public, rather than making a pointed announcement to all within earshot about her ordering her chicken breaded and fried. Most important, do it with a sense of humor and a lot of love.

Accentuate the Positive. Nothing will undermine her willpower like a faltering ego. So make a point of building her up, admiring her new pregnant shape, commenting often on how pregnancy becomes her.

Exercise with Her. It's much more fun for two to tango—or to follow a pregnancy exercise program. Proper exercise during pregnancy is important not only for keeping your wife (and you) trim, but also for getting her in good shape for labor and delivery.

FALLING APART DURING LABOR

"I'm afraid I'll faint or become ill during the delivery."

Few fathers enter the delivery room without fear. Even obstetricians who've assisted at births of thousands of other people's babies can experience a sudden loss of self-confidence when confronted with their own baby's delivery.

Yet very few of these fears—of freezing, falling apart, fainting, or becoming sick to the stomach while watching the delivery—are ever realized. And though being prepared for the birth (by taking childbirth education classes, for instance) generally makes the experience more satisfying, even most unprepared fathers come through labor and delivery better than they'd thought they would. One study of fathers who attended their babies' births with no previous preparation found that though 70% expected that the delivery would be a frightening, unpleasant, and negative experience, all described it afterward in highly positive terms.

But like anything new and unfamiliar, childbirth becomes less frightening and intimidating if you know what to expect. So become an expert on the subject. Read the entire chapter on labor and delivery, beginning on page 288. Attend childbirth education classes, watching the labor and delivery films with your eyes open. Visit the hospital ahead of time so that you'll be acquainted with the technology that's used in labor and delivery rooms. Talk to friends who have recently become first-time parents. You will probably find they had the same anxieties beforehand but came through feeling terrific.

Though it's important to get an education, it's also important to remember that childbirth isn't the final exam in your childbirth education course. Don't feel that you must perform perfectly (as some women feel obligated to) at the delivery. Nurses and doctors won't be evaluating your every move or comparing you to the husband next door. More important, neither will your wife. She won't care if you forget every coaching technique you learned in class. Your being beside her, holding her hand, urging her on, providing the comfort of a familiar face and touch, will do her more good than having Drs. Lamaze, Bradley, and Dick-Reade themselves at her bedside.

"I would really rather not be at the birth, but I feel pressured to be there."

Just because it's currently in vogue in the birthing business for fathers to attend births doesn't mean it's mandatory. Studies have shown that fathers who don't attend births don't have less meaningful relationships with their offspring than fathers who do; just as fathers who don't bond with their babies immediately after birth don't seem automatically to become less loving parents. What's important is that you do what's right for you and your wife. If it doesn't feel right for you to attend the delivery, for whatever reason, you would probably do more harm than good to all concerned by being there. Ignore those who try to pressure you into a decision that would be wrong for you. Remember, more generations of fathers *haven't* seen their babies born than *have*—with no ill effects.

However, that's not to say that attending the birth of your child is not a worthwhile experience, or one you should forgo without careful consideration. Though it's important that you not let anyone else make up your mind for you, it's equally important that you not make up—and close—your mind until the last minute. Go through all the preparations: accompany your wife on her prenatal visits, take childbirth classes, do extensive reading. Many once-hesitant fathers find that familiarity with labor and delivery breeds a new perspective, which allows them to feel comfortable enough with childbirth to attend and participate fully.

Others, however, still end up deciding that being at the birth would be counterproductive for themselves and their spouses. Still others decide to give labor a try but find, sometime before or during delivery, that they'd rather step outside. All should feel free to follow their instincts, with the reassurance that doing so won't reflect in any way on their capacity for fathering.

"My wife is having a planned cesarean. Hospital regulations won't allow me to be there, and I'm afraid that our new family won't get off to the best start."

If you made the decision to be at the birth only to discover that the decision wasn't yours to make (as in the case of a cesarean in a hospital that doesn't permit husbands to attend), don't give up without a civilized fight. With the support of your wife's obstetrician (if such support is forthcoming), try first to persuade hospital officials to bend—or even change—the regulations. (It may help to remind them that a majority of hospitals now allow fathers to be present at non-emergency surgical deliveries.) If your campaign is unsuccessful (or if a hasty delivery precludes your presence), you have every right to be disappointed. But you have no right to let that disappointment taint the joy that should surround the birth of your child. Your not being at the birth can threaten your relationship with your baby only if you let it, by harboring feelings of guilt, resentment, or frustration.

BONDING

"My wife had a last-minute cesarean and I wasn't allowed to be with her. I didn't hold the baby for 24 hours and I'm afraid I didn't bond with him."

Until the 1960s, few fathers ever witnessed the birth of their children, and since the word "bonding" originated only in the 1970s, none were ever even aware that the possibility of bonding with their offspring existed. But such a lack of enlightenment didn't stop generations of loving father-son and father-daughter relationships from developing. Conversely, every father who attends his child's birth and is allowed to hold him or her immediately isn't automatically guaranteed a lifetime of closeness with his offspring.

Being with your wife during delivery is ideal, and being deprived of that opportunity is reason for disappointment—particularly if you spent months training together for childbirth. But it's no reason to expect a less than fulfilling relationship with your baby. What really bonds you with your baby is daily loving contact—changing diapers, giving baths, feeding, cuddling, lullabying. Your child will never know that you didn't share in the moment of birth, but will know if you aren't there when he or she needs you from then on.

EXCLUSION DURING BREASTFEEDING

"My wife is breastfeeding our son. There's a closeness between them that I can't seem to share, and I feel left out."

There are certain immutable biological aspects of parenting that exclude the father: he can't be pregnant, he can't labor and deliver, and he can't breastfeed. But, as millions of new fathers discover each year, a man's natural physical limitations don't have to relegate him to spectator status. You can share in nearly all the joys, expectations, trials, and tribulations of your wife's pregnancy, labor, and delivery—from the first kick to the last push—as an active, supportive participant. And though you'll never be able to put your baby to the breast (at least not with the kind of results the baby's looking for), you *can* share in the feeding process:

Be Your Baby's Supplementary Feeder. There's more than one way to feed a baby. And though you can't nurse, you can be the one to give any supplementary bottles. Not only will it give your wife a break (whether in the middle of the night or in the middle of dinner), it will give you extra opportunities for closeness with your baby. Don't waste the opportunity by propping the bottle up to the baby's mouth. Strike a nursing position, with the bottle where your wife's breast would be and your baby snuggled close to you.

Don't Sleep Through the Night Until Your Baby Does. Sharing in the joys of feeding also means sharing in the sleepless nights. Even if you're not giving supplementary bottles, you can become a part of nighttime feeding rituals. You can be the one to take the baby out of the crib, do any necessary diaper changing, deliver him for his feeding, and return him to bed once he has fallen asleep again.

Watch in Wonder, and Appreciate. There can be enormous satisfaction in simply watching the miracle of breastfeeding—as there is in watching the miracle of birth. Instead of feeling left out, feel privileged to be a witness to the love that passes between your wife and your baby as they nurse.

Participate in All Other Daily Rituals. Nursing is the *only* daily chore limited to mothers. And chances are that if you make at least one other chore your responsibility (or as many as possible) you'll be too busy to be jealous.

FEELING UNSEXY AFTER DELIVERY

"The delivery was absolutely miraculous to watch. But seeing our baby come out

of my wife's vagina seems to have turned me off sexually."

Human sexual response, compared to that of other animals, is extremely delicate. It's at the mercy not only of the body but of the mind as well. And the mind can, at times, play merciless havoc with it. One of those times, as you probably already know, is during pregnancy. Another, as you seem to be discovering, is during the postpartum period.

It's very possible that the cause of your sudden sexual ambivalence has nothing to do with having seen your baby delivered. Most brand-new fathers find both the spirit and the flesh somewhat less willing after delivery (although there's nothing abnormal about those who don't), for many very understandable reasons: fatigue, especially if the baby still isn't sleeping through the night; uneasiness about having a third person in your home; fear that he or she will awake crying at the first caress (particularly if the baby is sharing your room); concern that you may hurt your wife by having intercourse before her body is thoroughly healed; and finally, a general physical and mental preoccupation with your newborn, which sensibly concentrates your energies where they are most needed at this stage of your lives.

In other words, it's probably just as well that you aren't feeling sexually motivated, particularly if your wife (like many women in the immediate postpartum period) isn't feeling emotionally or physically up to it either. Just how long it will take for your interest, and hers, to return is impossible to predict. As with all matters sexual, there is a wide range of what is "normal." For some couples, desire will precede even the doctor's go-ahead at six weeks. For others, six months can pass before l'amour and le bébé begin to coexist harmoniously in

the same home. (Some women find desire lacking until they stop breast-feeding, but that doesn't mean they can't enjoy the intimacy of intercourse with the man they love.)

Some fathers, even if they've been prepared for the childbirth experience, do come out of it feeling that their "territory" has been "violated," that the special place that had been meant for loving has suddenly taken on a practical purpose. But as the days pass, that feeling usually does too. The father begins to realize that the vagina has two functions, equally important and miraculous. Neither excludes the other, and in fact they are very much interconnected. He also comes to recognize that the vagina is a vehicle for childbirth only briefly, while it is a source of pleasure for himself and his wife for a lifetime.

If the sexual urge doesn't return and its absence begins to cause tension, professional counseling is probably needed.

"Before the baby, my wife's breasts were a focus of sexual pleasure—for both of us. Now that she's breastfeeding, they seem too functional to be sexy."

Like the vagina, breasts were designed to serve both a practical and a sexual purpose (which, from a strictly procreative standpoint, is also practical). And though these purposes aren't mutually exclusive in the long run, they can conflict temporarily during lactation.

Some couples find breastfeeding a sexual turn-on. Others, for esthetic reasons (leaking milk, for instance) or because they feel uncomfortable about using the baby's source of nourishment for their sexual pleasure, find it a very definite turn-off.

Whatever turns you on—or off—is what is normal for you. If you feel that your wife's breasts are too functional to be sexy now, don't try to force yourself to feel otherwise. Leave them out of sexual foreplay for now, with the reassurance that you will feel differently once the baby has been weaned. Be sure, however, to be open and honest with your wife; taking a sudden, unexplained hands-off approach to her breasts could leave her feeling unappealing. Be careful, also, not to harbor any resentment against the baby for using "your" breasts; try to think of nursing as a temporary "loan" instead.

21
Preparing for the Next Baby

I n the best of all possible worlds, we would be able to plan life to our precise specifications. In the real world, where most of us live, the best-laid plans often give way to the unexpected twists and turns of fate, over which we have precious little control—leaving us to accept, and to make the best of, what comes our way.

In the best of all possible pregnancies, we would know in advance when we would conceive and could make all the changes and adjustments in our lifestyle to help ensure that our baby has the best of all possible odds of being born alive and well. Such advance planning is a luxury that many women (because of menstrual irregularity and/or the frailties of contraception) may never be able to indulge in. And as has been stressed throughout this book, what a woman does before she realizes she's pregnant (a few drinks, a few dietary indiscretions, a dental x-ray) ordinarily does little to affect her baby's odds. Few women act pregnant from the moment of conception, and yet the vast majority give birth to normal, healthy babies.

But it would be remiss not to outline a plan for the best of all possible pregnancies—because the possibility does exist for an increasing number of women, as family planning techniques become more reliable. The plan is appropriate whether you're already in the process of trying to conceive or you're just thinking ahead. Although it's never too late to start taking care of your body, it's also never too early. And in fact, your good prepregnancy care will benefit not only your own children but your children's children. Act now, and:

Get a Thorough Physical. Both you and your husband should see your internist or family doctor. An exam will pick up any problems that need to be corrected beforehand, or that will need to be monitored during pregnancy. Also take care of allergy shots, minor elective surgery, and anything else medical—major or minor—that you've been putting off. (If you start allergy desensitization now, you will probably be able to continue once you conceive.)

See Your Dentist. Make an appointment for a thorough examination and cleaning. Have any necessary work, including x-rays, fillings, and dental or periodontal surgery, completed now.

Select a Practitioner—and Have a Prepregnancy Exam. It's easier to choose a practitioner now, in an unhurried manner, than when that first prenatal checkup is hanging over your head. (See Chapter 1 for your options.) Even if you think you might like to use a certified nurse-midwife, you should still have a gynecologist or family physician whose medical opinion you respect perform this examination to screen your planned pregnancy for high-risk potential. If your history and/or the physical findings suggest such potential, you will need the care of an obstetrician or even a maternal-fetal medicine subspecialist during your pregnancy. See page 8 for tips on choosing a practitioner.

Correct any Gynecological or Other Health Problems. Now is the time to be checked and/or treated for conditions that might interfere with pregnancy, such as polyps, cysts, benign tumors, an over- or underactive thyroid, endometriosis, or recurrent urinary tract infections. If you know, or suspect, that your mother took diethylstilbestrol (DES) when she was pregnant with you, tell the doctor, so your reproductive organs can be carefully examined—with colposcopy (which allows close visual examination of vagina and cervix) if necessary. If you've had a previous pregnancy problem, such as a miscarriage or premature delivery, discuss the measures that can be taken to head off a repeat. Even if you're sure you couldn't have a sexually transmitted disease, ask for tests for syphilis, gonorrhea, chlamydia, and herpes. Get treatment, if needed. If it is appropriate, have a test for HIV (the AIDS virus), but be sure to arrange for counseling in the unlikely event the results are positive.

Other tests that may be recommended before you conceive include hemoglobin or hematocrit (to test for anemia); Rh (to see if you are positive or negative); urine (to check for protein or sugar); TB skin test (if you live in a high-incidence area); hepatitis B (if you are in a high-risk category, such as a health care worker); possibly, cytomegalovirus and varicella antibody titer (to determine whether or not you are immune to CMV and chicken pox). If a test shows a medical problem, make certain that you get appropriate treatment before you try to conceive.

If you have a cat or regularly eat raw or rare meat or drink unpasteurized milk, a toxoplasmosis antibody titer may also be recommended. If you are found to be immune, you needn't worry about this problem now or during your pregnancy. If you're not, start taking the precautions on page 65 now.

Start Keeping Track. Your chances of conceiving when you want to will be much greater if you have intercourse during the fertile part of your cycle. Knowing exactly when you conceived will also make establishing an estimated date of delivery easier. To keep track, note the first day of each menstrual period on a handy calendar or diary; also try to note when you ovulate. Ovulation generally occurs at the midpoint of the cycle (on the 14th day of a 28 day cycle, for instance), but is less easy to predict in women with irregular cycles. The physical signs of ovulation are readily apparent to some women, more elusive to others (your basal body temperature, taken first thing in the morning, reaches its low point of the month then abruptly rises; your vaginal mucus is clear, jelly-like, and can be pulled into strings; your normally pink cervix turns bluish; and you may experience mittelshmerz—a brief period of pain on one side of your back or the other). If you're among the latter, appear to be ovulating irregularly, or are having trouble conceiving, home ovulation predictor kits are available to help you pinpoint ovulation; check with your practitioner for a recommendation.

Update Immunizations. If you haven't had a tetanus shot in the past ten years, have one now. You should also be sure you are immune to rubella (German measles), either through having had the disease or through vaccination. Ask your doctor for the appropriate blood test before you conceive. If you turn out not to be immune, you should get immunized and then wait three months before attempting to conceive (but don't panic if you accidentally conceive earlier—any risk is purely theoretical; see page 313). If you have never been immunized for measles and haven't had the disease or if you are at high risk for hepatitis B, it may also be recommended that you be immunized now.

Have a Genetic Screening. If either of you has any genetic disorder (for example cystic fibrosis, Down syndrome, muscular dystrophy, PKU, spina bifida, or other birth defects) in your personal history or among blood relatives, see a genetic counselor or a maternal-fetal medicine subspecialist. You should also be tested for any genetic disease common to your ethnic background: Tay-Sachs disease if either of you is of Jewish-European (Ashkenazi) or French Canadian descent; sickle-cell trait if you are of African descent; one of the thalassemias if you are of Greek, Italian, Southeast Asian, or Philippino origin. Previous obstetrical difficulties (such as two or more miscarriages, a stillbirth, a long period of infertility, or a child with a birth defect) or being married to a cousin or other blood relative are also reasons to seek genetic counseling.

Evaluate Your Birth Control Method. If you are using a method of birth control that might present some risk (however slight) to a future pregnancy, change it before you start trying to conceive. Birth control pills should be discontinued several months before conception, if possible, to allow your reproductive system to go through at least two normal cycles before you start making a baby. The IUD should be removed before you begin trying. Since the risks of spermicides are as yet unclear, playing it extra safe means discontinuing their use (alone or with a diaphragm or condom) one month to six weeks before you want to become pregnant. The birth control method to switch to for the interim: the condom (used with care and without spermicide).

Get Any Other Medical Condition Under Control. If you have diabetes, asthma, a heart condition, or any other chronic illness, be sure that you have your doctor's okay to become pregnant, that your condition is under control before you conceive, and that you start taking optimum care of yourself now (see Chapter 16). If you were a PKU baby (ask your mother if you aren't sure, or check your medical records), then begin a phenylalanine-free diet (distasteful as it may be) before conceiving (see page 336) and continue it through pregnancy.

Improve Your Diet. Start eliminating junk food and refined sugars from your diet, and increase whole grains and fiber. Since it's best to embark on your pregnancy at as close to normal weight as possible, try to get there before conceiving. Add or cut calories as necessary. (Use the Best-Odds Diet, page 80, for a good basic food plan; but you will need only two calcium and two protein servings daily until you conceive.) Any weight loss should be achieved sensibly, however, even if it means putting off conception for another couple of months. Strenuous dieting can result in a nutritional deficit, something you don't want to start pregnancy with. If you've been on a crash diet recently, give yourself a few months to get your body back into balance before you try to conceive.

If you have any unusual dietary habits (such as a taste for laundry starch or clay), suffer or have suffered from an eating disorder (such as anorexia nervosa or bulimia), or are on a special diet (macrobiotic, diabetic, or any other), inform your practitioner.

Improve Your Husband's Diet. The better your husband's nutrition, the healthier his sperm. His diet should mirror your prepregnancy diet, with caloric intake adjusted to accommodate his weight and activity. If he's a diabetic, he should get his blood sugar under control.

Take a Vitamin-Mineral Supplement Formulated for Pregnancy. Some studies show that taking a pregnancy supplement containing folic acid before conception and in the first months of pregnancy reduces even further the already small risk of having a baby with a neural-tube defect (such as spina bifida). In addition, the supplement will ensure that your baby will be getting necessary vitamins and minerals in the early days of development. If you are taking any other nutritional supplement, however, stop taking them before conception. Excesses can be hazardous.

Shape Up, But Keep Cool. An exercise program will tone and strengthen your muscles in preparation for the challenging tasks of carrying and delivering your baby-to-be. It will also help you take off excess weight. Avoid becoming overheated during workouts, however, when you begin trying to conceive, since this can lead to a potentially harmful increase in body temperature. Avoid hot tubs and direct exposure to heating pads and electric blankets for the same reason. Keep in mind, too, that while exercise is good for you, you *can* get too much of a

good thing. Excessive exercise can interfere with ovulation—and if you don't ovulate, you can't conceive.

Avoid Unnecessary Exposure to Radiation. If x-rays are necessary for medical reasons, be sure that your reproductive organs are protected (unless they are being targeted) and that the lowest doses possible are used. Once you start trying to conceive, keep in mind that you might have succeeded. Inform any physician treating you with radiation, or technicians taking x-rays, that you could be pregnant, and ask them to take all necessary precautions. Only radiation exposure that is absolutely required for your health or the baby's should be permitted (see page 66).

Avoid Excessive Exposure to Hazardous Chemicals. Some (though far from all) chemicals, usually only in very large doses, are potentially harmful to your husband's sperm and your ova before conception, and later to a developing embryo or fetus. Though the risk is in most cases slight, both of you should play it safe by avoiding potentially hazardous exposure on the job. Special care should be taken in certain fields (medicine and dentistry, art, photography, transportation, farming and landscaping, construction, hairdressing and cosmetology, dry cleaning, and some factory work). Contact the Occupational Safety and Health Administration for the latest information on job safety and pregnancy; also see page 72. In some cases it may be wise to change jobs or to take special precautions before trying to conceive.

Because elevated lead levels when you conceive could pose problems for your baby, you should be tested if you have been exposed to lead in the workplace or elsewhere, such as in your water supply. If your blood levels are high, experts recommend chelation therapy to remove the lead from the blood, and then reduced exposure before conception is attempted. Avoid, too, excessive exposure to household toxins (see page 67).

Cut Back on Caffeine. Moderating (and gradually cutting out, if possible) your intake of coffee, tea, and colas now will spare you the symptoms of withdrawal once you're pregnant. In addition, there's some recent evidence that women who consume more than one cup of brewed coffee or the equivalent in other caffeinated beverages (tea or soft drinks containing caffeine) daily are less likely to become pregnant. Whether this is because caffeine has a biological effect on fertility or because caffeine use is often part of the type of high-stress lifestyle that can compromise a couple's chances of conceiving is unclear. Regardless, it's a good idea to cut down.

Limit Your Intake of Over-the-Counter Drugs. Since most nonprescription medications carry warnings about use in pregnancy, consult your physician before taking them once you start trying to conceive.

Check the Safety of Any Prescription Drugs You Take. Certain medications used in the treatment of chronic illnesses or disorders are linked with the development of birth defects; if you're taking any medication now, consult with your physician. Potentially harmful drugs should be discontinued at least a month (for some, three to six months) before you begin trying to have a baby, with a safe alternative therapy standing in until pregnancy is over (or the baby is weaned if the drug also poses a threat to the nursing infant).

Avoid Illicit Drugs. All so-called recreational drugs, including cocaine, crack, marijuana, and heroin, can be dangerous to your pregnancy. To vary-

ing degrees they can prevent your conceiving, and then if you do succeed, they are potentially harmful to the fetus and also increase the risks of miscarriage, prematurity, and stillbirths. If you use drugs, casually or regularly, stop all use immediately. If you can't stop, seek help (see Appendix) before trying to conceive.

Get Your Husband to Give Up Illicit Drugs and Reduce Alcohol Consumption. All the answers are not yet in, but research is beginning to show that the use of drugs (including excessive amounts of alcohol) by the father prior to conception could prevent pregnancy or lead to a poor pregnancy outcome. The mechanisms aren't clear, but drugs can apparently damage sperm as well as reduce their number, can alter testicular function and reduce testosterone levels, and are excreted in the semen. If your husband is unable to quit, he should seek help through Alcoholics Anonymous or in- or outpatient treatment.

Cut Down on Alcohol Consumption. Although a daily cocktail or glass of wine will not be harmful in your pregnancy-preparation phase, avoid heavy drinking, which can interfere with fertility by disrupting your menstrual cycle. Once you start trying to conceive, stop drinking altogether (see page 52).

Quit Smoking. Both of you. Recent studies indicate that tobacco not only is hazardous to pregnancy, it can also prevent pregnancy from occurring by reducing fertility in both men and women. A smoke-free environment is one of the best birth-day gifts you can give your baby.

Relax. This is perhaps the most important of all. Getting tense and uptight about conception could prevent you from conceiving at all.

Appendix

COMMON TESTS DURING PREGNANCY*

TEST AND WHEN PERFORMED	PROCEDURE	REASON
Blood type; first visit, unless already known from previous pregnancy or test	Examination of blood drawn from your arm.	To determine blood and Rh type in case blood transfusion is needed at some point, and to be prepared for the possibility of Rh incompatibility (see page 37). Testing will also be done for the Kell factor; Kell factor incompatibility is much rarer.
Sugar (glucose) in the urine; at each visit	A specially treated stick, dipped in a specimen of your urine, shows presence of sugar.	While an occasional increase in sugar is normal in pregnancy (see page 152), persistent high levels could indicate hyperglycemia; further tests will determine if gestational diabetes is present, requiring special diet and care.
Albumin (protein) in the urine; at each visit	A special strip, dipped in a urine specimen, shows presence of albumin (protein).	High albumin levels could be related to toxemia; if routine test shows increase, a 24-hour test may be ordered.
Bacteria in urine; first visit	Urine specimen is examined in lab.	Bacteria in urine could indicate susceptibility to infection; treatment may be initiated.

*Your practitioner may omit some of these tests or add others, depending upon your condition and his or her professional opinion.

TEST AND WHEN PERFORMED	PROCEDURE	REASON
Blood pressure; at each visit	Blood pressure is measured with cuff and stethoscope, or with an electronic device.	A sudden rise in your normal blood pressure of more than 30 points in the upper (systolic) range, or 15 in the lower (diastolic) range, could be warning of complication such as pre-eclampsia (pages 204, 351).
Hematocrit or hemoglobin; first visit and often fourth month (repeated if values are low or anemia diagnosed)	Blood drawn from arm or from pricked finger is examined.	Values are slightly reduced in pregnancy, but abnormally low levels require further examination and treatment.
Rubella titer; first visit	Blood drawn from your arm is tested for levels of antibodies to rubella.	High levels of rubella (German measles) antibodies in your blood indicate you are immune to the disease; if you aren't immune, it is important to avoid exposure to the disease—particularly in your first trimester—and to be immunized before another pregnancy.
Pap smear; first visit	Cervical secretions are collected on a swab and examined under a microscope for abnormal cells.	Abnormal cells could, on further study, turn out to be malignant, requiring treatment.
Glucose tolerance test; fifth month; usually earlier and more often in diabetics	Examination of a series of blood samples, taken before and after a special glucose drink.	Abnormal levels of glucose in blood may indicate inadequate insulin and the presence of diabetes.
VDRL; first visit, sometimes again in seventh or eighth month	Blood drawn from your arm is tested.	To test for syphilis infection; if present, prompt treatment will prevent harm to fetus.
Gonorrhea culture; first visit†	Vaginal secretions are collected on a swab and cultured in the lab.	If gonococcus is present, treatment will prevent eye infection in baby at birth.

†Tests for genital herpes may also be done at the first visit.

TEST AND WHEN PERFORMED	PROCEDURE	REASON
Test for chlamydia; preconception or first visit	Area around cervix, urethra, or rectum is swabbed to pick up possible infectious organisms.	Chlamydia in the mother must be treated to prevent infection in newborn.
Test for Acquired Immune Deficiency Syndrome (AIDS); preconception or first visit	Blood drawn from your arm is examined for antibodies to the HIV virus.	Presence of antibodies does not mean AIDS is present, but that it may develop; HIV can be passed to fetus.
Drug screen; preconception or first visit	Urine specimen is examined for signs of illicit drug use. Sometimes a blood sample is used.	Any abuse of drugs during pregnancy is hazardous to the fetus and should be promptly treated.
Group B streptococcus swab; 26 to 28 weeks	A sample of material from cervix is examined for strep B.	If strep B is present, mother is treated as labor begins or when membranes rupture, to prevent infection of newborn.
Hepatitis B screen; usually late in second trimester	Blood sample drawn from your arm is evaluated.	To uncover hepatitis B infection, so mother can be treated prenatally and infant immediately after birth.

See individual conditions (diabetes, hepatitis B, etc.) for more information.

NON-DRUG TREATMENTS DURING PREGNANCY

SYMPTOMS	TREATMENT	PROCEDURE
Aching back	Warmth	Take a long warm (not hot-as-you-can-stand-it) bath, morning and evening. Apply a heating pad wrapped in a towel for up to 20 minutes, 3 or 4 times a day.
	Preventive measures	Exercise, proper body mechanics, good posture; see page 174.

SYMPTOMS	TREATMENT	PROCEDURE
Bruises due to injury	Ice pack	Use a commercial ice pack you store in the freezer; a plastic bag filled with ice cubes and a few paper towels to absorb the melting ice, closed with a twist tie or rubber band; or an unopened can of frozen juice or package of vegetables. Apply for 30 minutes; repeat 30 minutes later if swelling or pain persists, and as needed.
	Cold compresses	Dip a soft cloth in a basin of ice cubes and cold water, wring it out, and place over affected site. Re-chill when cold dissipates.
Bruises on hands, wrists, feet	Cold soaks	Place a tray or two of ice cubes in a basin (a Styrofoam bucket or cooler is best) of cold water and immerse the injured part for 30 minutes; repeat 30 minutes later if necessary.
Burns	Cold compresses	See Bruises. Do not apply ice directly to a burn.
Burns on hands, wrists, feet	Cold soaks	See Bruises.
Colds	Saline nose drops	Use a commercial preparation or a solution of ¼ teaspoon salt in 8 ounces water (measure carefully). Put a few drops in each nostril, wait 5 to 10 minutes and blow your nose.
	Vicks VapoRub	Follow package directions.
	Additional fluids	Drink 8 ounces liquid every hour, including water, juices, soups. Hot

SYMPTOMS	TREATMENT	PROCEDURE
		fluids, particularly chicken soup, are best. Limit milk intake only if recommended by your doctor.
	Inhalation	Use a steam vaporizer, humidifier, or steaming kettle; prepare a tent by draping a sheet over an open umbrella which is resting on a chair back; place humidifier on chair.

Keeping Moist

Hot dry air can contribute to dry skin, coughing, and possibly to an increase in colds and other respiratory ailments. Adding moisture to your home can help reduce this problem, but how you do this can make a difference. Sometimes the suggested cure can do more harm than good.

Vaporizers and humidifiers, for example, have to be chosen and used with caution. Steam vaporizers manufactured since the 1970s are safe and effective, although if young children are around, the vaporizer must be carefully positioned out of reach. Cold-mist humidifiers, which became popular because they didn't present a burn hazard, encourage bacterial growth and spread germs, and should not be used at all. Ultrasonic humidifiers spew tiny particles of bacteria and other impurities from the water into the air and can cause allergic reactions or illness if they are not cleaned daily, and if plain tap water (rather than unfiltered or undistilled water) is used in them. Pans of water on radiators can add small amounts of moisture to the air but, again, could be a burn risk for small children. A steaming kettle under a tent also presents a burn problem and should be used with care for brief periods only.

Manufacturers have been attempting to produce safer humidifiers. Warm-mist humidifiers (which boil the water before mixing it with cool water to produce a mist) and wicking humidifiers (which use wicks to remove impurities) appear to release fewer germs than older cool-mist units. All humidifiers should be drained and cleaned before storing, and should be thoroughly cleaned before being used again.

No matter which method you use to add humidity to your home, limit the time of operation. Don't humidify around the clock—among other things, this can encourage the growth of molds on plants and furniture. Instead, try not to let the air in your home become dry and overheated in the first place. To do this, keep the indoor temperature under 68 degrees in cold weather. And don't make your home totally airtight—allow some leakage through windows or doors, for example, by eliminating weather-stripping. (This will also minimize hazards from indoor pollutants, such as radon.)

SYMPTOMS	TREATMENT	PROCEDURE
Colds (con't.)		Spend 15 minutes 3 or 4 times a day under tent; extend the time to 30 minutes if you aren't too uncomfortable. (Don't stay under tent if you become uncomfortably warm.) Keep the humidifier near your bedside when you are sleeping or resting.
Coughing, due to colds or flu	Inhalation	See Colds.*
	Additional fluids	See Colds.
Diarrhea	Additional fluids	Drink 8 ounces liquid every hour, including water, diluted fruit juice (but not prune juice), soups. Take milk as recommended by your practitioner. (See page 311.)
Fever	Cooling bath	Use a tub of tepid water and gradually cool it by adding ice cubes—stopping immediately if shivering begins.
	Sponge bath	Soak towels in bowl containing 2 quarts water, 1 pint rubbing alcohol, and 1 quart ice cubes; apply cold towels to the skin. Use a plastic sheet to catch drips. Stop if shivering begins.
		Call your doctor immediately for fevers of 102°F or higher.
Hemorrhoids	Sitz bath	Sit in enough hot water (hotter than your usual

*See "Keeping Moist," page 433. Though steam inhalation has long been a standard in treating coughs and colds, there is now some question as to whether it is really effective.

SYMPTOMS	TREATMENT	PROCEDURE
		bath) to cover the affected area for 20 to 30 minutes, 2 or 3 times daily.
Itchy abdomen or skin elsewhere	Baking soda and ammonia paste	Mix ½ cup baking soda with enough household ammonia to make a paste (avoid breathing the fumes); apply to itchy skin. Check any persistent skin problems with your practitioner.
	Preventive measures	Avoid long hot showers and baths, and soaps that are drying. Use a good moisturizer, spread on while you are still damp from the shower. For moisturizing indoor air, see page 433.
Itchy eye discharge	Warm soaks	Use a cloth dipped in warm, not hot, water (test it for comfort on your inner forearm), and apply to your eye for 5 or 10 minutes every 3 hours.
Muscle soreness, injury	Ice pack, cold compresses, or cold soaks for first 24 to 48 hours	See Bruises.
	After 48 hours, hot soaks, warm baths, or heating pad	Wet a towel thoroughly in warm water, then wring it out and place it over the affected site, covering all completely with a plastic bag. Place a heating pad over the plastic at a medium setting, being careful that it does not touch the wet towel. Apply for 1 hour twice daily.
Nasal congestion due to colds	Saline nose drops	See Colds.

SYMPTOMS	TREATMENT	PROCEDURE
	Additional fluids	See Colds.
Sinusitis	Alternating hot and cold compresses	Dip a cloth in hot water, wring it out, and apply to the painful area until the heat dissipates, about 30 seconds; then apply a cold compress until the cold dissipates. Continue alternating heat and cold for 10 minutes, 4 times daily.
Sore or scratchy throat	Gargle	Dissolve 1 teaspoon salt in 8 ounces hot water (the temperature of tea) and gargle for 5 minutes; repeat as needed, or every 2 hours.

BEST-ODDS CALORIE AND FAT REQUIREMENTS

Calorie and fat requirements vary according to an individual's weight and level of activity; factors such as metabolism also come into play. Though the following are merely rough guidelines, they can help you plan your daily fat intake during pregnancy. These servings take into account the fact that you will get at least one fat serving a day in dribs and drabs from "low-fat" foods.

Your Ideal Weight (pounds)	Your Activity Level*	Daily Calorie Needs†	Maximum Fat Intake (grams)	Maximum Full Fat Servings
100	1	1,500	50	2 ½
100	2	1,800	60	3 ½
100	3	2,500	83	5
125	1	1,800	60	3 ½
125	2	2,175	72	4
125	3	3,050	101	6
150	1	2,100	70	4
150	2	2,550	85	5
150	3	3,600	120	7 ½

*Score your activity level this way: 1 sedentary, 2 moderately active, 3 extremely active; very few pregnant women will fall into the extremely active category.
†See page 83.

Sources and Resources

Maternal and Child Health Center. Disseminates information to both the public and professionals: (202) 625-8410.

March of Dimes Birth Defects Foundation, Community Services Division. Provides information on prenatal hazards: 1275 Mamaroneck Avenue, White Plains, NY 10705; (914) 428-7100 or your local chapter.

Healthy Mother, Healthy Babies Coalition. Provides information on pregnancy safety: 409 12th Street SW, Washington, DC; (800) 424-8576.

City- or state-sponsored pregnancy, women's health, health, or environmental hotlines. Provides information and referrals: check your local telephone directory (avoid hotlines that are sponsored by private clinics unless referred by your practitioner).

Pesticide Hotline. Provides information on pesticides and their safe use, for the public and professionals: (800) 858-7378.

National Council on Alcoholism. Provides information and materials: 733 Third Avenue, New York, NY 10017; (800) NCA-CALL or your local or state affiliate.

Alcoholics Anonymous. Provides information and materials: 468 Park Avenue South, New York, NY 10016; for referral to nearby AA meetings, check Alcoholics Anonymous listing in your local directory.

National Cocaine Hotline. Information and referrals for cocaine users and their families: (800) COCAINE.

National Institute on Drug Abuse. Information and referrals for drug abusers and their families: (800) 662-HELP.

National Library of Medicine. Provides a list of 300 health hotlines: 8600 Rockville Pike, Bethesda, MD 20894; ATTN: Health Hotlines: (301) 496-6308.

INDEX

B

Baby
ambivalence about, 162, 383
anxiety about, 110, 115, 216
birth of, 301
bonding with, 382
condition of, at birth, 287
first look at, 302
life with, 189
loss of, 366
and maternal love, 383
responsibility for, 221
size, and diabetes, 329
size, and maternal weight gain, 235
Baby roulette, 76
Back
exercises to strengthen, 175
exercising on, 190
sleeping on, 173
Back pain, 173
in labor, 269, 276
lower, 222
non-drug treatments for, 431
prevention of, 174
relief of, 174
Bacteria in urine, testing for, 317, 429
Baking soda-ammonia paste, 434
Basic exercise position, 190
Baths
for fever, 434
in last six weeks, 249
postpartum, 407
Bed rest, living with, 339
Belly, sleeping on, 173
Bending and lifting, 174
Best-Odds Diet, 80
basic principles of, 81
for breastfeeding, 392
calorie and fat requirements in, 436
cheating on, 129
daily requirements in, 83
Food Selection Groups for, 89
Best-Odds Fries, 93

Beta-carotene
foods rich in, 91
need for, in pregnancy, 85
Bicycling, 197
Biophysical profile (BPP), 263
Biotin, 88
Birth control
altering, preconception, 426
need for, postpartum, 406
Birth control
altering, preconception, 426
need for, postpartum, 406
Birth control pills, and pregnancy, 39
Birth defects, 24
correction of, 43, 216
prenatal diagnosis of, 42
see also, Genetic defects, 24
Birth of baby (stages in), 301
Birthing
alternatives, 12
bed, 12
centers, 12
chair, 12
plan, 225
rooms, 12
Birthmarks, in newborn, 303
Bladder
after lightening, 260
in first trimester, 107
postpartum, 377
Bleeding
in early pregnancy, 344
in mid or late pregnancy, 345
in ninth month, 259
postpartum, 365, 375
rectal, 203
related to sexual intercourse, 166
vaginal, 117, 344, 345, 375
Blood
banking your own, 241
concern about transfusions of, 241
at delivery, 283
Blood clot, in vein, 360
Blood pressure
changes in, during pregnancy, 152

chronic high, 330
high, in preeclampsia, 352
low, 172
measuring of, 430
Blood sugar
and fainting or dizziness, 172
and fatigue, 103
and morning sickness, 105
in gestational diabetes, 153, 350
low, 103, 105, 172
regulation of, in diabetes, 328
Blood type, Rh, 33
Blood type, tests for, 429
Bloody show, 269, 270, 271
Bonding
father-baby, 420
mother-baby, 382
Boron, 86
Bottle feeding
benefits of, 253
succeeding at, 255
Bowel movement, postpartum, 378
Bradley method of childbirth, 213
Bran Muffins, 94
Braxton Hicks contractions, 248
Breast milk
adequacy of, 380
benefits of, 251
contamination of, 401
Breastfeeding, 251
after cesarean, 394
as birth control, 406
basics, 389
benefits of, 251
Best-Odds Diet for, 392
contraindications for, 254
deciding about, 253
getting started, 388
and medication, 254
positions for, 389
twins, 395
Breast changes
in first trimester, 108
postpartum, 108
as a sign of pregnancy, 3
in subsequent pregnancies, 108

Afterword

Now that you have read *What to Expect When You're Expecting,* you can see that every pregnancy (like every expectant parent) is different, that there are few hard and fast rules about what you can (or should) expect. You have learned that today we can control much of what happens in our pregnancies and childbirths—through the way we utilize medical care, the way we eat, through our lifestyles—making our chances of having a healthy baby better than those of any generation of parents in history. And we hope you have benefited from the fact that, though all of us worry, accurate information can go a long way toward easing our anxieties.

We hope that this book will answer all of your questions, quiet your fears, help you sleep better at night. We hope that by knowing what you can *really* expect, both the expectation and the reality will become more manageable, more exciting, and more truly fulfilling.

In our preparation and research for this book, we strove to leave no question unanswered. We relied not only on our personal experiences but also on those of the hundreds of pregnant parents we surveyed and interviewed. But since the variations of what expectant couples worry about are great, we're likely to have missed a few questions. If we overlooked any of yours, we'd like to know. That way we'll be able to include your concerns (and reassurances for them) in our next edition—in plenty of time, we hope, for *your* next edition.

Wishing you the happiest of pregnancies and the most joyous of outcomes,

Arlene Eisenberg
Heidi E. Murkoff
Sandee E. Hathaway